Veterinary Science: Clinical Research and Advances

Veterinary Science: Clinical Research and Advances

Edited by Naomi Bell

AMERICAN
MEDICAL PUBLISHERS
www.americanmedicalpublishers.com

American Medical Publishers,
41 Flatbush Avenue,
1st Floor, New York,
NY 11217, USA

Visit us on the World Wide Web at:
www.americanmedicalpublishers.com

ISBN: 978-1-63927-530-4

Cataloging-in-Publication Data

Veterinary science : clinical research and advances / edited by Naomi Bell.
p. cm.
Includes bibliographical references and index.
ISBN 978-1-63927-530-4
1. Veterinary medicine. 2. Veterinary medicine--Research. 3. Animals--Diseases--Treatment.
4. Animal health. I. Bell, Naomi.
SF745 .V48 2022
636.089--dc23

Table of Contents

Preface

Veterinary science is the scientific field that is involved in the health and well-being of animals. Some of the aspects which are dealt within veterinary science are livestock management, microbiology, genetics, pharmacology and surgery. Veterinary medicine is a sub-field of veterinary science which focuses on the prevention, treatment and diagnosis of diseases in animals. Some of the common procedures performed under this field are docking of tails, debarking on dogs, declawing of cats, etc. Veterinary science is also involved in the promotion of human health through monitoring and controlling zoonotic diseases. These are infectious diseases that are transmitted from non-human animals to humans. They can be caused by viruses, bacteria and parasites. This book is a valuable compilation of topics, ranging from the basic to the most complex discoveries in the field of veterinary science. It will prove to be immensely beneficial to students and researchers in this field. The book aims to shed light on some of the unexplored aspects of veterinary science and the recent researches and advances in this field.

The information shared in this book is based on empirical researches made by veterans in this field of study. The elaborative information provided in this book will help the readers further their scope of knowledge leading to advancements in this field.

Finally, I would like to thank my fellow researchers who gave constructive feedback and my family members who supported me at every step of my research.

Editor

1

Diagnosis of diabetes insipidus observed in Swiss Duroc boars

Alexander Grahofer[1], Natalie Wiedemar[2], Corinne Gurtner[3], Cord Drögemüller[2] and Heiko Nathues[1*]

Abstract

Background: Diabetes insipidus (DI) is a rare disease in humans and animals, which is caused by the lack of production, malfunction or dysfunction of the distal nephron to the antidiuretic effect of the antidiuretic hormone (ADH). Diagnosis requires a thorough medical history, clinical examination and further laboratory confirmation. This case report describes the appearance of DI in five Duroc boars in Switzerland.

Case presentation: Two purebred intact Duroc boars at the age of 8 months and 1.5 years, respectively, with a history of polyuric and polydipsic symptoms had been referred to the Swine Clinic in Berne. Based on the case history, the results of clinical examination and the analysis of blood and urine, a tentative diagnosis of DI was concluded. Finally, the diagnosis was confirmed by findings from a modified water deprivation test, macroscopic examinations and histopathology. Following the diagnosis, three genes known to be involved in inherited DI in humans were analyzed in order to explore a possible genetic background of the affected boars.

Conclusion: The etiology of DI in pigs is supposed to be the same as in humans, although this disease has never been described in pigs before. Thus, although occurring only on rare occasions, DI should be considered as a differential diagnosis in pigs with polyuria and polydipsia. It seems that a modified water deprivation test may be a helpful tool for confirming a diagnosis in pigs. Since hereditary forms of DI have been described in humans, the occurrence of DI in pigs should be considered in breeding programs although we were not able to identify a disease associated mutation.

Keywords: Polydipsia, Polyuria, Hyposthenuria, Pig, Antidiuretic hormone, Vasopressin, Water deprivation test

Background

Primary disorders of water balance, such as diabetes insipidus (DI) or psychogenic polydipsia, belong to the 'polyuric and polydipsic complex'. DI is characterized by polyuria, a markedly decreased urine specific gravity and compensatory polydipsia without other findings. Combining a thorough clinical examination with specific laboratory testing for particular causes (e.g., diabetes mellitus, hyperthyroidism, pyelonephritis, chronic renal failure), the diagnosis can be established and several other differential diagnoses can be ruled out [1, 2]. In order to verify a presumptive diagnosis, a water deprivation test, an antidiuretic hormone (ADH) stimulation test as well as measurement of endogenous ADH have been described [1–4].

DI is caused by an inadequate secretion, release or activity of ADH [5–8]. The ADH, also known as vasopressin, is a neurohypophyseal peptide hormone and its most important function, maintained through interaction with the V2-receptor in the kidney, is to increase water reabsorption [9]. Any distinction of the several forms of DI cannot solely relay on clinical examination, because symptoms are rather unspecific. A central DI (CDI) occurs due the inadequate secretion of ADH, whereas nephrogenic DI (NDI) is characterized by an insufficient or absent response of the distal nephron to the antidiuretic effect of vasopressin [6–8, 10]. The gestational DI (GDI) is caused by the enzyme 'cysteine aminopeptidase', which is produced in the placenta and degrades ADH [6–8].

DI has rarely been reported in pets and farm animals [10, 11]. In humans the disease occurs with a prevalence

* Correspondence: heiko.nathues@vetsuisse.unibe.ch
[1]Clinic for Swine, Department of Clinical Veterinary Medicine, Vetsuisse Faculty, University of Berne, Bremgartenstrasse 109a, CH-3012 Bern, Switzerland
Full list of author information is available at the end of the article

of 1:25,000 [8]. From these cases less than 10 % can be attributed to a hereditary background. In this context, three different genes are often analyzed in order to identify the form of DI [14]: the arginine vasopressin gene (*AVP*), the arginine vasopressin receptor 2 gene (*AVPR2*) and the vasopressin-sensitive water channel gene (*AQP2*).

In most of the human CDI cases the disease is acquired and can have various underlying etiologies, such as tumors, trauma, infections or central nervous system malformations [12, 13]. There are also familial forms caused by mutations in *AVP*. Most of these mutations are inherited in a dominant manner [14] though recessive cases have been reported [15]. The time of onset of first clinical symptoms in familial CDI shows huge variation and it usually occurs after one year of age [14]. The acquired forms of NDI are often secondary diseases following other metabolic disorders (e.g. diabetes mellitus), urinary tract diseases or drug abuse [12]. Familial NDI can either be caused by mutations in the *AVPR2* or *AQP2* gene [10, 14]. In both circumstances, symptoms usually manifest themselves in the first weeks after birth [14]. Two particular *AVPR2* mutations [14] are responsible for about 90 % of familial NDI cases [10], they cause an X-linked recessive form of NDI and therefore mainly affect male individuals [14] with a frequency of 4–8 per 1 million man born alive [16]. Furthermore, there are autosomal dominant and recessive variants of NDI [17]. Mutations in *AQP2* are the least frequent cause of familial DI. In most of the cases it is inherited in an autosomal recessive way [10].

This case report describes the findings in Duroc boars with DI. The clinical symptoms were partly in accordance with case reports in other animal species. To the authors' knowledge, this is the first report of the DI in pigs and specifically in Duroc boars.

Case history

Two purebred Duroc boars were referred to the Swine Clinic Berne, Vetsuisse-Faculty, for further investigation of polyuric and polydipsic symptoms combined with reduced growth despite maintenance of appetite. Owners of the Duroc boars were informed about the possible examinations in written form and they agreed upon Terms of Services that include the intention to publish descriptions of clinical cases in reports. Both animals had a significant drop of semen quality and were excluded from the semen collection process in a boar stud. The first symptoms appeared around a month before referral to the clinic and no other relevant medical history was reported. No treatment was administered by the herd attending veterinarian or animal care taker prior to presentation of the case in the clinic. The boars were kept in individual pens interspersed with straw. In the boar stud, the animals were fed with commercial feed and were provided with fresh water from the public supplier. Water was freely available through a nipple drinker system. The vaccination program included an immunization against *Erysipelothrix rhusiopathiae* twice and *porcine parvovirus* once a year. A yearly deworming of all boars was not conducted, because of negative results from regular examinations of faeces. According to the EU-regulations the boar stud was also tested for Classical swine fever, *Brucella spp.* and *Foot-and-mouth disease virus* and in addition for *Porcine reproductive and respiratory syndrome virus*, *Porcine herpesvirus 1* and *African swine fever virus*. During the interview with the herd attending veterinarian and the thorough clinical history three very similar cases were further identified, where some years ago Duroc boars had shown identical signs. In these three cases the herd attending veterinarian had performed on-farm necropsies. Furthermore, samples from each boar had been sent to a laboratory for diagnostic purpose including the histopathology and bacteriological investigation of the urinary tract system. Also a physical-chemical urinalysis was conducted. At necropsy and the histopathological examination no distinctive gross lesions were found that could explain the polyuric and polydipsic disorders. Apart from this, pathogens not specific for urinary tract infection were found with low quantity in culture, likely due to environmental contamination. All of the urine samples from these three pigs showed a highly decreased specific gravity without other abnormalities.

Case #1

Case #1 was a 1.5 year old intact Duroc boar with a body weight of 172 kg. Clinical examination revealed the boar was alert and in a moderate body condition. The boar showed a dull, ruffled bristled coat and the integument had multiple superficial skin wounds. The boar had several lesions with an exudative inflammatory process on the ears as well as lateral to the left carpal joint and lateral to the right tarsus. The rectal body temperature was 38.6 °C. The heart rate was 116 beats per minute and the heart sound was slightly muffled. The respiratory rate was 16 breaths per minute, with the animal showing a costoabdominal, abdominal breathing type and a moderate expiratory as well as a slight inspiratory respiratory noise. Based on the examination of the mucous membrane there was currently no evidence that the animal had a circulatory insufficiency. The neurological examination revealed no pathological findings.

During abdominal ultrasonography, the cranial part of the urinary bladder could not be identified, because the *vesica urinaria* extended below the ribs. The bladder was completely distended with echogenic urine. No sediment was observed in the urine. The thickness, the regularity of the bladder wall and mucosal relief, all dependent on the bladder's volume, i.e. filling, were evaluated and assessed as being physiological. During the clinical examination no urination could be observed.

The genitals were evaluated visually, by digital palpation and by ultrasound examination. The two testes were located in and freely moveable within the scrotum. The scrotum had several skin abrasions and a hard thickening of the skin around 10×4cm on the left lateral side. There was a physiological asymmetry of the testes with both being around 1.5 fists big, but one being slightly bigger than the other one. The tissue was soft and elastic and no pain reaction could be recognized by palpation. No abnormality was found during the ultrasound scan.

Results from the concurrent blood examination and the urine analysis are listed in Tables 1 and 2.

Macroscopic examination and histopathology were performed and are described in the section 'gross examination and histopathological findings'.

Case #2

Case #2 was an 8 months old intact Duroc boar with a body weight of 133 kg. The clinical examination revealed the boar was alert and in a moderate body condition. The bristles and integument were in a good condition, although there were multiple marble sized, firm nodules on both ears and decubitus ulcerations on both carpi and the left tarsus. The rectal body temperature was 37.8 °C. The heart rate was 100 beats per minute and the heart sound was slightly muffled. The respiratory rate was 20 breaths per minute, with the animal showing a costoabdominal, abdominal breathing type and a moderate expiratory respiratory noise. Based on the examination of the mucous membrane there was currently no evidence that the animal had a circulatory insufficiency. The animal showed a slightly arched back and tripling in hindquarters. The neurological examination revealed no pathological findings, except of proprioceptive deficits in hindquarters. Moreover, the panniculus reflex was slightly decreased from pelvis until thorax and thereafter moderately increased.

During abdominal ultrasonography, the cranial part of the urinary bladder could not be identified, because the *vesica urinaria* extended into the ribcage. The bladder was completely distended with echogenic urine and no sediment was observed in the urine. The thickness, regularity of the bladder wall and mucosal relief, all dependent on bladder's volume, were evaluated and assessed as being physiological. During the clinical examination urination could be observed nearly every half hour.

The genitals were evaluated visually, by digital palpation and by ultrasound examination. Both testes were located and freely moveable within the scrotum. There was a physiological asymmetry of the two fist-sized testes. The tissue was soft and elastic and no pain reaction could be recognized by palpation. No abnormality was found during the ultrasound examination. The caudal part of the paired bulbourethral gland was manually

Table 1 Blood parameters of case #1

Parameter	Unit	Patient's value	Reference value
Hematocrite	l/L	0.33	0.33–0.45
Erythrocytes	10e12/L	6.24	6.3–8.8
Leukocytes	10e9/L	**18.74**	7.9–18.5
Sodium	mmol/L	127	129–150
Potassium	mmol/L	4.54	4.26–6.99
Chloride	mmol/L	**87**	96–110
Calcium	mmol/L	2.35	2.32–2.92
Phosphorus	mmol/L	**1.59**	2.06–3.25
Magnesium	mmol/L	**0.75**	0.86–1.21
Iron	µmol/L	17.2	9.5–29.1
Glucose	mmol/L	6.01	4.0–6.6
Total protein	g/L	66.4	54–83
Albumin	g/L	36.6	27.3–39.5
Urea	mmol/L	5.47	3.15–8.07
Creatinine	µmol/L	95	39–130
Bilirubin	µmol/L	1.1	1.0–6.4
ALAT (GPT)	IU	102	41–160
ALP	IU	20	50–303
ASAT (GOT)	IU	37 °	30–139
CK	IU	1020	0–2687
GLDH	IU	**1** °	2–11
LDH	IU	1172	909–2172
SQR	IU	0 °	0–8

°possible interference due to haemolysis
Values not within the physiological range are marked in bold

Table 2 Urine parameters of case #1

Parameter	Patient's value
Colour	diluted
Transparency	clear
Specific weight	1002
Nitrite	negativ
pH-Value	6.0
Protein	negativ
Glucose	negativ
Ketone bodies	negativ
Urobilinogen	negativ
Bilirubin	negativ
Blood	negativ
Squamous epithelium	(+)

palpated. The consistency and the size of the gland revealed no pathological findings.

A blood sample was taken and a complete blood count was performed. Furthermore, the concentration of Thyroxin (T4) was determined in order to exclude hyperthyroidism. The results are listed in Table 3. For further diagnostic examinations and as a support for the final diagnosis an 'abrupt water deprivation test' was conducted. The body weight was measured and a urine sample was taken and examined immediately prior to the trial (Table 4). Then the animal was completely deprived of water and food for 6 h. During the test, the general condition was monitored every 30 min. After the water deprivation test a 6.7 % loss of body weight was assessed and the urine specific gravity was marginally increased from 1.001 to 1.008.

Based on the results of the abrupt water deprivation test it was decided to try a therapy with 3-5 drops of Desmopressinacetat (Minirin® solution for intranasal application) into the conjunctival sac every 8 h for 5 days. During the treatment period a clinical examination and measurement of the urine specific gravity was conducted daily. Just a slightly increase of the urine specific gravity was observed (Fig. 1). Five days after the last treatment with Desmopressinacetat, a blood sample was taken and analyzed for Copeptin with an immunoassay for humans. The concentration of Copeptin was lower than 0.8 pmol/l in the serum.

For further diagnostics a necropsy was performed and completed by histopathological examinations. The results are described in the section below.

Table 3 Blood parameter of case #2 including Thyroxin (T4)

Parameter	Unit	Patient's value	Reference value
Hematocrite	l/L	0.33	0.33–0.45
Erythrocytes	10e12/L	6.60	6.3–8.8
Leukocytes	10e9/L	**20.98**	7.9–18.5
Sodium	mmol/L	140	129–150
Potassium	mmol/L	4.53	4.26–6.99
Chloride	mmolL	100	96–110
Calcium	mmol/L	2.44	2.32–2.92
Phosphorus	mmol/L	**1.93**	2.06–3.25
Magnesium	mmol/L	**0.76**	0.86–1.21
Iron	μmol/L	17.5	9.5–29.1
Glucose	mmol/L	**7.37**	4.0–6.6
Total protein	g/L	68.3	54–83
Albumin	g/L	37.1	27.3–39.5
Urea	mmol/L	3.88	3.15–8.07
Creatinine	μmol/L	79	39–130
Bilirubin	μmol/L	**0.8**	1.0–6.4
ALAT (GPT)	IU	75	41–160
ALP	IU	**34**	50–303
ASAT (GOT)	IU	46 °	30–139
CK	IU	278	0–2687
GLDH	IU	2 °	2–11
LDH	IU	**900** °	909–2172
SQR	IU	**1** °	0–8
Thyroxin (T4)	ug/L	44	42–66 *

°possible interference due to haemolysis
*reference range from Anderson et al. [36]
Values not within the physiological range are marked in bold

Table 4 Comparing urine parameter before and after the water deprivation test

Parameter	*Before water deprivation test*	*After water deprivation test*
Body weight (kg)	133	124
Colour	diluted	bright yellow
Transparency	clear	turbid
Specific weight	1.001	1.008
Nitrite	negativ	negativ
pH-Value	5.8	6.1
Protein	negativ	negativ
Glucose	negativ	negativ
Ketone bodies	negativ	negativ
Urobilinogen	negativ	negativ
Bilirubin	negativ	negativ
Blood	0-1	negativ
Squamous epithelium	+	+++
Round cell	(+)	+
Amorphic crystal	-	+++

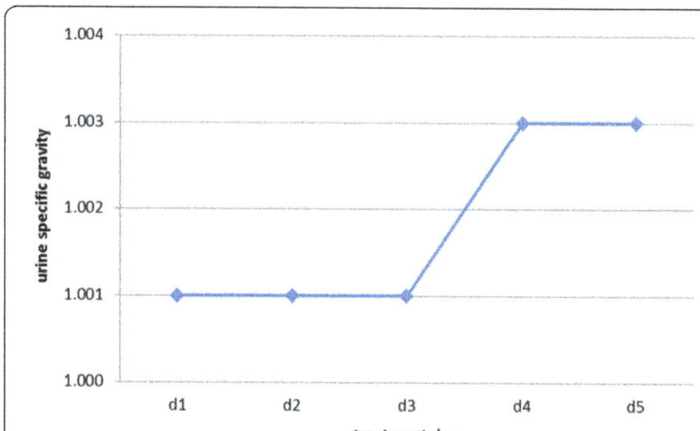

Fig. 1 Line diagram displaying the development of the urine specific gravity over treatment time. Data were obtained during desmopressin administration with a Duroc boar suffering from polydipsia and polyuria

Gross examination

Case #1

The boar showed multiple skin abrasions on various parts of the body. The soles of all claws showed fissures.

Bilateral the cranial lung lobes were affected by a chronic suppurative bronchopneumonia and about 20 % of the lung tissue was affected. The pericardium contained 0.1 l (L) of clear, serous fluid.

The urinary bladder contained approximately 9 L of clear yellowish urine (Fig. 2). The mucosal lining of the urinary bladder was intact and the lumen of the urethra was free from obstruction. The testes were softer than normal on palpation.

Case #2

Like the first animal, the boar showed multiple skin abrasions and the claws showed fissures. The boar also suffered from a bilateral chronic suppurative bronchopneumonia which affected about 20 % of the lung tissue. The pericard contained about 1 L of serous and clear fluid. The boar had multiple renal cysts in both kidneys of up to 0.5 cm in diameter. The urinary bladder was filled with 3 L of clear yellowish urine and the mucosa was without changes. The lumen of the urethra was free. Both testes were softer than normal on palpation.

Histological findings for both boars

The macroscopically affected parts of the lung showed a severe infiltration with degenerated neutrophils into the lumen of bronchi and bronchioli and extending into the alveoli. Additionally, there was exudation of fibrin admixed with necrotic debris and proliferation of fibroblasts.

In both pigs the tubuli seminiferi were mostly devoid of mature spermatids and contained a reduced amount of spermatogonia. Additionally, there was also a multifocal reduced amount of sertoli cells. The interstitium of the testes contained few foci of lymphocytes with a mild amount of edema.

In the gray and white matter of the spinal cord of case #1, there were multiple swollen and hypereosinophilic axons (spheroids). Additionally, in the white substance along the whole length of the spinal cord there were few glial nodules.

In the interstitium of the kidneys of boar 1, there were few foci composed of lymphocytes and a lesser amount of macrophages. Some renal tubuli of case #1 contained a small amount of eosinophilic proteinaceous material. Few tubuli of case #2 showed mild multifocal degeneration of epithelial cells.

The corpus of the urinary bladder showed no histological changes.

Multifocal in the hypophysis there were small amounts of mineralized colloid. No special findings were present in the hypothalamus.

Bacteriological investigation

A bacteriological examination of the affected lung from case #1 yielded a moderate to high concentration of *Trueperella pyogenes* and *Pasteurella multocida subsp. multocida*.

Genetic analysis

With the aim of examining a possible genetic background of the disease, the pedigrees of the five affected boars were analyzed. All cases can be traced back to a total of 101 common ancestors, the closest of them 3, to 6 generations away from the affected animals (Fig. 3). According to the knowledge about the genetic causes of DI in humans, the annotated exons of the three functional candidate genes *AVP*, *AVPR2* and *AQP2* were sequenced in material obtained from the

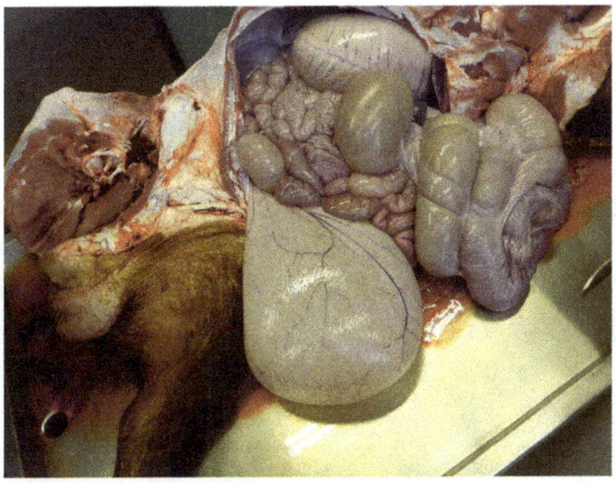

Fig. 2 Macroscopic examination of a Duroc boar suffering from polydipsia and polyuria: enlarged urinary bladder

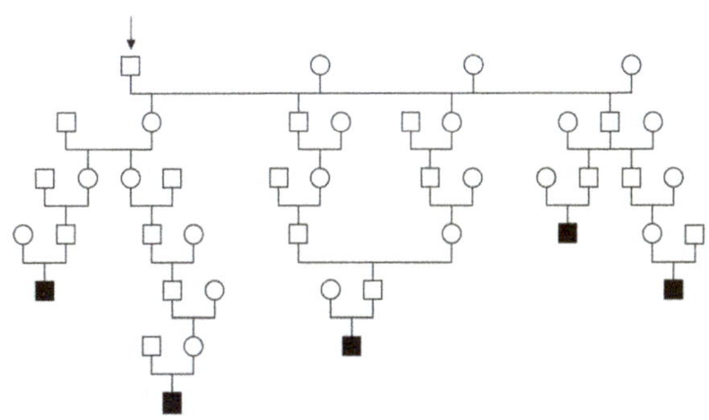

Fig. 3 Pedigree of five Duroc boars affected by polydipsia and polyuria. All the cases (shown in black) can be traced back to a particular number of common ancestors. The closest common ancestor is shown in the figure (*labelled with an arrow*). It's a boar which is 3, 4, 4, 5 and 6 generations away respectively

affected boars and from healthy animals serving as controls, which have been collected in our laboratory in the course of other ongoing studies. The DNA was isolated either from EDTA-blood using the Nucleon Bacc2 kit (GE Healthcare) or from ear punch biopsies using QIAGEN's DNeasy spin kit according to the manufacturers' instructions. Exon-spanning primers (Table 5) were designed using Primer3 software [17] after masking of repetitive sequences with RepeatMasker [18]. PCR reactions were carried out in 10 μl volumes with 5 pmol primer, 5 μl Amlitaq Gold 360 Master Mix (LifeTechnologies), 1 μl 360 GC Enhancer (LifeTechnologies) and ~20 ng of genomic DNA. PCR-products were amplified using GeneAmp 9700 thermocycler (LifeTechnologies), the amplification conditions were 10 min at 95 °C, 32 cycles of 30 s denaturation at 95 °C, 30 s annealing at 60 °C and 1 min elongation at 72 °C, followed by a 7 min hold at 72 °C. To remove redundant primers and nucleotides PCR-products were purified with 1 unit exonuclease I (Roche) and 0.5 units of shrimp alkaline phosphatase (New England BioLabs) in a 30 min incubation step at 37 °C, followed by a 15 min inactivation step at 80 °C. Subsequently the PCR-products were sequenced with the BigDye Terminator v.3.1 cycle sequencing kit (LifeTechnologies) at the following conditions: a hold of 96 °C, followed by 25 cycles of 10 s at 96 °C, 5 s at 50 °C and 2 min at 60 °C. Sequencing-products were resolved on an ABI 3730 capillary sequencer (LifeTechnologies) and the obtained sequence data was analyzed with Sequencher 5.1 software. The sequences were compared to the pig reference sequence and deviations from the reference (variants) were searched for in the affected animals (Table 6). As the mode of inheritance is not defined, both homozygous and heterozygous variants were considered. Subsequently, variants, which were present in the healthy controls, were excluded. In *AVP* three exonic single nucleotide polymorphisms (SNPs) were found in the cases, but all of them were also present in homozygous state in control animals. In *AVPR2* two exonic SNPs were found in four of the cases but all of them were present in healthy control animals as well. In *AQP2* no variants were found in the cases.

Discussion

Clinical signs, findings of the physical examination and results of further diagnostic methods confirmed the diagnosis of DI in two Duroc boars originating from a semen collection centre. There are several forms of DI described, but in the present study it was not possible to classify the type of DI accurately, as there are some limitations in diagnostics for pigs.

With a clinical history characterized by polyuria and polydipsia in pigs several differential diagnoses have to be kept in mind and each one has to be excluded from the list of differential diagnosis. Therefore, clinical examination and further tests are essential and need to be performed sequentially. During the physical examination the urinary bladder of both boars were extremely full and distended, but dehydration, which is often reported in DI [19], could not be observed. It is noteworthy that in pigs there is no adequate method to measure the hydration status and therefore experimental studies in DI use diuretic medication [20] or fluid restricted pigs [21] for evaluation. As a next step, analysis of the urine was performed and revealed a hyposthenuria with a specific gravity of 1.001 in one boar and 1.002 in the other boar. The specific gravity in pigs, which is the lowest among animals, usually is 1.020 on average and can range between 1.010 and 1.050 [22, 23]. No further abnormalities such as glucosuria or inflammatory signs were detected. Several blood compounds are able to provoke

Table 5 Primer used for sequencing of DNA from Duroc boars affected by polydipsia and polyuria and from negative controls

Gene	Chr	Position exons	Exon	Forward primer	Reverse primer	Length
AVP	17	36950915-36951078	1	CATCTTGACCACACCACTGC	TGTCCTAGTCCACCCGACA	576 bp
		36952271-36952472	2	CCGAGCGAATCAGTAGCTTT	TCGGTCACGCAGCTCTCT	546 bp
		36952626-36952826	3	GCTGCCAGGAGGAGAACTAC	ATCGCTTCCCCTACAGGATT	628 bp
AVPR2	X	142203295-142203330	1	CAGGAAGGGAAGCAGAGGA	CTACGCTCCTCTCGGGACT	390 bp
		142203810-142203859	2	CAAACCTGGTCAGGCTAAGG	CTGCCAGCAGAACACACATC	496 bp
		142204155-142205039	3a	GCCTCTCCCCAGTAAGATGA	GCTGAGAAGCAGCGAGAAG	747 bp
			3b	GTGGCTCTGTTCCAAGTGCT	CGTAGATCCAGGGGTTGGTA	848 bp
		142205173-142205695	4	GAAGGTGGGTGTGGCTGT	ACTGCTCAAGGCCAGCTC	848 bp
AQP2	5	16095902-16095541	1	AACTCCACCTCCAACTCACG	ATGTGTCTGGCTCCAGCATT	683 bp
		16092242-16092078	2	CAGGAAGAAGGCATCCGTAG	CCCCAGGAGGAGGACTGT	828 bp
		16091774-16091694	3			
		16091033-16090821	4	TTACATGGATGCGCCTTTG	CTCAGGGCAGGGGATCTT	497 bp

Table 6 Sequence variants detected in two candidate genes from Duroc boars suffering from polydipsia and polyuria

Gene	Chr	Position	dbSNP NCBI_ss#	Genotypes cases			Genotypes controls		
				ref/ref	ref/var	var/var	ref/ref	ref/var	var/var
AVP	17	36952357A > G	1966414018			2			1
		36952471 T > C	1966414019		3	2		1	1
		36952785 T > C	1966414020		3	2		1	1
AVPR2	X	142204712A > C	1966414021	1		4			2
		142205642C > T	1966414022	1		4	9		11

The positions of the variants are given based on the current assembly (SGSC Sscrofa10.2/susScr3). All the variants are single nucleotide polymorphisms (SNP) whereas the first letter represents the reference nucleotide and the second letter represents the variant (e.g. A > G means a nucleotide exchange from an adenine to a guanine). The SNPs were submitted to dbSNP (www.ncbi.nlm.nih.gov/SNP/) and the submitted SNP (ss) number is reported and will be publicly available with the dbSNP Build 147 release. The genotypes of the cases are displayed separately from the genotypes of the control animals, whereas the number of animals carrying a specific genotype is given. Ref/ref means homozygous for the reference allele, ref/var heterozygous and var/var homozygous for the variant/SNP

dysfunction of the renal system, hence a complete blood count was conducted and showed a slight chronic inflammation, which might have been caused by the pneumonia.

As a further diagnostic approach a modified water deprivation test was performed. The test is designed to determine, whether ADH is released in response to dehydration and if the kidneys are able to respond normally to the hormone [1–3]. The aim of the test is to achieve maximal ADH secretion and thereby higher concentrated urine. This commonly occurs after a 3 to 5 % loss of body weight due to water loss, which makes it necessary to measure the body weight several times. Additionally, emptying of the bladder with a catheter is required [1]. Due to the characteristic anatomy of the urethra of male pigs, transurethral catheterization of the bladder is impossible [24]. The endpoint of the water deprivation test is a loss of body weight greater than 5 % or a specific gravity of the urine higher than 1.030 [1]. A more accurate measurement is the assessment of the urine's osmolality [1]. Unfortunately, this was not feasible throughout the whole water deprivation test, because of logistical and financial reasons. The osmolality of urine can also be approximated by multiplying the last two digits of the urine specific gravity by 36 [25]. There was one single measurement of urine's osmolality of case #2, which was performed during the trial and revealed a result of 32.5 mOsm/Kg. Comparing the measured value with the calculated urine osmolality of 36 mOsm/Kg, there was a good correlation, which can also be observed in other species, e.g. in dogs.

The pig is a good model for renal research. The ratio between urine and serum osmolality in healthy pigs and healthy humans is 3.3 [21]. In the literature, there are numerous different equations described to calculate serum osmolarity in humans. One group reported an equation (Eq. 1) derived from results of an experiment in pigs, where concentrations are expressed in mEq/L [26].

Equation 1:

$$\begin{aligned}\text{Serum osmolarity (mEq/l)} &= 1.8177 * [\text{Na}]\ (\text{mEq/L}) + [\text{Urea}]\ (\text{mEq/L}) \\ &\quad + [\text{Glucose}]\ (\text{mEq/L}) + 26.05\end{aligned}$$

A baseline of 294.9 with a SD of ± 1.8 mOsm/Kg in 10–40 kg femal Yorkshire-Duroc crossbred pigs was reported [27]. Furthermore, in fattening pigs 284.74 ± 5.73 mOsm/Kg [26] was described. In order to get an indication for serum osmolarity in boars, additional three Duroc boars at the age of 8 month to 1.1 year from the semen collecting centre were tested. A reference range from 321 to 326 was measured. The calculated value of serum osmolarity in case #2 was 290.9 mOsm/Kg and, thus, within the above mentioned reference values taken from the literature. In contrast, the calculated value was significantly lower than those measured in the control boars. However, the result generally must be interpreted with caution, because there is a significant bias by food and water intake [28], which can have an impact on the level of osmolarity. If we compare the ratio of serum osmolarity with urine osmolality it is almost three times higher than the average value of healthy pigs.

After the water restriction test a therapeutic attempt was tried, as it is commonly performed with small animals and also with horses. The animals are treated with desmopressin acetate (DDAVP), a synthetic analogue of ADH. There are several routes of administration available, but most often the conjunctival route is chosen. Therefore, one to two drops are applied into the conjunctival sac of both eyes every 12 to 24 h [3, 29]. The eye drop method is a non-invasive, practical and effective way of hormone administration [30]. An oral application of desmopressin is possible, but the bioavailability is lower compared to the afore mentioned method [19, 31]. The duration of the effect of DDAVP varies from eight to 24 h [3]. Since no specific dosage regime was available for pigs, a treatment of the boar

2-3 times per day with 3–5 drops in the conjunctival sac of one eye was proposed. Only a slight decrease of the urine specific gravity was observed. In small animals this result would lead to diagnosis of primary NDI. However, the porcine vasopressin contains a lysine residue in position 8 (lysine-vasopressin), which makes the pig quite different from other mammalian species, where vasopressin contains an arginine residue in position 8 (arginine-vasopressin) [9]. Therefore the porcine V2 receptor has less sensitivity to desmopressin than human V2 receptors. In the literature a two hundred times lower affinity of desmopressin on porcine V2 receptor is described [32]. Even in high doses desmopressin did not induce any hematological response [33]. The authors clinical interpretation is that desmopressin cannot be recommended for diagnostics or treatment in pigs due to the implications mentioned above.

Unfortunately, we performed both diagnostic approaches, therapeutic attempt and modified water deprivation test, only in one boar, because it was only possible to keep one boar in our facilities, regarding to Swiss legislation. To prove the efficiency for both tests in a larger number of pigs with DI, warrants further investigation.

Another diagnostic tool for the confirmation of the disease's aetiology is the measurement of endogenous ADH in plasma, where in case of diseases osmotic and cardiovascular homeostasis are disturbed [4]. However, the reliability of assessments of plasma ADH levels is poor because the hormone is unstable, largely attached to platelets, and rapidly cleared from plasma [34, 35]. Therefore, the level of a precursor of ADH, Copeptin, which is stable for days, is usually measured in plasma samples [35]. Test kits, specifically designed for pigs, are available for the purpose of clinical research, but they are rarely used and in the presented case the authors could not find a laboratory offering the determination of Copeptin in swine plasma.

The genetic analysis revealed that all the candidate variants in the three DI candidate genes were obviously not associated with the disease and therefore no genetic explanation of the phenotype was found by sequencing of these three genes. Pedigree analysis showed a large number of common ancestors among the affected cases indicating inbreeding. But these shared ancestors are some generations ago which decreases the likelihood of a common inherited simple recessive mutation. Nevertheless, a dominantly inherited mutation with a late onset of clinical signs could also be the cause of the disease, as for example human CDI is caused by dominant mutations of *AVP* [14]. A recessive inheritance analogue to *AQP2* mutations in humans [10] with inbreeding loops further behind in the pedigree is possible as well as an X-linked disease like NDI caused by *AVPR2* mutations in humans [14]. Even though, both types of mutations usually manifest in the first weeks after birth in humans. As the phenotype in the boars was recognized later in life one can also hypothesize that a dominant mutation in one of these three genes which is located in the upstream, intronic, or downstream regions affecting the expression level is causing the disease. The used approach is only appropriate to detect variants in the coding region and therefore other more comprehensive methods like genome-wide-association mapping in combination with sequencing of the genome of one case could be useful to map the responsible locus in the swine genome and finally to find the causative mutation.

Conclusions

This case report provides a description of a diagnostic approach to confirm DI in pigs. The report also addresses the limitations and pitfalls while diagnosing DI due to the limited availability of different tests and methods for pigs.

To the author's knowledge, this report is the first describing DI in Duroc boars. Severe polyuria and polydipsia as major clinical signs indicated an inclusion of Diabetes insipidus in the differential diagnosis. Failure to differentiate polyuric syndromes from other conditions may lead to an incorrect or inconclusive diagnosis of DI. Importantly, a response to ADH administration cannot be used as a diagnostic approach in pigs, because the chemical structure of the product commonly used in humans, cats and dogs is not stimulating the V2 receptors in swine. The observed relationship of the affected animals suggest a possible genetic cause. Although coding mutations in three DI candidate genes can be excluded a genetic background of the disease could not be ruled out and should be carefully investigated in future using more comprehensive methods.

Competing interests

There are no competing interests of any of the authors that could inappropriately influence or bias the content of the paper.

Authors' contributions

AG performed the clinical examination, developed the diagnosis, designed the treatment of the boars, summarized the results of the cases and drafted the manuscript. NW planned and performed the genetic analysis and drafted parts of the manuscript. CG conducted the macroscopic examination and the histopathology. HN and CD supervised and coordinated the project. All authors contributed to the development and the revisions of the manuscript and approved the final version.

Acknowledgments

The authors gratefully acknowledge Dr. Thierry Francey, Small Animal Clinic, Vetsuisse Faculty University of Berne, for his continuous support during this study. The authors also thank the veterinarians from the boar stud for the provision of data.

Author details
[1]Clinic for Swine, Department of Clinical Veterinary Medicine, Vetsuisse Faculty, University of Berne, Bremgartenstrasse 109a, CH-3012 Bern, Switzerland. [2]Institute of Genetics, Department of Clinical Research and Veterinary Public Health, Vetsuisse Faculty, University of Berne, Bremgartenstrasse 109a, CH-3012 Bern, Switzerland. [3]Institute of Animal Pathology, Department of Infectious Diseases and Pathobiology, Vetsuisse Faculty, University of Berne, Länggassstrasse 122, CH-3012 Bern, Switzerland.

References

1. Nichols R. Polyuria and polydipsia. Diagnostic approach and problems associated with patient evaluation. Vet Clin North Am Small Anim Pract. 2001;31:833–44.
2. Grünbaum EG, Moritz A. The diagnosis of nephrogenic diabetes insipidus in the dog. Tierarztl Prax. 1991;19:539–44.
3. Nichols R, Hohenhaus AE. Use of the vasopressin analogue desmopressin for polyuria and bleeding disorders. J Am Vet Med Assoc. 1994;205:168–73.
4. Robertson GL. The use of vasopressin assays in physiology and pathophysiology. Semin Nephrol. 1994;14:368–83.
5. Braun U, Feller B, Gerber A, Ossent P. Diabetes insipidus bei einem Braunviehrind mit Hydrocephalus internus. Schweiz Arch Tierheilkd. 2008;150:409–12.
6. Fenske W, Allolio B. Clinical review: Current state and future perspectives in the diagnosis of diabetes insipidus: a clinical review. J Clin Endocrinol Metab. 2012;97:3426–37.
7. Shapiro M, Weiss JP: Diabetes & Metabolism Diabetes Insipidus : A Review. J Diabetes Metab 2012:1–11.
8. Di Iorgi N, Napoli F, Allegri AEM, Olivieri I, Bertelli E, Gallizia A, et al. Diabetes insipidus–diagnosis and management. Horm Res pædiatrics. 2012;77:69–84.
9. Petersen MB. The effect of vasopressin and related compounds at V1a and V2 receptors in animal models relevant to human disease. Basic Clin Pharmacol Toxicol. 2006;99:96–103.
10. Wesche D, Deen PMT, Knoers NVAM. Congenital nephrogenic diabetes insipidus: the current state of affairs. Pediatr Nephrol. 2012;27:2183–204.
11. Burnie AG, Dunn JK. A case of central diabetes insipidus in the cat: diagnosis and treatment. J Small Anim Pract. 1982;23:237–41.
12. Baylis PH, Cheetham T. Diabetes insipidus. Arch Dis Child. 1998;79:84–9.
13. Al-Agha AE, Thomsett MJ, Ratcliffe JF, Cotterill AM, Batch JA. Acquired central diabetes insipidus in children: a 12-year Brisbane experience. J Paediatr Child Health. 2001;37:172–5.
14. Fujiwara TM, Bichet DG. Molecular biology of hereditary diabetes insipidus. J Am Soc Nephrol. 2005;16:2836–46.
15. Willcutts MD. Autosomal recessive familial neurohypophyseal diabetes insipidus with continued secretion of mutant weakly active vasopressin. Hum Mol Genet. 1999;8:1303–7.
16. Bichet DG. Vasopressin receptor mutations in nephrogenic diabetes insipidus. Semin Nephrol. 2008;28:245–51.
17. Homepage Primer3 [http://bioinfo.ut.ee/primer3-0.4.0]
18. Homepage Repeat Masker Server [http://www.repeatmasker.org]
19. Aroch I, Mazaki-Tovi M, Shemesh O, Sarfaty H, Segev G. Central diabetes insipidus in five cats: clinical presentation, diagnosis and oral desmopressin therapy. J Feline Med Surg. 2005;7:333–9.
20. Fahlman A, Dromsky DM. Dehydration effects on the risk of severe decompression sickness in a swine model. Aviat Sp Env Med. 2006;77:102–6.
21. Hess JR, MacDonald VW, Winslow RM. Dehydration and shock: an animal model of hemorrhage and resuscitation of battlefield injury. Biomater Artif Cells Immobilization Biotechnol. 1992;20:499–502.
22. Kahn CM, editor. The Merck veterinary manual. 10th ed. Merck: Whitehouse Station; 2010.
23. Drolet R. Urinary system. In: Zimmermann JJ, Karriker LA, Ramirez A, Schwartz KJ, Steveson GW, editors. Dis Swine. 10th ed. Chichester: Wiley-Blackwell; 2012. p. 363–79.
24. Holliman CJ, Kenfield K, Nutter E, Saffle JR, Warden GD. Technique for acute suprapubic catheterization of urinary bladder in the pig. Am J Vet Res. 1982;43:1056–7.
25. Hendriks HJ, de Bruijne JJ, van den Brom WE. The clinical refractometer: a useful tool for the determination of specific gravity and osmolality in canine urine. Tijdschr Diergeneeskd. 1978;103:1065–8.
26. Căpriţă R, Căpriţă A. Experimentally-derived formula for computing serum osmolarity in pigs. Sci Pap Anim Sci Biotechnol. 2009;42:537–42.
27. Houpt TR, Anderson CR. Spontaneous drinking: is it stimulated by hypertonicity or hypovolemia? Am J Physiol. 1990;258:143–8.
28. Houpt TR, Yang H. Water deprivation, plasma osmolality, blood volume, and thirst in young pigs. Physiol Behav. 1995;57:49–54.
29. Harb MF, Nelson RW, Feldman EC, Scott-Moncrieff JC, Griffey SM. Central diabetes insipidus in dogs: 20 cases (1986-1995). J Am Vet Med Assoc. 1996;209:1884–8.
30. Kranenburg LC, Thelen MHM, Westermann CM, de Graaf-Roelfsema E, van der Kolk JH. Use of desmopressin eye drops in the treatment of equine congenital central diabetes insipidus. Vet Rec. 2010;167:790–1.
31. Critchley H, Davis SS, Farraj NF, Illum L. Nasal absorption of desmopressin in rats and sheep. Effect of a bioadhesive microsphere delivery system. J Pharm Pharmacol. 1994;46:651–6.
32. Ufer E, Postina R, Gorbulev V, Fahrenholz F. An extracellular residue determines the agonist specificity of V2 vasopressin receptors. FEBS Lett. 1995;362:19–23.
33. Bowie EJ, Solberg LA, Fass DN, Johnson CM, Knutson GJ, Stewart ML, et al. Transplantation of normal bone marrow into a pig with severe von Willebrand's disease. J Clin Invest. 1986;78:26–30.
34. Scollan KF, Bulmer BJ, Sisson DD. Validation of a commercially available enzyme immunoassay for measurement of plasma antidiuretic hormone concentration in healthy dogs and assessment of plasma antidiuretic hormone concentration in dogs with congestive heart failure. Am J Vet Res. 2013;74:1206–11.
35. Morgenthaler NG, Struck J, Alonso C, Bergmann A. Assay for the measurement of copeptin, a stable peptide derived from the precursor of vasopressin. Clin Chem. 2006;119:112–9.
36. Andersson H, Wallgren M, Rydhmer L, Lundström K, Andersson K, Forsberg M. Photoperiodic effects on pubertal maturation of spermatogenesis, pituitary responsiveness to exogenous GnRH, and expression of boar taint in crossbred boars. Anim Reprod Sci. 1998;54:121–37.

2

Detection and measurement of alpha-amylase in canine saliva and changes after an experimentally induced sympathetic activation

María Dolores Contreras-Aguilar[1], Fernando Tecles[1*], Silvia Martínez-Subiela[1], Damián Escribano[1,2], Luis Jesús Bernal[1] and José Joaquín Cerón[1]

Abstract

Background: Salivary alpha-amylase (sAA) is considered a biomarker of sympathetic activation in humans, but there is controversy regarding the existence of sAA in dogs. The hypothesis of this study was that sAA exists in dogs and it could change in situations of sympathetic stimulation. Therefore, the aims of this study were: 1) to demonstrate the presence of alpha-amylase in saliva of dogs by Western-Blot, 2) to validate an spectrophotometric method for the measurement of sAA activity and 3) to evaluate the possible changes in sAA activity after the induction of an ejaculation in dogs which is known to produce a sympathetic activation.

Results: Western-Blot demonstrated a band in dog saliva specimens between 60 kDa and 50 kDa, similar to purified sAA. The spectrophotometric assay validated showed an adequate inter- and intra-assay precision, and a high correlation coefficient ($r = 0.999$) in the linearity under dilution study. sAA median activity significantly increased just after ejaculation compared with just before the ejaculation (2.06-fold, $P = 0.005$).

Conclusions: This study demonstrated the existence of alpha-amylase in saliva of dogs and that this enzyme can be measured by a spectrophotometric assay. In addition, results showed that sAA increase after a sympathetic activation and could be potentially used as non-invasive biomarker of sympathetic activity in this species.

Keywords: Salivary alpha-amylase, Dog, Saliva, Sympathetic activation

Background

Salivary alpha-amylase (sAA) is considered in humans as a biomarker of sympathetic activation [1, 2], increasing not only in exercise [3], but also after psychological stressors [4]. This biomarker is measured in saliva, which can be obtained easily and in a non-invasive way [5, 6].

sAA has been also evaluated in other animal species such as pigs [7], Bonobos and other simians [8], horses [9] and sheep [10]. However, in dogs despite the growing interest in the evaluation of stress [11–13], there is controversy regarding the existence of sAA. Some authors described a lack of sAA [14, 15], whereas others identified sAA by sodium dodecyl sulphate polyacrylamide gel electrophoresis (SDS-PAGE) following liquid chromatography coupled with tandem mass spectrometry (LC-MS/MS) approaches [16]. In addition, to the authors' knowledge there are no validated assays for alpha-amylase measurement in dogs saliva, as well as it is unknown whether sAA increases in those situations producing sympathetic activation in this species.

The hypothesis of this study was that sAA exists in dogs and it could show changes in situations of sympathetic stimulation. To test this hypothesis, firstly a Western-Blot was performed to detect the presence of alpha-amylase in canine saliva. Then, a method for sAA measurement based on its enzymatic activity was validated in dogs, and the changes of sAA activity after an experimental model of sympathetic activation consisting on the induction of an ejaculation were studied.

* Correspondence: ftecles@um.es
[1]Interdisciplinary Laboratory of Clinical Analysis (Interlab-UMU), Veterinary School, Campus of Excellence Mare Nostrum, University of Murcia, 30100, Espinardo, Murcia, Spain
Full list of author information is available at the end of the article

Methods

Saliva sampling

Saliva specimen was collected introducing a small sponge around the mouth until it was thoroughly moist. Sponges were placed in collection devices (Salivette, Sarstedt, Aktiengesellschaft & Co, Nümbrecht, Germany) and stored with ice until arrival at the processing laboratory, where devices were centrifuged at *3.000 g* for 10 min at 4 °C. Saliva was transferred into 1.5 mL Eppendorf tubes and stored at −80 °C until analysis that were performed 1 week later.

SDS-PAGE and Western-Blot

Twenty five µg of total protein from a pool integrated by four canine saliva specimens obtained from the sympathetic activation pilot situation with high sAA activity and 10 µg of total protein from a concentrated saliva specimen from a healthy dog were used for this approach. To concentrate saliva, an Amicon 50 K molecular weight cut-off (MWCO) filter (Millipore Corp., Billerica, MA) was used as previously reported [17] because the molecular mass of sAA is higher than 50 kDa [18]. Purified human sAA (ab 77,875, Abcam, Cambrigde, UK) and a human saliva specimen (10 µg protein each) were used as positive controls. Total protein was determined using the bicinchoninic acid method [19]. Proteins were separated in mini polyacrylamide gels containing 0.1% (*w*/*v*) sodium dodecyl sulphate (SDS-PAGE), with a separating gel prepared in 10% (*w*/*v*) and a stacker gel prepared in 4% (*w*/*v*) according to the methodology described by Laemmli [20], stained with 1% *w*/*v* coomassie Brillant Blue for 5 min, followed by distaining with 5% *v*/v ethanol 7% *v*/v acetic acid for 24 h. Western-Blot were carried out as described previously [21] using an indirect detection. Proteins separated in SDS-PAGE were transferred to nitrocellulose membrane (Bio-Rad Laboratories Inc., Hercules, CA, USA). Rabbit polyclonal antibody against human sAA (ab 173,163, Abcam, Cambridge, UK) at 1:500 dilution were used as primary antibody, while horseradish peroxidase (HRP)-conjugated goat polyclonal antibody anti-rabbit (ab 6721, Abcam, Cambrigde, UK) at 1:2000 were employed as secondary antibody, which one was detected using Pierce ECL2 kit (Pierce, Thermo Fisher Scientific, USA) and Thyphoon 9410 scanner (GE Healthcare, Wilmington, MA, USA).

sAA enzymatic assay

sAA activity was determined by a commercial kit (alpha-Amylase, Beckman Coulter Inc., Fullerton, CA, USA) using the International Federation of Clinical Chemistry and Laboratory Medicine method [22]. This assay is a spectrophotometric assay that uses 4,6-ethylidene (G7)-p-nitrophenol (G1)-alpha-D- maltoheptaoside (G7PNP) as a substrate of the enzyme. The intermediate product of substrate hydrolysis reacts with a-glucosidase, giving p-nitrophenol as the final product of the reaction. The rate of p-nitrophenol formation was directly proportional to the alpha-amylase activity of the sample and could be determined by measuring the absorbance at 405 nm. The assay was adapted to an automatic analyzer (Olympus UA600, Olympus Diagnostica GmbH, Ennis, Ireland), according to the manufacturer's indications regarding reagent and specimen volumes.

Analytical validation of sAA enzymatic assay

The following characteristics were evaluated for the analytical validation of the method:

- Reproducibility. Three canine saliva specimens from the sympathetic activation pilot situation described below with low, medium and high sAA activity were used. Intra-assay precision was evaluated by measuring 6 times each of the selected specimens in the same analytical series. Inter-assay precision was calculated by measuring each of the specimens once a day for 5 days; the possible effect of repetitive thawing and freezing was removed by storing of the samples in separate vials (aliquots) and using a new one for each measurement. Results were expressed as the coefficient of variation (CV): standard deviation divided by mean of the replicates times 100%.
- Accuracy. It was evaluated by linearity under dilution (indirect method), because no reference assay is available for sAA activity in dogs. Two specimens with different sAA activity were serially diluted (75%, 50%, 25%, 12.5%) with deionized water. The results were compared with those expected by linear regression analysis.
- Limit of detection. It was defined as the lowest concentration of the analyte that could be distinguished from a specimen of zero value, and it was calculated on the basis of data from 13 replicate determinations of the zero standard (deionized water) as mean value plus three standard deviations.
- The lower limit of quantification. It was calculated as the lowest sAA activity that could be measured above the limit of detection with a CV <20%. A saliva specimen was serially diluted in deionized water and each dilution was analyzed in five replicates in the same run. CVs for each dilution were estimated as previously described.

Experimental model of sympathetic activation

The model for sympathetic activation consisted on semen collection in 10 healthy male beagles of a research colony of the Animal Resources Center of Murcia University (average age = 13.0 ± 3.9 months). All of them were inside kennels in-groups of two individuals. Semen specimens were taken by digital manipulation [23], using a latex semen

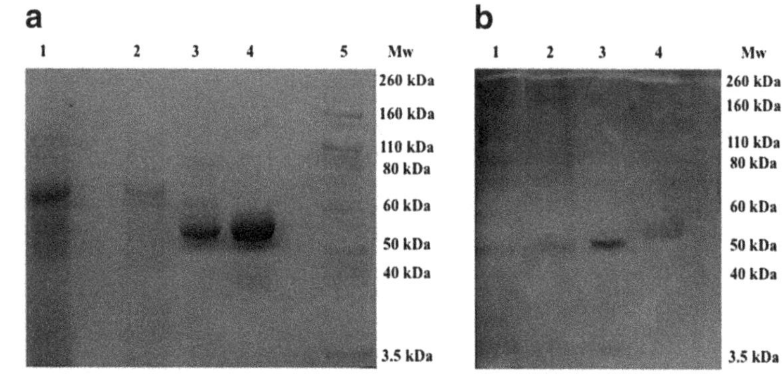

Fig. 1 SDS-PAGE (**a**) and Western-Blot (**b**). Lane 1: 10 μg dog saliva specimen concentrated; Lane 2: 25 μg pool of canine saliva; Lane 3: 10 μg human saliva; Lane 4: 10 μg purified human sAA (ab 77,875, Abcam, Cambrigde, UK); Lane 5: Molecular weight markers (Novex Sharp Pre-Stained, Invitrogen, Carlsbad, California)

collection cone (artificial vagina) and 15 mL sterile centrifuge tubes. Artificial vagina was washed with water between each dog to avoid sperm contamination. Saliva specimens were collected at least 30 min before the ejaculation at basal time (TB), just starting the ejaculation (T-0), just after ejaculation (T + 0), and 30 min later (T + 30). The heart rate was also measured at TB, T + 0 and T + 30, and the dogs' sexual behaviour during the semen collection (pelvic thrusting, engorgement of the bulbus glandis and full erection) was evaluated [23]. The experimental situation lasted from 8:30 to 10:35 a.m. To perform the entire procedure, each dog was taken out of its original kennel and passed to a close empty kennel.

To guarantee the presence of the second fraction (sperm-rich), semen specimens were evaluated as Toro-Montoya [24] describes.

Statistical analysis

Arithmetic means, medians, CVs and linear regression analyses were calculated using routine descriptive statistical procedures by spreadsheet (Excel 2000, Microsoft Corporation, Redmond, Washington, USA). Normality was evaluated by using Shapiro-Wilk test showing non-parametric distribution in sAA activity results, therefore they were transformed logarithmically by applying the formula ln x = ln (x + 1) before the statistical analyses [25, 26]. Analyses of variance of repeated measures with Fisher's LSD tests were used to determine if the values at different times were significantly different. The significance level used in each case was $P < 0.05$. These statistical analyses were calculated using Graph Pad Prism 6 (GraphPad Software, San Diego, CA, USA).

Results

SDS-PAGE and Western-Blot

SDS-PAGE and Western-Blot results are shown in Fig. 1. In SDS-PAGE (Fig. 1a), human saliva and purified human sAA (ab 77,875, Abcam) showed two bands between 60 kDa and 50 kDa, while an undefined band could be intuited in concentrated dog saliva. This band did not appear in the pool of canine non-concentrated saliva. Western-Blot (Fig. 1b) showed a band with high intensity between 60 kDa and 50 kDa in the human saliva specimen and the purified human sAA (ab 77,875, Abcam). This band also appeared in both canine specimens, although the intensity was lower compared to human saliva.

Analytical validation of sAA enzymatic assay

Results from the precision study are shown in Table 1. Intra-assay and inter-assay CVs (%) for sAA were <4% for specimens with low, medium and high sAA activity. The linearity under dilution study yielded a coefficient of correlation of 0.999 for both, specimen 1 and 2 (Fig. 2). In both specimens, slopes [0.99 (0.98; 1.02) and 1.00 (0.98; 1.01), respectively] were not significantly different from one, and intercepts [−2.11 (−11.63; 7.40) and 0.03 (−1.28; 1.35), respectively] were not significantly different from zero. The limit of detection, as well as lower limit of quantification, was set at 1.6 U/L, since CVs of all dilutions tested were below 20% (Fig. 3).

Experimental model of sympathetic activation

All dogs showed erection signs (pelvic thrusting and engorgement of the bulbus glandis) and ejaculated. The ejaculation's average duration was 50.7 ± 22.2 s. sAA median activity (Fig. 4a) showed significant increases at T + 0 when compared with TB (1.84-fold, $P = 0.004$)

Table 1 Intra- and inter-assay coefficients of variation (CVs) in saliva specimens with different alpha-amylase activity

	Intra-assay		Inter-assay	
Specimens	Mean (U/L)	CV (%)	Mean (U/L)	CV (%)
Low	40.3	2.00	33.4	2.60
Medium	160.0	2.27	130.0	1.38
High	765.7	1.27	656.3	3.47

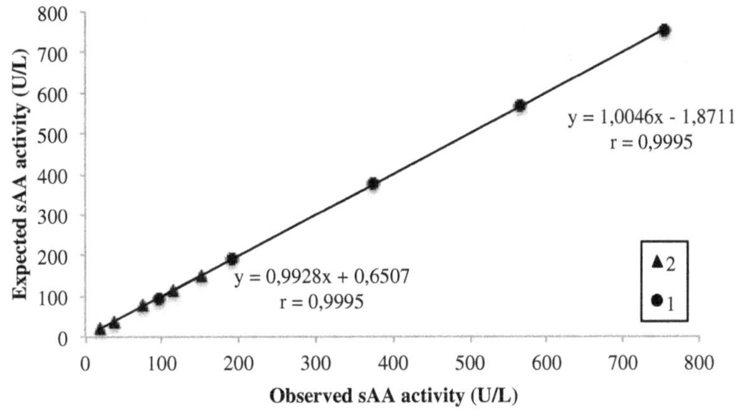

Fig. 2 Linearity under dilution of two specimens with different activity of salivary alpha-amylase (sAA): 755.2 and 152.1 U/L, specimen 1 and 2 respectively. The 'x' expressed sAA activity measured and 'y' sAA expected level at the particular dilution. r = Pearson r-value of linear correlation

and T-0 (2.06-fold, P = 0.005). Heart rate (Fig. 4b) did not show any significant change.

Discussion

Western-Blot findings corroborated the results obtained with the enzymatic assay and indicated that alpha-amylase exists in dog saliva, reacting with the sAA antibody used in this study and producing a band between 50 and 60 kDa as occurs in humans. This band was observed in both concentrated and un-concentrated canine saliva with similar intensity between them, but having lower intensity compared to human saliva probably due to a lower immunological cross-reactivity of the antibody against canine alpha-amylase or to the lower alpha-amylase concentration that exists in canine saliva compared to human. The later is in accordance with the SDS-PAGE findings and with enzymatic activity results obtained in our study, since sAA enzymatic activity in human saliva could reach ranges of 200–300 × 10^3 U/L after psychological stress [5, 25] or even 1441 ± 262 × 10^3 U/L after post intense exercise [3], which is much higher that the median values (89.5 U/L) observed in the dogs of our study. The low alpha-amylase concentration in saliva was the possible reason why Chauncey et al. [14] could not quantitate its levels in the dog. It is interesting to point out that the values of alpha-amylase in saliva of dogs were lower than the values that can be found in serum of healthy dogs (our reference interval for serum alpha-amylase is 250–1300 U/L).

Analytical validation of the sAA enzymatic method showed an acceptable intra- and inter-assay imprecision, being in all cases lower than 15%, which is the limit recommended for method validation [27]. In addition, it is lower than the within-subject biologic variation reported by Ricos et al. for sAA in human [28]. The assay showed high correlation coefficients (r = 0.999) and a good linearity (slopes were not significant different of one, and

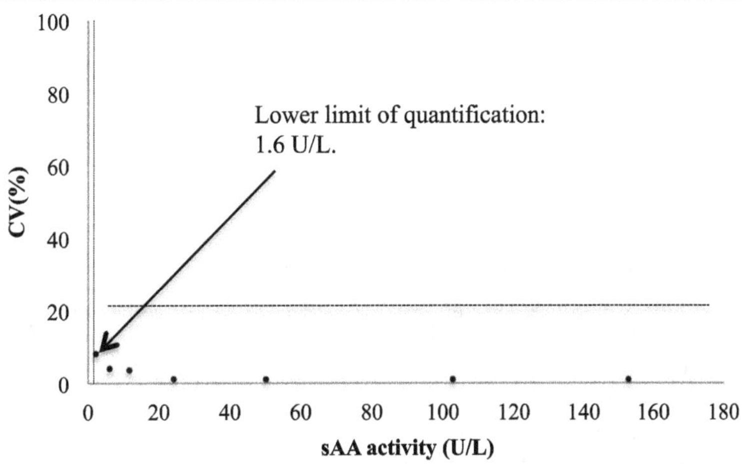

Fig. 3 Limit of quantification graph for detection of salivary alpha-amylase (sAA) activity. Horizontal line show the highest coefficient of variation (CV) accepted (20%) for the limit of quantification calculation. The vertical line reflects the analytical limit of detection (1.6 U/L)

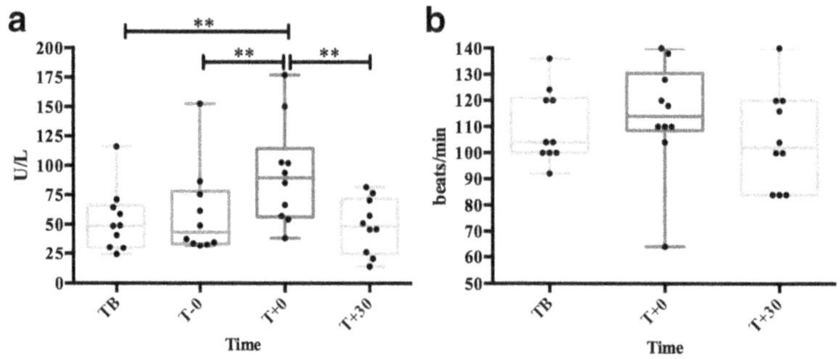

Fig. 4 Salivary alpha-amylase (sAA) activity (**a**) and heart rate (**b**) during an experimental model of sympathetic activation in dogs. TB: basal time; T-0: just starting the ejaculation; T + 0: just after ejaculation; T + 30: 30 min later. The plots show medians (line within box), 25th and 75th percentiles (boxes), min and max values (whiskers) and individual values (points). Asterisk indicates statistically significant difference (**$P < 0.01$) between times

the intercepts were not of zero) in serially diluted saliva pools. These results demonstrate that the activity–response relationship is similar in the calibration curve and the specimens, and the sample matrix and calibrator diluent did not affect the response in signal [29]. All the measurements made by sAA enzymatic assay in this study were higher than the limits of detection and quantification of the assay (set at 1.6 U/L), with a minimum recorded value of 15.2 U/L.

In this study, the induction of an ejaculation was selected as a model of sympathetic activation to evaluate sAA behavior, since it has been described that ejaculation is caused by stimulation of the sympathetic nerves which stimulate bulbocavernosus and ischiocavernosus muscles to expel semen and prostatic fluid by peristaltic contractions [23]. A prompt sAA raise at the end of the ejaculation in dogs was observed. These results could indicate that sAA increases after sympathetic activation in this species.

Heart rate has been also proposed as a marker of sympathetic nervous system activation [30, 31]. However, there were not significant increases in heart rate in our study. This is in agreement to Beerda et al. [32], who did not find a significant response in dogs to different stress stimulus (sound blasts, short electric shocks, a falling bag, an opening umbrella and two forms of restraint) when heart rate was evaluated.

It is described that alpha-amylase in human saliva is produced in the salivary glands and not diffuse into saliva from blood [25]. Probably in dogs could occur the same process. However the very low although measurable alpha-amylase activity found in dog's salivary glands and other organs, but the very high activity found in pancreas [33, 34] could open the possibility that alpha-amylase in dog saliva could be produced in the salivary gland (salivary isoenzyme) but also be partially of plasmatic origin (plasmatic isoenzyme) by diffusion from plasma into saliva as it is reported for other salivary enzymes [35].

The limited number of dogs employed in this study, and the fact that they were only male beagles from a research colony, makes difficult to extrapolate these results to the entire canine population or to real conditions. Therefore, this report should be considered as a pilot one and further studies in dogs of different sexes, breeds and living conditions, as well as using others stimulating models should be performed in order to fully evaluate the possible use of saliva alpha amylase as a stress marker.

Conclusions

This study demonstrates that there is alpha-amylase in saliva of dogs and validates a reliable spectrophotometric assay to measure this enzyme in this specie with a good precision, sensitivity and accuracy. In addition, it reports a sAA activity increase after an experimental model of sympathetic activation in the dog and suggests that sAA could be potentially used as non-invasive biomarkers of sympathetic activation in this species.

Abbreviations

CV: Coefficient of variation; G7PNP: 4, 6-ethylidene (G7)-p-nitrophenol (G1)-alpha-D- maltoheptaoside; HRP: Horseradish peroxidase; LC-MS/MS: Liquid chromatography coupled with tandem mass spectrometry; MWCO: Molecular weight cut-off; sAA: Salivary alpha-amylase; SDS-PAGE: One-dimensional sodium dodecyl sulphate polyacrylamide gel electrophoresis

Acknowledgements

D. Escribano was granted by the postdoctoral program 'Juan de la Cierva' of the 'Ministerio de Economía y Competitividad', Spain. María Dolores Contreras-Aguilar was granted by the predoctoral contract 'FPU' of University of Murcia, Spain. This study has been founded by Seneca Foundation of Murcia Region (grant number: 19894/GERM/15). We wish to thank Josefa Hernández, Luis Pardo, Sandra Valverde and Susana Ros for their technical assistance.

Funding

Seneca Foundation of Murcia Region (grant number: 19,894/GERM/15).

Authors' contributions
JJC conceived and designed the study. MDCA and LJB collected the data. MDCA were involved in the chemical analysis. MDCA, FT, SMS, DE, LJB and JJC were involved in the data interpretation. MDCA drafted the manuscript and FT, SMS, DE, LJB and JJC critically read and edited the manuscript. All authors read and approved the final manuscript.

Consent for publication
Not applicable.

Competing interests
None of the authors has any financial or personal relationships that could inappropriately influence or bias the content of the paper.

Author details
[1]Interdisciplinary Laboratory of Clinical Analysis (Interlab-UMU), Veterinary School, Campus of Excellence Mare Nostrum, University of Murcia, 30100, Espinardo, Murcia, Spain. [2]Department of Food and Animal Science, School of Veterinary Medicine, Universitat Autònoma de Barcelona, 08193, Bellaterra, Barcelona, Spain.

References

1. Bosch JA, Veerman ECI, de Geus EJ, Proctor GB. Alpha-amylase as a reliable and convenient measure of sympathetic activity: Don't start salivating just yet! Psychoneuroendocrinology. 2011;36:449–53.
2. Nater UM, La Marca R, Florin L, Moses A, Langhans W, Koller MM, et al. Stress-induced changes in human salivary alpha-amylase activity – associations with adrenergic activity. Psychoneuroendocrinology. 2006;31: 49–58.
3. Koibuchi E, Suzuki Y. Exercise upregulates salivary amylase in humans. Exp Ther Med. 2014;7:773–7.
4. Contreras-Aguilar MD, Escribano D, Martínez-Subiela S, Martínez-Miró S, Rubio M, Tvarijonaviciute A et al. Influence of the way of reporting alpha-Amylase values in saliva in different naturalistic situations: A pilot study. PLoS One. 2017;12(6):e0180100.
5. Nater UM, Rohleder N. Salivary alpha-amylase as a non-invasive biomarker for the sympathetic nervous system: current state of research. Psychoneuroendocrinology. 2009;34:486–96.
6. Granger DA, Kivlighan KT, El-Sheikh M, Gordis EB, Stroud LR. Salivary alpha-amylase in biobehavioral research - recent developments and applications. Ann N Y Acad Sci. 2007;1098:122–44.
7. Fuentes M, Tecles F, Gutierrez A, Otal J, -Subiela M, Ceron J. Validation of an automated method for salivary alpha-amylase measurements in pigs (Sus Scrofa Domesticus) and its application as a stress biomarker. J Vet Diagnostic Investig. 2011;23:282–7.
8. Behringer V, Deschner T, Möstl E, Selzer D, Hohmann G. Stress affects salivary alpha-amylase activity in bonobos. Physiol Behav. 2012;105:476–82.
9. Fuentes-Rubio M, Fuentes F, Otal J, Quiles A, Tecles F, Cerón JJ, et al. Measurements of salivary alpha-amylase in horse: comparison of 2 different assays. J Vet Behav Clin Appl Res. 2015;10:122–7.
10. Fuentes-Rubio M, Fuentes F, Otal J, Quiles A, Luisa HM. Validation of an assay for quantification of alpha-amylase in saliva of sheep. Can J Vet Res Can Rech Vet. 2016;80:197–202.
11. Bragg RF, Bennett JS, Cummings A, Quimby JM. Evaluation of the effects of hospital visit stress on physiologic variables in dogs. J Am Vet Med Assoc. 2015;246:212–5. D P.
12. Travain T, Colombo ES, Heinzl E, Bellucci D, Prato Previde E, Valsecchi P. Hot dogs: Thermography in the assessment of stress in dogs (Canis Familiaris)-a pilot study. J Vet Behav Clin Appl Res. 2015;10:17–23.
13. Part CE, Kiddie JL, Hayes WA, Mills DS, Neville RF, Morton DB, et al. Physiological, physical and behavioural changes in dogs (Canis Familiaris) when kennelled: testing the validity of stress parameters. Physiol Behav. 2014;133:260–71.
14. Chauncey HH, Henriques BL, Tanzer JM. Comparative enzyme activity of saliva from the sheep, hog, dog, rabbit, rat, and human. Arch Oral Biol. 1963;8:615–27.
15. Hudson EB, Strombeck DR. Effects of functional nephrectomy on disappearance rates of canine serum amylase and lipase. Am J Vet Res. 1978;39:1316–21.
16. de Sousa-Pereira P, Cova M, Abrantes J, Ferreira R, Trindade F, Barros A, et al. Cross-species comparison of mammalian saliva using an LC-MALDI based proteomic approach. Proteomics. 2015;15:1598–1607.
17. Peng Y, Chen X, Sato T, Rankin SA, Tsuji RF, Ge Y. Purification and high-resolution top-down mass spectrometric characterization of human salivary alpha-amylase. Anal Chem. 2012;84:3339–46.
18. Deutsch O, Fleissig Y, Zaks B, Krief G, Aframian D, Palmon A. An approach to remove alpha amylase for proteomic analysis of low abundance biomarkers in human saliva. Electrophoresis. 2008;29:4150–7.
19. Noble JE, Bailey MJA. Quantitation of protein. In: Burgess RR, Deutscher M, editors. Guide to protein purification. Second edi. San Diego: Elsevier Academic Press Inc; 2009. p. 73–95.
20. Laemmli UK. Cleavage of structural proteins during assembly of head of bacteriophage-T4. Nature. 1970;227:680.
21. Towbin H, Staehelin T, Gordon J. Electrophoretic transfer of proteins from polyacrylamide gels to nitrocellulose sheets - procedure and some applications. Proc Natl Acad Sci U S A. 1979;76:4350–4.
22. van der Heiden C, Bais R, Gerhardt W, Lorentz K, Rosalki S. IFCC methods for measurement of catalytic concentration of enzymes - part 9. IFCC method for alpha-amylase {[]1,4-alpha-D-glucan 4-glucanohydrolase, EC 3.2.1.1]. Clin Chim Acta. 1999;281:S5–S39.
23. Kutzler MA. Semen collection in the dog. Theriogenology. 2005;64:747–54.
24. Toro-Montoya A. Espermograma Med Lab. 2009;15:145–70.
25. Rohleder N, Nater UM. Determinants of salivary α-amylase in humans and methodological considerations. Psychoneuroendocrinology. 2009;34:469–85.
26. Nater UM, Rohleder N, Schlotz W, Ehlert U, Kirschbaum C. Determinants of the diurnal course of salivary alpha-amylase. Psychoneuroendocrinology. 2007;32:392–401.
27. FDA. Guidance for industry: bioanalytical method validation. Rocckville: US Department of Health and Human Service; 2001. http://www.fda.gov/downloads/Drugs/GuidanceComplianceRegulatoryInformation/Guidances/ucm070107.pdf. Accesed 16 Sept 2011.
28. Ricos C, Alvarez V, Cava F, Garcia-Lario JV, Hernandez A, Jimenez CV, et al. Current databases on biological variation: pros, cons and progress. Scand J Clin Lab Invest. 1999;59:491–500.
29. Andreasson U, Perret-Liaudet A, van Waalwijk van Doorn LJC, Blennow K, Chiasserini D, Engelborghs S, et al. A practical guide to immunoassay method validation. Front Neurol. 2015;6:1–8.
30. Anderson DE, Brady JV. Differential preparatory cardiovascular responses to aversive and appetitive behavioral conditioning. Cond Reflex. 1972;7:82–96.
31. Galosy RA, Clarke LK, Mitchell JH. Cardiac changes during behavioral stress in dogs. Am J Phys. 1979;236:H750–8.
32. Beerda B, Schilder MBH, Van Hooff JARAM, De Vries HW, Mol JA. Behavioural, saliva cortisol and heart rate responses to different types of stimuli in dogs. Appl Anim Behav Sci. 1998;58:365–81.
33. Keller P. Enzyme activities in the dog: tissue analyses, plasma values, and intracellular distribution. Am J Vet Res. 1981;42:575–82.
34. Keller P, Freudiger U. Enzyme activities in urine, cerebrospinal fluid, bile, saliva and ejaculate of dogs. Kleintierpraxis. 1984;29:15-&.
35. Tvarijonaviciute A, Barranco T, Rubio M, Carrillo JM, Martinez-Subiela S, Tecles F, et al. Measurement of Creatine kinase and Aspartate aminotransferase in saliva of dogs: a pilot study. BMC Vet Res. 2017;13:168.

3

Bile components and lecithin supplemented to plant based diets do not diminish diet related intestinal inflammation in Atlantic salmon

Trond M. Kortner[1*], Michael H. Penn[1,4], Ingemar Björkhem[2], Kjell Måsøval[3] and Åshild Krogdahl[1]

Abstract

Background: The present study was undertaken to gain knowledge on the role of bile components and lecithin on development of aberrations in digestive functions which seemingly have increased in Atlantic salmon in parallel with the increased use of plant ingredients in fish feed. Post smolt Atlantic salmon were fed for 77 days one of three basal diets: a high fish meal diet (HFM), a low fishmeal diet (LFM), or a diet with high protein soybean meal (HPS). Five additional diets were made from the LFM diet by supplementing with: purified taurocholate (1.8 %), bovine bile salt (1.8 %), taurine (0.4 %), lecithin (1.5 %), or a mix of supplements (suppl mix) containing taurocholate (1.8 %), cholesterol (1.5 %) and lecithin (0.4 %). Two additional diets were made from the HPS diet by supplementing with: bovine bile salt (1.8 %) or the suppl mix. Body and intestinal weights were recorded, and blood, bile, intestinal tissues and digesta were sampled for evaluation of growth, nutrient metabolism and intestinal structure and function.

Results: In comparison with fish fed the HFM diet fish fed the LFM and HPS diets grew less and showed reduced plasma bile salt and cholesterol levels. Histological examination of the distal intestine showed signs of enteritis in both LFM and HPS diet groups, though more pronounced in the HPS diet group. The HPS diet reduced digesta dry matter and capacity of leucine amino peptidase in the distal intestine. None of the dietary supplements improved endpoints regarding fish performance, gut function or inflammation in the distal intestine. Some endpoints rather indicated negative effects.

Conclusions: Dietary supplementation with bile components or lecithin in general did not improve endpoints regarding performance or gut health in Atlantic salmon, in clear contrast to what has been previously reported for rainbow trout. Follow-up studies are needed to clarify if lower levels of bile salts and cholesterol may give different and beneficial effects, or if other supplements, and other combinations of supplements might prevent or ameliorate inflammation in the distal intestine.

Keywords: Gut health, Intestinal inflammation, Fish feed, Plant ingredients, Cholesterol, Bile

* Correspondence: trond.kortner@nmbu.no
[1]Department of Basic Sciences and Aquatic Medicine, Faculty of Veterinary Medicine and Biosciences, Norwegian University of Life Sciences, Oslo, Norway
Full list of author information is available at the end of the article

Background

Levels of plant protein ingredients in feeds for salmonids and several other cultivated species have gradually increased over the last two decades, replacing fish meal. Substitution of marine with plant protein in feed for carnivorous fish, especially when using less refined plant protein sources such as full-fat or extracted soybean meal (SBM), will in many cases result in reduced body pools of cholesterol and bile acids [1–6]. In severe cases, the reduced levels of cholesterol and bile acids may be observed in concert with reduced fish growth and gastro-intestinal problems such as intestinal inflammation and steatosis [2, 7]. These conditions may be related to, or influenced by reduced levels of cholesterol and bile components, or disturbances in lipid digestion and metabolism. The apparent drain of bile acids in Atlantic salmon suffering from SBM-induced enteritis (SBMIE) [2, 3, 8, 9] is likely caused by a combination of the reduced dietary cholesterol load and specific action of soy antinutrients such as saponins, which may impair cholesterol and bile acid uptake from the intestinal lumen [10–13].

Recent reports suggest that bile salts, in addition to their key role in lipid digestion, have important anti-inflammatory effects in the gut, and can preserve the intestinal barrier in inflammatory bowel disease (IBD) models [14–17]. Similarly, studies with rainbow trout indicate that dietary inclusion of bile salts or soybean lecithin may prevent distal intestinal inflammation induced by SBM or plant antinutrients [5, 18, 19]. In Atlantic salmon, the SBMIE has been established as an excellent and reproducible intestinal inflammation model, and the Atlantic salmon is more susceptible to SBMIE than the rainbow trout. However, it has not yet been investigated if supplementation with bile components or lecithin can prevent or reduce diet related intestinal inflammation in Atlantic salmon.

The work presented here is part of a larger experimental series with the main objective to develop knowledge needed to produce sustainable, healthy and cost efficient fish feeds with low fish meal inclusion, based on plant and other alternative nutrient sources, and to identify indicators of feed related health effects. Specifically, the present study aimed at increasing knowledge on relationships between plant induced intestinal inflammation and deficiencies of bile components in Atlantic salmon. Based on the above mentioned studies in rainbow trout, we hypothesized that dietary supplementation with bile components or lecithin to plant protein based diets would improve performance and gut health in Atlantic salmon. For that purpose, a 77 day feeding trial was conducted. At termination of the feeding trial, the weights of body and intestines were recorded, and blood, bile, intestinal tissues and digesta were sampled for evaluation of effects on growth, nutrient metabolism and intestinal structure (histomorphological changes) and function (digestive enzyme activities and faecal dry matter).

Methods

Experimental animals, diet and sampling

Atlantic salmon (*Salmo salar* L.) post smolts of the Sunndalsøra breed with mean weight of 362 ± 95 g (mean ± SD) were weighed, pit tagged and randomly allocated into 20 cylindrical fiberglass tanks (200 L, 35 fish pr tank) with flow-through seawater (6–7 L min^{-1}). Two replicate tanks per diet were used. Water temperature varied between 7 and 14 °C. Oxygen content and salinity of the outlet water were monitored to ensure saturation above 85 % and stability, respectively. A 24 h lighting regime was employed during the experimental period. The fish were weighed individually when allocating the fish to the experimental units to assure similar biomass in all tanks.

Ten experimental diets were formulated (Table 1). A fish meal based diet (high fish meal; HFM) was used as a control. A low fish meal (LFM) combination of soy protein concentrate (SPC) and pea protein concentrate, or high protein soya (HPS) provided the bulk of dietary protein in the two other diets. Conjugated bile salts, taurine, lecithin and cholesterol were added to these diets singly or in combination as described in Table 1. Supplementation levels were based on levels used in rainbow trout as previously reported [5, 18, 19]. Feed intake was not recorded. Diets were formulated to contain 41 % crude protein and 30 % lipid (DM basis). They were supplemented with a standard vitamin and micro-mineral premix and limiting essential amino acids (lysine, methionine) as necessary to provide required amounts as suggested by NRC guidelines [20]. Diets also contained 100 mg kg-1 yttrium oxide as an inert marker for calculation of nutrient apparent digestibilities. Chemical analysis of the diets is shown in Table 1. Feed was produced by extrusion at the BioMar AS production facility in Brande, Denmark. Diets were extruded with a feed pellet size of 6 mm.

The feeding trial ran for 77 days. Tank sampling order and fish sampling were conducted randomly. Fifteen fish were sampled from each tank and euthanized by anaesthetization with tricaine methane-sulfonate (MS-222) followed by a sharp blow to the head. From ten fish per tank, blood was sampled by venipuncture of the caudal vein. Blood was collected in Vacutainers containing lithium heparin and stored on ice until centrifugation. Plasma was separated and immediately frozen in liquid nitrogen and stored at −80 °C until analysis. After blood withdrawal, fish were dissected to remove the viscera. Intestinal contents (digesta) were collected from the pyloric, mid and distal intestines. The contents from the pyloric intestines were

Table 1 Diet formulation and chemical analysis

	HFM	LFM	LFM + Tauro-cholate	LFM + Bovine bile salt	LFM + Taurine	LFM + Lecithin	LFM + Suppl Mix	HPS	HPS + Bovine bile salt	HPS + Suppl Mix
Ingredient (g 100 g^{-1})										
SA SP Sara Rousing[a]	15.00	5.00	5.00	5.00	5.00	5.00	5.00	7.50	7.50	7.50
Nordic LT 94 fishmeal[b]	15.00	5.00	5.00	5.00	5.00	5.00	5.00	7.50	7.50	7.50
Soya HP 48[c]								20.00	20.00	20.00
Soya 60 % (SPC)[d]	10.00	19.03	19.03	19.03	19.03	19.03	19.03	3.52	3.52	3.52
Corn Gluten[e]	5.34	15.00	15.00	15.00	15.00	15.00	15.00	10.19	10.19	10.19
Pea Protein 50[f]	6.00	13.00	13.00	13.00	13.00	13.00	13.00	0.40	0.40	0.40
Dehulled Beans[g]	14.58	14.00	14.00	14.00	14.00	14.00	14.00	14.00	14.00	14.00
Sunflower expeller[h]	10.00									
Wheat Gluten[i]		1.97	1.97	1.97	1.97	1.97	1.97	10.00	10.00	10.00
Fishoil (Standard)[j]	7.45	7.67	7.67	7.67	7.67	7.67	7.67	7.82	7.82	7.82
Rapeseed oil[k]	17.09	17.60	17.60	17.60	17.60	17.60	17.60	17.94	17.94	17.94
Sodium taurocholate[l]			1.80							
Bovine bile salt[l]				1.80			1.80		1.80	1.80
Cholesterol[l]							1.50			1.50
Taurine[l]					0.40					
Lecithin[l]						1.50	0.40			0.40
MCP	0.70	1.82	1.82	1.82	1.82	1.82	1.82	1.56	1.56	1.56
Lysine	0.20	0.81	0.81	0.81	0.81	0.81	0.81	0.98	0.98	0.98
Methionine	0.11	0.32	0.32	0.32	0.32	0.32	0.32	0.25	0.25	0.25
Threonine		0.11	0.11	0.11	0.11	0.11	0.11	0.14	0.14	0.14
Barox (antioxidant)	0.03	0.03	0.03	0.03	0.03	0.03	0.03	0.03	0.03	0.03
Vitamin-Mineral mix[m]	0.30	0.30	0.30	0.30	0.30	0.30	0.30	0.30	0.30	0.30
Yttrium[n]	0.05	0.05	0.05	0.05	0.05	0.05	0.05	0.05	0.05	0.05
Lucantin Pink CWD 10 %	0.04	0.04	0.04	0.04	0.04	0.04	0.04	0.04	0.04	0.04
Chemical analysis[o]										
Dry matter (%)	95.0	95.0	95.0	95.0	95.0	95.0	95.0	95.0	95.0	95.0
Ash (%)	7.0	5.0	5.0	5.0	5.0	5.0	5.0	5.2	5.2	5.2
Fat (%)	29.8	29.2	29.2	29.2	29.2	29.2	29.2	29.6	29.6	29.6
Protein (%)	40.8	40.4	40.4	40.4	40.4	40.4	40.4	41.4	41.4	41.4
D Protein (%)	36.0	36.0	36.0	36.0	36.0	36.0	36.0	36.0	36.0	36.0
DE (MJ/kg)	20.3	20.3	20.3	20.3	20.3	20.3	20.3	20.3	20.3	20.3
GE (MJ/kg)	24.4	24.4	24.4	24.4	24.4	24.4	24.4	24.6	24.6	24.6
Cholesterol (g/kg)	2.1	0.8	0.7	0.6	0.7	0.7	19.1	1.0	1.0	17.8
Bile salts (g/kg)	0.3	0.2	16.3	n/a	n/a	n/a	11.0	n/a	10.58	n/a

[a]Superprime, supplied by Köster Marine Proteins GmbH, Hamburg, Germany
[b]Supplied by Norsildmel AS, Bergen, Norway
[c]Supplied by Scan Mills, Germany
[d]Supplied by Selecta S/A, Av. Jamel Ceilio, 2496 – 12th region, Goiania, Brazil
[e]Supplied by Cargil Nordic, SAS van Gent, Holland
[f]Supplied by DLG Food Grain, Roslev, Denmark
[g]Supplied by HC Handelscenter, Skibby, Denmark
[h]Supplied by DLA agro, Denmark
[i]Supplied by Roquette, Beinheim, France
[j]Supplied by FF Skagen, Skagen, Denmark
[k]Supplied by Emmelev, Otterup, Denmark
[l]Supplied by Sigma-Aldrich, Broendby, Denmark
[m]Supplied to meet requirements. Composition is intellectual property of BioMar AS
[n]Inert marker for the evaluation of nutrient digestibility
[o]Complete chemical analysis was conducted only for the basal diets (HFM, LFM, HPS). Cholesterol content was analyzed in all diets, bile salt content was analyzed in five diets as shown in table

divided into two equal portions labelled as PI1 and PI2 where PI1 constituted the most proximal located portion. A similar separation was performed for the contents of the distal intestines and labelled as DI1 and DI2. Intestinal contents were frozen in liquid nitrogen and stored at −80 °C until analysis. For analysis of leucine amino peptidase enzymatic activity, the entire pyloric caeca and distal intestine tissues were immediately frozen in liquid nitrogen in pre-weighed tubes and stored at −80 °C before further processing. From five additional fish per tank, distal intestine tissues were fixed in 10 % neutral buffered formalin (4 % formaldehyde) for 24 h and subsequently transferred to 70 % EtOH for storage until processing for histological examination. The remaining fish in each tank were stripped for faeces and continued on feeds for an additional week at which time they were stripped again. Faecal samples were pooled and frozen until analysis.

Chemical analyses

Diet and faecal samples were analyzed for dry matter (after heating at 105°C for 16–18 h), ash (combusted at 550 °C to constant weight), nitrogen (crude protein) (by the semi-micro-Kjeldahl method, Kjeltec-Auto System, Tecator, Höganäs, Sweden), fat (diethylether extraction in a Fosstec analyzer (Tecator) after HCl-hydrolysis), starch (measured as glucose after hydrolysis by alpha-amylase (Novo Nordisk A/S, Bagsvaerd, Denmark) and amyloglucosidase (Bohringer Mannheim GmbH, Mannheim, Germany), followed by glucose determination by the 'Glut-DH method' (Merck, Darmstadt, Germany)), gross energy (using the Parr 1271 Bomb calorimeter, Parr, Moline, IL, USA), and yttrium (by inductivity coupled plasma (ICP) mass-spectroscopy as described by Refstie et al. [21]).

Plasma variables and bile salt levels

All diets were analyzed for cholesterol by isotope dilution mass spectrometry as described by Schaffer et al. [22]. Plasma was analyzed for cholesterol following standard procedures at the Central Laboratory of the Norwegian University of Life Sciences, Faculty of Veterinary Medicine and Biosciences, Oslo. Total intestinal bile salt levels were measured in plasma and pooled freeze dried gastrointestinal contents from PI1, PI2, MI, DI1, and DI2. Bile salt concentration was determined using the enzyme cycling amplification/Thio – NAD method (Inverness Medical, Cheshire, UK) in the ADVIA®1650 Chemistry System (Siemens Healthcare Diagnostics Inc.) at the Central Laboratory. In diet samples and bile taken directly from the gall bladder, glycine and taurine conjugated bile acids were analyzed by HPLC-MS-MS by a modification of the method described by Tagliacocci et al. [23] using deuterium labeled glycine derivatives of bile acids as internal standards. Total bile acids in plasma and in intestinal contents were also analyzed by isotope dilution and combined GC-MS after addition of deuterated cholic acid, chenodeozycholic acid and deoxycholic acid as internal standards followed by deconjugation as described by Björkhem and Falk [24]. The two methods have been shown to give almost identical results. Plasma oxysterols were analyzed by isotope dilution and combined GC-MS after hydrolysis as described by Dzeletovic et al. [25]. Sitosterol and campesterol were assayed by isotope dilution and combined GC-MS after hydrolysis as described by Acimovic et al. [26]. Lathosterol was analyzed by isotope dilution mass spectrometry as described by Lund et al. [27]. 7α-hydroxy-4-cholesten-3-one (C4) was analyzed by isotope dilution and use of combined HPLC-MS as described by Lövgren-Sandblom et al. [28]. Lipoprotein profiles in plasma were conducted employing size exclusion chromatography and measurements of cholesterol on-line using microliter sample volumes as described by Parini et al. [29].

Histology

Formalin fixed DI tissue samples were processed using standard histological techniques and stained with haematoxylin and eosin (H&E). Examination was conducted blinded and in randomized order. The degree of histomorphological change (i.e., deviation from normal) was assessed and assigned to one of four categories: normal, slight, moderate or marked. The following histological characteristics were evaluated: length and fusion of mucosal folds, cellular infiltration and width of the lamina propria and submucosa, enterocyte vacuolization, nucleus position within the enterocytes and the relative number of goblet cells [30, 31].

Calculations

Crude protein (CP) was calculated as N x 6.25. Thermal-unit growth coefficient (TGC) was calculated as: TGC = $1000*(FBW^{1/3} - IBW^{1/3}) \times (\Sigma D°)^{-1}$, where IBW and FBW are the initial and final body weights (tank means) and ΣD° is the thermal sum (feeding days × average temperature in °C). The specific growth rate (SGR) was calculated using the tank means for initial body weight (IBW) and final body weight (FBW) as follows: SGR = [(ln FBW − ln IBW) /number of days] × 100. Organo-somatic indices were calculated as percentages of the weight of the organ in relation to body weight.

Statistical analyses

Data was analyzed using one-way ANOVA followed by Duncan's test for post hoc comparison. Tank means were used as the statistical unit. Histology data from individual fish were analyzed using Chi-square test. The level of significance was set to $p < 0.05$ for all analyses.

Results

Diet content of cholesterol and bile salts

As expected, among the diets used in this experiment cholesterol level was higher in the HFM diet than in the LFM and HPS basal diets. Supplementation with cholesterol (suppl mix) increased diet cholesterol concentration (Table 1). Bile salt concentrations were determined in five diets: HFM, LFM, LFM + taurocholate, LFM + suppl mix, and HPS + bovine bile salt diets (Table 1). Unsupplemented diets contained very little bile salts, and as expected the LFM had lower levels than the HFM diet. Supplementation with bile salts, either taurocholate or bovine bile salt, markedly increased dietary bile salt level. The taurocholate supplement was more than 98 % pure, a result that was confirmed by direct analysis (data not shown). The bovine bile salt used as supplement contained a range of bile acids and bile salts. Free bile acids, tauroconjugates and glycoconjucates comprised about 45, 25 and 30 % respectively of this bovine bile preparation.

Fish growth, organ indices and nutrient digestibilities

Final fish weights, thermal growth coefficients (TGC) and specific growth rates (SGR) are presented in Table 2. TGC and SGR values were significantly lower in fish in the groups fed the LFM and HPS diets compared to those receiving the HFM diet. None of the supplements improved TGC or SGR significantly. The lowest TGC and SGR values were found in the fish fed the bovine bile salt supplemented diets (LFM + bovine bile salt, LFM + suppl mix, HPS + bovine bile salt, and HPS + suppl mix). When supplemented to the LFM diet, the reductions in TGC and SGR values were significant.

Organosomatic indices of the pyloric (PI), mid (MI) and distal (DI) intestines are shown in Table 2. For PI somatic indices significant different treatment effects were observed. The LFM fed fish had significantly higher PI somatic index compared to those fed the HFM and HPS diets. Among the LFM groups of fish, lecithin supplementation led to lower relative PI weights. No differences due to supplementation were observed among the HPS groups. Similar results were observed in the MI, increased weights in the LFM groups compared to HFM and HPS groups, except for the lecithin supplemented groups, which showed similar values as HFM and HPS groups. The opposite situation was observed in the distal intestine. LFM fed fish had similar DI somatic index as those fed HFM, but the HPS groups had a significantly lower DI relative weight. Among the LFM groups, fish fed diets supplemented with bovine bile salt (LFM + bovine bile salt and LFM + suppl mix) had lower DI somatic indices compared to the non-supplemented fish (LFM). The supplementations to the HPS diet did not significantly affect relative weight of DI.

Table 3 shows the results of the digestibility analyses. Only small differences were observed for the protein and lipid digestibilities. Interestingly enough, the LFM diets showed significantly higher protein digestibility than the HFM diet. No significant differences were observed between the LFM and HPS diets. Likewise, no significant differences in lipid digestibility were observed between these diets.

Morphology of the distal intestine

Slight to moderate inflammatory changes were observed in several samples. See Fig. 1 for numbers of samples from each treatment classified by severity of changes and Fig. 2 for representative histological images. All fish fed the HFM diet appeared normal. Eight out of ten fish fed the LFM diet appeared normal, whereas 2 fish showed slight changes. Supplementing the LFM diet with taurocholate increased the number of samples with slight changes, whereas supplementing the LFM diet with bovine bile salt or the suppl mix clearly increased the number of samples with moderate changes. Other LFM diets did not significantly affect the number of samples with inflammatory changes, or the severity of changes. Varying degrees of accumulation of eosinophilic material within enterocytes (Fig. 3) were frequently observed in fish fed LFM diets. Fish fed the LFM + taurocholate diet had the highest frequency of eosinophilic inclusions, in 8 out of 10 samples.

Table 2 Growth and relative organ weights of Atlantic salmon during the feeding period

	HFM	LFM	LFM + Tauro-cholate	LFM + Bovine bile salt	LFM + Taurine	LFM + Lecithin	LFM + Suppl Mix	HPS	HPS + Bovine bile salt	HPS + Suppl Mix	Pooled SEM
BW (g)	789^{a}	709^{bcd}	678^{cd}	656^{cd}	704^{bcd}	758^{ab}	638^{d}	681^{cd}	669^{cd}	667^{cd}	17
TGC	3.04^{a}	2.54^{bcd}	2.36^{cde}	2.09^{e}	2.52^{bcd}	2.75^{ab}	2.08^{e}	2.37^{bcde}	2.24^{cde}	2.16^{de}	0.09
SGR	1.02^{a}	0.87^{bc}	0.81^{bcd}	0.72^{d}	0.86^{bc}	0.92^{ab}	0.72^{d}	0.81^{bcd}	0.77^{cd}	0.74^{d}	0.03
Organosomatic indicies											
PI	2.02^{c}	2.52^{a}	2.37^{ab}	2.30^{abc}	2.33^{abc}	2.12^{bc}	2.41^{ab}	2.01^{c}	2.09^{bc}	2.09^{bc}	0.08
MI	0.17^{ef}	0.21^{ab}	0.22^{a}	0.21^{abc}	0.19^{cd}	0.17^{f}	0.19^{cd}	0.17^{ef}	0.19^{de}	0.19^{def}	0.005
DI	0.48^{ab}	0.49^{a}	0.47^{abcd}	0.43^{de}	0.48^{abc}	0.49^{ab}	0.44^{bcde}	0.39^{e}	0.43^{cde}	0.40^{e}	0.01

Abbreviations: *BW* body weight, *TGC* thermal growth coefficient, *SGR* specific growth rate, *PI* pyloric intestine, *MI* mid intestine, *DI* distal intestine. Different letters denote diet groups that are significantly different

Table 3 Apparent digestibility of crude protein and lipid

	HFM	LFM	LFM + Tauro-cholate	LFM + Bovine bile salt	LFM + Taurine	LFM + Lecithin	LFM + Suppl Mix	HPS	HPS + Bovine bile salt	HPS + Suppl Mix	Pooled SEM
Protein	88.3[c]	90.0[ab]	89.4[abc]	89.0[bc]	90.1[ab]	90.7[a]	89.5[abc]	90.2[a]	90.0[ab]	89.3[bc]	0.25
Lipid	96.5[a]	95.7[abc]	95.0[bc]	95.7[abc]	95.2[abc]	96.2[ab]	94.5[c]	95.1[bc]	96.2[ab]	94.6[c]	0.25

Different letters denote diet groups that are significantly different

Inflammatory responses varied between fish fed HPS-containing diets. When present, changes were typical of soy enteropathy, including decreased enterocyte vacuolization, apical displacement of enterocyte nuclei, leukocyte infiltration of the epithelia and submucosa, and hyperplastic connective tissue in the lamina propria and submucosa. Supplementation of the HPS diet with either the bovine bile salt or the suppl mix did not significantly affect the number of fish showing inflammatory changes, or the severity of changes.

Blood plasma biochemistry

Blood plasma variables are presented in Table 4. Total plasma cholesterol levels were higher in fish fed cholesterol supplemented diets (suppl mix). No significant differences were observed between fish fed the other diets. Most of the plasma cholesterol was present in the HDL lipoprotein fraction, except in the fishes fed with the cholesterol supplemented diets (suppl mix). In these, most of the cholesterol was present in the LDL fraction and much less in the HDL fraction.

Plasma bile salt concentrations differed between treatments. The individual variation of plasma bile salt was, however, greater than expected, in particular for the groups fed bovine bile salt. The variation was largely reflective of dietary supplementation with bile acids. Although the One-Way ANOVA did not show significant differences between fish fed any of the basal diets, taking the results of all the LFM treatments without bile salt supplementation together it is clear that fish fed LFM diet had lower plasma total bile salt levels than fish fed the HFM diet. The HPS groups had the lowest plasma bile salt concentration. In fish fed both LFM and HPS, the bovine bile salt and suppl mix groups had higher levels of plasma bile acids compared to groups fed their respective basal diets.

Lathosterol is an intermediate in cholesterol synthesis and the circulating level of this steroid reflects cholesterol synthesis in the liver. As expected, the cholesterol-containing diets (suppl mix) depressed circulating lathosterol. Lower lathosterol levels were also observed in the LFM groups as compared to HFM and HPS groups. The cholesterol supplemented diets caused markedly increased plasma levels of 7α-Hydroxy-4-cholesten-3-one (C4), indicative of conversion of excess cholesterol to bile acids. No significant differences in C4 levels were observed between fish fed the other diets. Marked reduction in plasma levels of the plant sterols sitosterol and campesterol were observed for fish fed the cholesterol-containing diets (suppl mix). Supplementation with taurocholate, taurine and the bovine bile salt also reduced plasma plant sterol levels, but

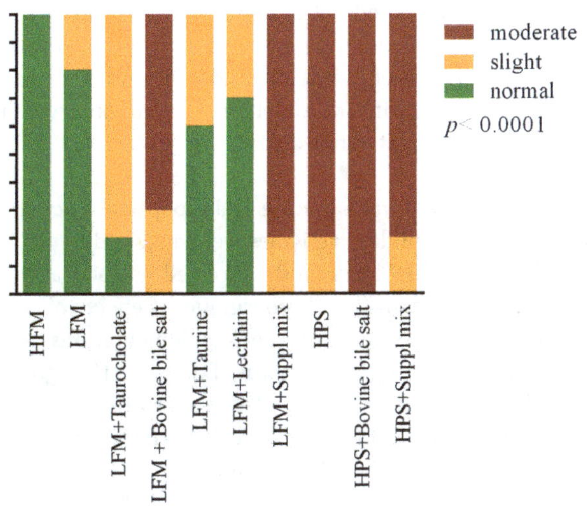

Fig. 1 Number of samples in each diet group classified by severity of inflammatory changes in the distal intestine. The *P* value for the Chi-square test is given

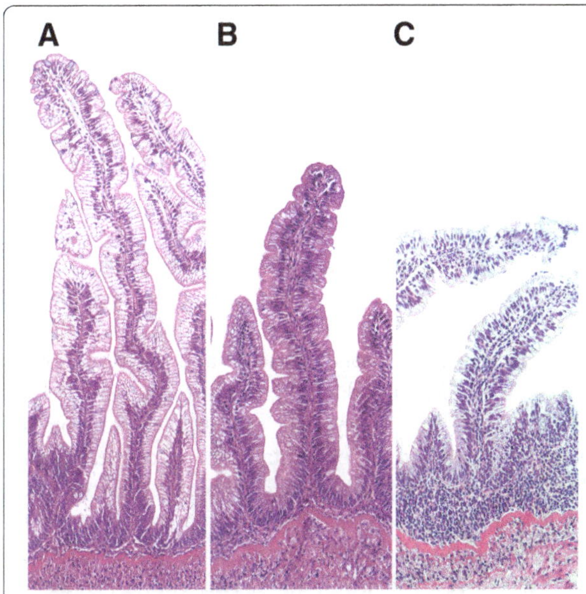

Fig. 2 Distal intestinal histolomorphology showing representative appearance of sections that were graded as (**a**) normal, (**b**) mild, or (**c**) moderate changes characteristic of soybean meal-induced distal intestinal enteritis

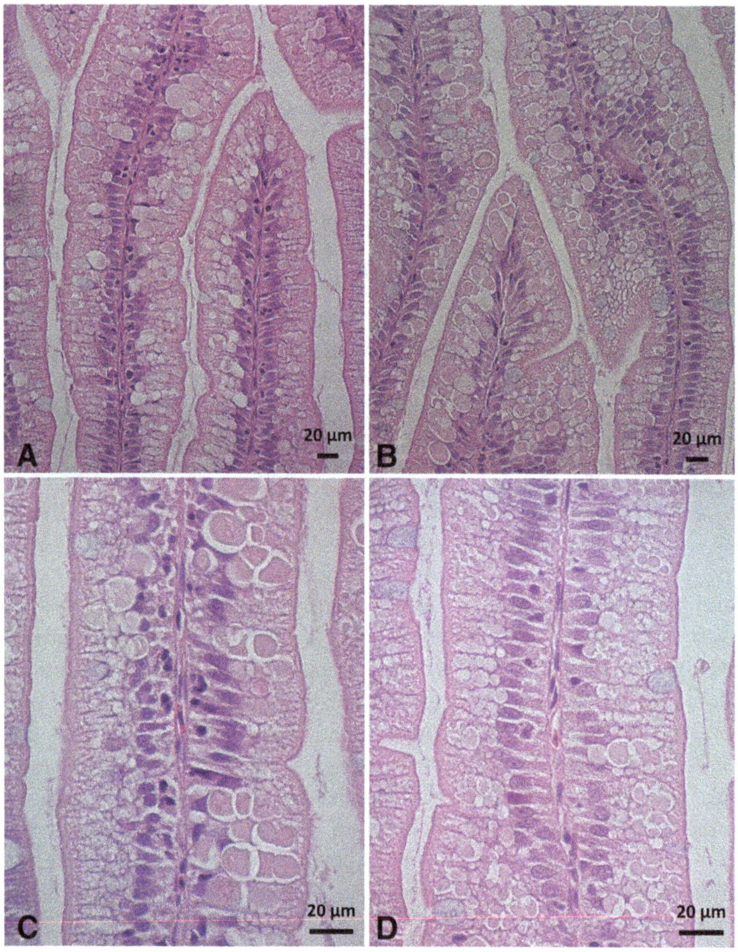

Fig. 3 Eosinophilic inclusions within distal intestine enterocytes in (**a**) LFM, (**b**) LFM + taurocholate, (**c**) LFM, and (**d**) LFM + taurocholate fed fish

to a lesser extent. Plasma levels of oxysterols were markedly higher in the two cholesterol supplemented groups, whereas few differences were observed between fish fed the other diets.

Gall bladder bile

Bile taken directly from the gall bladder was analyzed for individual bile salts. Total, conjugated and unconjugated bile salt concentrations are shown in Table 5. No significant differences in total concentrations were found between the LFM and HPS fed groups of fish compared to the HFM fed fish. Bovine bile salt supplementation increased or tended to increase total bile acid concentrations when added to both the LFM and HPS diets. The majority of bile acids in the gallbladder bile were conjugated; the only unconjugated bile acid found was cholic acid which was detected at low concentration. The taurine conjugated bile acids were the predominant form of bile acids found in the bile, with taurocholic acid being the predominant individual bile acid. Taurodeoxycholic acid was higher in the bile of fish groups fed diets supplemented with the bovine bile salt. The glycine conjugated bile acids were detected at very low concentrations except for the groups fed diets supplemented with bovine bile salt. The glycine conjugated bile acids were also largely responsible for differences observed in total bile acid concentrations since no statistically significant differences were observed in total taurine conjugated bile acids.

Brush border membrane leucine aminopeptidase activity

Leucine aminopeptidase activities were analyzed in pyloric and distal intestine tissue and expressed as total activity per kg fish weight. In the PI, no significant effects of basal diet formulation or any of the supplementations were found (data not shown). In the DI, the HPS groups showed lower enzyme activity compared to the HFM and LFM groups (Fig. 4). Groups fed diets with the suppl mix, i.e., both the LFM and HPS groups, showed the lowest activities. Fish fed the diets with bovine bile salt also showed lower enzyme activity compared to the LFM control. Supplementation with either bovine bile salt or suppl mix to the HPS formulation did not result in

Table 4 Mean values (n = ten fish pr diet group) for blood plasma variables

	HFM	LFM	LFM+ Tauro cholate	LFM+ Bovine bile salt	LFM+ Taurine	LFM+ Lecithin	LFM+ Suppl mix	HPS	HPS+ Bovine bile salt	HPS+ Suppl mix	pooled SEM
Total CH (mmol/l)	10.7^{a}	8.3^{a}	8.5^{a}	8.4^{a}	8.4^{a}	9.5^{a}	24.6^{b}	8.6^{a}	8.9^{a}	24.6^{b}	1.1
VLDL-CH[a]	0.1	0.1	0.2	0.2	0.2	0.1	0.5	0.2	0.1	0.5	
LDL-CH[a]	1.6	1.3	0.9	1.0	0.9	0.9	19.9	0.9	1.0	23.5	
HDL-CH[a]	10.5	7.5	6.6	7.9	6.4	8.0	7.3	7.5	5.8	9.1	
Bile salts (μmol/l)	31^{abc}	20^{bc}	23^{abc}	48^{ab}	22^{bc}	15^{bc}	55^{a}	6^{c}	41^{ab}	23^{abc}	7
Lathosterol (μg/ml)	6.6^{b}	3.8^{cd}	3.2^{de}	3.5^{d}	4.7^{c}	4.6^{c}	2.4^{ef}	5.8^{b}	3.6^{d}	2.5^{ef}	0.4
C4 (ng/ml)	13^{a}	10^{a}	10^{a}	10^{a}	13^{a}	11^{a}	200^{b}	12^{a}	9^{a}	180^{b}	8
Sitosterol(μg/ml)	67^{ab}	74^{a}	47^{cd}	52^{bcd}	44^{d}	64^{ab}	6^{e}	64^{ab}	40^{d}	6^{e}	4
Campesterol(μg/ml)	229^{a}	188^{ab}	151^{b}	160^{b}	133^{b}	220^{a}	14^{c}	239^{a}	162^{b}	18^{c}	16
Oxysterols (ng/ml)[a]											
7α-hydroxy-CH	124	130	111	116	172	116	1800	103	591	2110	
7β-hydroxy-CH	52	37	40	42	66	29	238	32	404	285	
7-keto-hydroxy-CH	130	101	122	125	201	59	730	89	1915	554	
24-hydroxy-CH	3.6	2.2	1.8	2.0	3.3	3.5	7.1	3.8	5.3	11.5	
25-hydroxy-CH	5	5	7	8	9	7	36	5	15	40	
27-hydroxy-CH	34	21	14	17	42	22	64	32	22	92	

[a]Lipoprotein and oxysterol profiles were measured in a pooled sample of n = ten animals pr diet group. CV for the different assays, i.e., the analytical variance, as estimated by analyzing a control sample over 10 consecutive days: VLDL-CH: 8.1 %, LDL-CH: 3.4 %, HDL-CH: 5.0 %, VLDL-TAG: 13.1 %, LDL-TAG: 10.5 %, HDL-TAG: 9.7 %. CVs for all oxysterol assays are <8 %, except for 25-hydroxy-CH (11 %) [(25)]. Different letters denote diet groups that are significantly different

significant effects regarding this enzyme activity compared to the respective unsupplemented diets.

Dry matter, trypsin activity and bile salt levels in intestinal content

Dry matter (DM) of digesta in the intestinal sections (PI1, PI2, MI, DI1, DI2) are presented in Table 6. No statistically significant differences were found in DM of digesta from the PI and MI. However, the trends observed in these regions became significant in the DI. The digesta DM of fish fed the LFM diet did not differ significantly from those fed the HFM diet, but the HPS groups showed significantly lower digesta DM in both the DI segments. For the LFM fed groups, bile salt supplementation tended to decrease DM. No differences due to any of the supplementation were observed among the HPS diets. Trypsin activities in intestinal regions are shown in Table 6. In the distal half of the DI, trypsin activities in fish fed the LFM diet were low and similar to fish fed the HFM diet. Fish fed the HPS diet showed significantly higher trypsin activity as compared to the other controls. Fish fed bile salt (taurocholate, bovine

Table 5 Mean values (n = ten fish pr diet group) for gall bladder bile acid levels

	HFM	LFM	LFM+ Tauro cholate	LFM+ Bovine bile salt	LFM+ Taurine	LFM+ Lecithin	LFM+ Suppl mix	HPS	HPS+ Bovine bile salt	HPS+ Suppl mix	pooled SEM
Total bile acids	99^{cd}	117^{bcd}	112^{bcd}	137^{ab}	104^{bcd}	95^{d}	139^{ab}	112^{bcd}	161^{a}	134^{abc}	9
Total conjugated	99^{cd}	117^{bcd}	112^{bcd}	136^{ab}	104^{bcd}	95^{d}	138^{ab}	112^{bcd}	161^{a}	133^{abc}	9
Total unconjugated	$<0.1^{c}$	$<0.1^{c}$	$<0.1^{c}$	0.6^{b}	$<0.1^{c}$	$<0.1^{c}$	1.2^{a}	$<0.1^{c}$	0.3^{bc}	1.0^{a}	<0.1
Taurine conjugated	99^{cd}	117^{bcd}	112^{bcd}	97^{cd}	104^{bcd}	95^{d}	113^{bcd}	112^{bcd}	122^{b}	107^{bcd}	8
T-CA	92^{ab}	110^{a}	108^{a}	66^{b}	99^{ab}	89^{ab}	92^{ab}	100^{ab}	87^{ab}	83^{ab}	9
T-CDCA	7^{bc}	6^{c}	2^{d}	6^{c}	5^{cd}	6^{c}	9^{bc}	13^{a}	7^{bc}	10^{ac}	1
T-DCA	$<0.1^{c}$	$<0.1^{c}$	2^{c}	25^{a}	$<0.1^{c}$	$<0.1^{c}$	12^{b}	$<0.1^{c}$	28^{a}	14^{b}	1
Glycine conjugated	$<0.1^{c}$	$<0.1^{c}$	$<0.1^{c}$	39^{a}	$<0.1^{c}$	$<0.1^{c}$	25^{b}	0.1^{c}	39^{a}	26^{b}	1
G-CA	$<0.1^{c}$	$<0.1^{c}$	$<0.1^{c}$	27^{a}	$<0.1^{c}$	$<0.1^{c}$	19^{b}	0.1^{c}	30^{a}	19^{b}	1
G-CDCA	$<0.1^{d}$	$<0.1^{d}$	$<0.1^{d}$	1.9^{a}	$<0.1^{d}$	$<0.1^{d}$	0.8^{c}	$<0.1^{d}$	1.4^{b}	0.9^{c}	<0.1
G-DCA	$<0.1^{d}$	$<0.1^{d}$	$<0.1^{d}$	9.8^{a}	$<0.1^{d}$	$<0.1^{d}$	5.3^{c}	$<0.1^{d}$	8.1^{ab}	6.1^{bc}	0.3

Abbreviations: *T-* tauro-, *G-* glyco, *CA* colic acid, *CDCA* chenodeoxycholic acid, *DCA* deoxycholic acid. Different letters denote diet groups that are significantly different

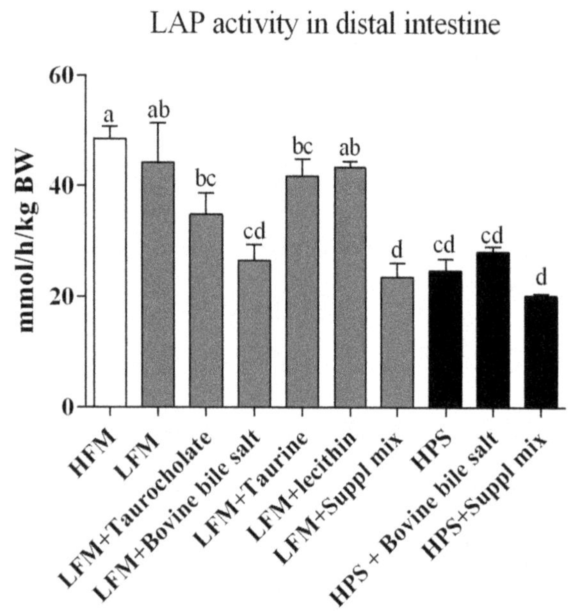

Fig. 4 Leucine aminopeptidase (LAP) activity in the distal intestinal tissue, expressed as per kg body weight. Values are means with standard errors represented by vertical bars. Different letters denote diet groups that are significantly different

bile salt and suppl mix) supplemented LFM diets had higher trypsin activity compared to their respective control and similar to the HPS groups. Levels were high in all HPS groups, and no effect of supplementation was observed. No statistically significant differences in digesta bile salt concentrations were observed for any of the treatments, in any of the intestinal regions (Table 6).

Discussion

Effects of basal diet

In the present study, the two plant based diets (LFM and HPS) suppressed fish growth performance as compared to the high fish meal control diet (HFM). Animal growth parameters are arguably among the most appropriate and practical response variables for examining the effects of variation in diet composition, and a large body of literature has described effects of inclusion of fish meal alternatives on fish growth performance (reviewed by [32, 33]). The lower growth rates observed for the LFM and HPS diets were probably related to, or directly caused by the observed histomorphological changes in the distal intestine and the accompanying signs of gut dysfunction. Slight to moderate signs of enteritis in the distal intestine were observed in 2 and 10 out of 10 fish in the LFM and HPS fed fish, respectively. The changes were typical of soybean meal induced enteritis (SBMIE), including decreased enterocyte vacuolization, apical displacement of enterocyte nuclei,

Table 6 Dry matter (DM) content, trypsin activity and bile salt levels in digesta of Atlantic salmon

	HFM	LFM	LFM + Tauro-cholate	LFM + Bovine bile salt	LFM + Taurine	LFM + Lecithin	LFM + Suppl Mix	HPS	HPS + Bovine bile salt	HPS + Suppl Mix	Pooled SEM
Digesta dry matter (mg/g)											
PI1	10.1	9.3	8.4	8.2	9.0	10.7	9.9	9.1	9.2	10.4	0.54
PI2	11.9	11.0	10.3	9.6	11.5	12.1	11.5	12.3	10.5	12.1	0.58
MI	14.1	12.9	12.2	11.2	12.6	13.8	13.1	13.2	12.8	14.0	0.54
DI1	14.0^{a}	12.9^{ab}	11.4^{bcd}	11.2^{cd}	12.3^{bcd}	13.1^{ab}	11.8^{bcd}	10.9^{c}	12.8^{abc}	11.6^{bcd}	0.38
DI2	11.8^{ab}	11.0^{bc}	9.3^{de}	9.7^{cde}	10.7^{bcd}	12.1^{ab}	10.0^{cd}	8.3^{e}	9.4^{cde}	8.1^{e}	0.32
Digesta trypsin activity (U/mg DM)											
PI1	308^{abc}	232^{bc}	221^{c}	293^{abc}	234^{bc}	226^{c}	234^{bc}	335^{a}	330^{ab}	344^{a}	29
PI2	182^{ab}	113^{bc}	132^{bc}	175^{abc}	108^{bc}	93^{c}	158^{bc}	155^{bc}	192^{ab}	249^{a}	24
MI	106	72	72	139	78	53	87	78	126	120	30
DI1	50^{abc}	38^{c}	47^{abc}	79^{a}	41^{bc}	37^{c}	67^{abc}	56^{abc}	74^{ab}	64^{abc}	10
DI2	7^{c}	8^{c}	25^{b}	48^{a}	6^{c}	10^{c}	37^{ab}	35^{ab}	37^{ab}	41^{a}	5
Digesta bile salt levels (mg/g DM)											
PI1	290	355	376	367	356	285	268	330	346	299	75
PI2	228	262	256	303	268	292	290	242	301	251	57
MI	171	218	205	207	275	220	275	159	183	204	44
DI1	78	74	98	103	124	63	83	97	99	92	34
DI2	5	10	11	11	16	5	15	15	14	17	7

Different letters denote diet groups that are significantly different

leukocyte infiltration of the epithelia and submucosa, and hyperplastic connective tissue in the lamina propria and submucosa [30, 31]. The histomorphological changes in the soya (HPS) fed fish were milder than what is typically observed in feeding trials with Atlantic salmon fed full-fat or extracted soya. The reason for this is not clear, but a likely explanation could be that the soy variant used in the current study contained lower levels of antinutrients, such as saponins.

The observed histomorphological alterations in fish fed the LFM and HPS diets were accompanied by alterations in a panel of indicators of gut function, most pronounced for the HPS groups. Decreased faecal dry matter, first reported in salmon by van den Ingh and co-workers [30], is frequently observed during distal intestinal inflammations and is probably a result of impaired ability to absorb water in the inflamed and damaged intestine. Decreased weight of the DI, as seen for fish fed the HPS diet, is also typically observed in concert with intestinal inflammation, apparently due to loss of intestinal mucosa [34]. Brush border membrane enzyme activity is a sensitive indicator of enterocyte dysfunction and changes may be present even in the absence of altered tissue histology. The lower LAP activity in fish fed HPS diets is in agreement with presence of SBMIE [3]. The higher trypsin activity, as seen for fish fed the HPS diet, is also commonly observed during intestinal inflammatory conditions. Trypsin activity in DI digesta typically shows a correlation with the severity of morphological changes associated with SBMIE [3, 35, 36]. Furthermore, the two plant diets tended to reduce blood plasma cholesterol and bile acid levels. This is a commonly observed response to plant feed ingredients, with their content of fibers, phytosterols, phytoestrogens and saponins that all may affect cholesterol and bile salt absorption from the intestine [37]. Increased levels of plant ingredients in formulated feeds will also reduce the dietary load of cholesterol and bile acids, as demonstrated in the present study. Dietary supplementation of plant based fish feeds with cholesterol and/or bile components have therefore been subject to systematic investigations, in order to assess if removal of marine based feed ingredients may create a deficiency of any of these compounds. These results are discussed in the following section.

Effects of supplements

The main finding of the present work was that supplementation with bile salts, either as pure taurocholate or as a mix of bovine bile salts did not reduce signs of enteritis in the distal intestine. Similarly, supplementation with lecithin, taurine or combinations of bile acids, cholesterol and lecithin were also ineffective in ameliorating enteritic changes. The results of the present investigation contrast previous reports in rainbow trout [5, 18, 19], where supplementation with bovine bile salts (1.5–2.0 %), taurocholate (1.0 %) or soybean lecithin (2.0 %) were reported to prevent SBM-induced morphological abnormalities in the DI. Bile salt supplementation was also interpreted to restore growth, feed efficiency and intestinal maltase activity to comparable levels reported in the control group [5]. In contrast, the present study clearly indicated that supplementation with bovine bile salt at similar levels (1.8 %), either alone or in the suppl mix, impaired intestinal function. The strongest responses were seen when the bovine bile salt was supplemented to the LFM diet, as witnessed by reduced DI relative weight and LAP activity, increased trypsin activity in DI digesta and clear signs of enteritis in the DI. A likely explanation for the observed negative effects would be cytotoxic actions of the bile salts on intestinal mucosa. Toxicity of bile acids is thought to be highly correlated with its hydrophobicity. Therefore, the high levels (45 %) of unconjugated, more hydrophobic bile acids in the bovine bile salt may be the reason for the observed negative responses. The bovine bile salt also reduced fish growth. Feed intake was not monitored during the trial, and therefore, supplementation effects on palatability cannot be assessed. However, it is possible that the bovine bile salt may have caused reduced palatability.

There are likely direct interactions between bile acids and intestinal immunity. For example, in mammalian IBD models, activation of the nuclear receptor farnesoid X receptor (FXR) by natural or synthetic ligands has been associated with immunosuppressive actions and preservation of intestinal epithelial barrier integrity [38]. Specifically, FXR activation has been shown to decrease epithelial permeability and suppress proinflammatory cytokine levels in murine intestinal mucosa [17]. Additionally, FXR activation is inhibited by proinflammatory stimuli in different model systems [16]. As bile acids are natural endogenous FXR ligands, this may point to a direct role of bile salts in modulation of immune responses via FXR. Whether a similar mechanism exists in fish is currently unknown. However, a recent study demonstrated that FXR mRNA levels are strongly induced in the DI of Atlantic salmon suffering from SBMIE, concurrent with a marked induction of proinflammatory cytokines and alterations in bile salt metabolism [2, 39].

Reported studies of dietary inclusion of bile salts to teleost fish feeds are, to our knowledge, limited to the above mentioned studies with rainbow trout and our present work with salmon. In contrast, many studies have investigated dietary supplementation with cholesterol, taurine and lecithin/phospholipids to formulated fish feeds, in order to estimate requirements (reviewed in [20, 40, 41]). Reported results are not consistent, but positive effects of inclusion on fish growth and feed intake have often been observed, most prominent during larval and early juvenile stages. For adult fish, reported studies are fewer, but requirements of dietary cholesterol, taurine and lecithin/phospholipids are probably species-specific and absorption along the gut dependent on diet formulation. Importantly, evaluation of gut health and function, for example by histological examination, has not been carried out in most of these studies. Given that future fish feeds most likely will contain lower levels of cholesterol, bile salts and marine phospholipids, more research within this area is clearly warranted.

Conclusions

In conclusion, dietary supplementation with bile components or lecithin in general did not improve endpoints regarding performance or gut health in Atlantic salmon, in clear contrast to what has been previously reported for rainbow trout. Thus, our work does not add to the understanding of a relationship between intestinal inflammation and deficiencies of bile acids and taurine. The reason why our results differ from previous observations in rainbow trout may be the general bile salt status of the fish and/or species differences. Follow-up studies are needed to clarify if lower levels of bile salts and cholesterol may give different and beneficial effects, and if other supplements and other combinations of supplements might improve the inflammation status of the distal intestine. The present study complements our previous report from the same feeding trial [42] and demonstrates how dietary cholesterol and bile salts are taken up and metabolized in Atlantic salmon, showing clear effects of the dietary supplements on gall bladder bile acid levels, cholesterol lipoprotein profiles and plasma levels of oxysterols and markers for cholesterol synthesis and breakdown.

Acknowledgements

The present paper publishes results of contract research mainly funded by BioMar AS. The Aquaculture Protein Centre (APC) at the Norwegian School of Veterinary Science, a Centre of Excellence under the Norwegian Research Council (Project no. 145949/120), was the main scientific partner of the work. The authors wish to thank the senior researcher Gerd Marit Berge and technicians at Nofima Research Station at Sunndalsøra, Norway for skillful animal care and scientific follow up, and APC's technicians Ellen K. Hage, Elin C. Valen and Gunn C. Østby for excellent technical assistance.

Funding

The present paper publishes results of contract research mainly funded by BioMar AS.
The funding body participated in study design, but had no role in data collection, analysis and interpretation, decision to publish, or preparation of the manuscript.

Authors' contributions

The authors' contributions were as follows: TMK: data evaluation and interpretation, manuscript development, MHP: experimental design, data evaluation and interpretation, IB: data evaluation and interpretation, KM: experimental design, data evaluation and interpretation, ÅK: leadership, experimental design, data evaluation and interpretation, manuscript development. All authors read and approved the final manuscript.

Competing interests

The present paper publishes results of contract research mainly funded by BioMar AS. Co-author Kjell Måsøval is employed by BioMar AS.

Consent for publication

Not applicable.

Author details

[1]Department of Basic Sciences and Aquatic Medicine, Faculty of Veterinary Medicine and Biosciences, Norwegian University of Life Sciences, Oslo, Norway. [2]Department of Laboratory Medicine, Division for Clinical Chemistry, Karolinska University Hospital, Huddinge, Sweden. [3]Biomar AS, Nordre gate 11, 7011 Trondheim, Norway. [4]Present Address: US Fish & Wildlife Service, Lamar, PA 16848, USA.

References

1. Kaushik SJ, Cravedi JP, Lalles JP, Sumpter J, Fauconneau B, Laroche M. Partial or total replacement of fish-meal by soybean protein on growth, protein-utilization, potential estrogenic or antigenic effects, cholesterolemia and flesh quality in rainbow-trout, *Oncorhynchus mykiss*. Aquaculture. 1995;133:257–74.
2. Kortner TM, Gu J, Krogdahl Å, Bakke AM. Transcriptional regulation of cholesterol and bile acid metabolism after dietary soybean meal treatment in Atlantic salmon, *Salmo salar* L. Br J Nutr. 2013;109:593–604.
3. Krogdahl Å, Bakke-McKellep AM, Baeverfjord G. Effects of graded levels of standard soybean meal on intestinal structure, mucosal enzyme activities, and pancreatic response in Atlantic salmon (*Salmo salar* L.). Aquaculture Nutr. 2003;9:361–71.
4. Sitja-Bobadilla A, Pena-Llopis S, Gomez-Requeni P, Medale F, Kaushik S, Perez-Sanehez J. Effect of fish meal replacement by plant protein sources on non-specific defence mechanisms and oxidative stress in gilthead sea bream (*Sparus aurata*). Aquaculture. 2005;249:387–400.
5. Yamamoto T, Suzuki N, Furuita H, Sugita T, Tanaka N, Goto T. Supplemental effect of bile salts to soybean meal-based diet on growth and feed utilization of rainbow trout *Oncorhynchus mykiss*. Fish Sci. 2007;73:123–31.
6. Yun BA, Mai KS, Zhang WB, Xu W. Effects of dietary cholesterol on growth performance, feed intake and cholesterol metabolism in juvenile turbot (*Scophthalmus maximus* L.) fed high plant protein diets. Aquaculture. 2011;319:105–10.
7. Gu M, Kortner TM, Penn M, Hansen AK, Krogdahl Å. Effects of dietary plant meal and soya-saponin supplementation on intestinal and hepatic lipid droplet accumulation and lipoprotein and sterol metabolism in Atlantic salmon (*Salmo salar* L.). Br J Nutr. 2014;111:432–44.
8. Romarheim OH, Skrede A, Gao YL, Krogdahl Å, Denstadli V, Lilleeng E, Storebakken T. Comparison of white flakes and toasted soybean meal partly replacing fish meal as protein source in extruded feed for rainbow trout (*Oncorhynchus mykiss*). Aquaculture. 2006;256:354–64.
9. Romarheim OH, Skrede A, Penn M, Mydland LT, Krogdahl Å, Storebakken T. Lipid digestibility, bile drainage and development of morphological intestinal changes in rainbow trout (*Oncorhynchus mykiss*) fed diets containing defatted soybean meal. Aquaculture. 2008;274:329–38.
10. Krogdahl A, Gajardo K, Kortner TM, Penn M, Gu M, Berge GM, Bakke AM. Soya Saponins induce enteritis in Atlantic Salmon (*Salmo salar* L.). J Agric Food Chem. 2015;63:3887–902.
11. Vinarova L, Vinarov Z, Atanasov V, Pantcheva I, Tcholakova S, Denkov N, Stoyanov S. Lowering of cholesterol bioaccessibility and serum concentrations by saponins: in vitro and in vivo studies. Food Funct. 2015;6:501–12.
12. Lee SO, Simons AL, Murphy PA, Hendrich S. Soyasaponins lowered plasma cholesterol and increased fecal bile acids in female golden Syrian hamsters. Expn Biol Med. 2005;230:472–8.
13. Malinow MR, Mclaughlin P, Papworth L, Stafford C, Kohler GO, Livingston AL, Cheeke PR. Effect of alfalfa saponins on intestinal cholesterol absorption in rats. Am J Clin Nutr. 1977;30:2061–7.

14. Fiorucci S, Cipriani S, Mencarelli A, Renga B, Distrutti E, Baldelli F. Counter-regulatory role of bile acid activated receptors in immunity and inflammation. Curr Mol Med. 2010;10:579–95.
15. Gadaleta RM, van Mil SWC, Oldenburg B, Siersema PD, Klomp LWJ, van Erpecum KJ. Bile acids and their nuclear receptor FXR: Relevance for hepatobiliary and gastrointestinal disease. Biochim Biophys Acta Mol Cell Biol Lip. 1801;2010:683–92.
16. Gadaleta RM, Oldenburg B, Willemsen ECL, Spit M, Murzilli S, Salvatore L, Klomp LWJ, Siersema PD, van Erpecum KJ, van Mil SWC. Activation of bile salt nuclear receptor FXR is repressed by pro-inflammatory cytokines activating NF-kappa B signaling in the intestine. Biochim Biophys Acta Mol Bas Dis. 1812;2011:851–8.
17. Gadaleta RM, van Erpecum KJ, Oldenburg B, Willemsen ECL, Renooij W, Murzilli S, Klomp LWJ, Siersema PD, Schipper MEI, Danese S, Penna G, Laverny G, Adorini L, Moschetta A, van Mil SWC. Farnesoid X receptor activation inhibits inflammation and preserves the intestinal barrier in inflammatory bowel disease. Gut. 2011;60:463–72.
18. Iwashita Y, Suzuki N, Yamamoto T, Shibata J, Isokawa K, Soon AH, Ikehata Y, Furuita H, Sugita T, Goto T. Supplemental effect of cholyltaurine and soybean lecithin to a soybean meal-based fish meal-free diet on hepatic and intestinal morphology of rainbow trout *Oncorhynchus mykiss*. Fish Sci. 2008;74:1083–95.
19. Iwashita Y, Suzuki N, Matsunari H, Sugita T, Yamamoto T. Influence of soya saponin, soya lectin, and cholyltaurine supplemented to a casein-based semipurified diet on intestinal morphology and biliary bile status in fingerling rainbow trout *Oncorhynchus mykiss*. Fish Sci. 2009;75:1307–15.
20. NRC. Nutrient requirements of fish and shrimp. Washington, D.C: The National Academies Press; 2011. p. 360.
21. Refstie S, Helland SJ, Storebakken T. Adaptation to soybean meal in diets for rainbow trout, *Oncorhynchus mykiss*. Aquaculture. 1997;153:263–72.
22. Schaffer R, Sniegoski LT, Welch MJ, White VE, Cohen A, Hertz HS, Mandel J, Paule RC, Svensson L, Bjorkhem I, Blomstrand R. Comparison of two isotope dilution/mass spectrometric methods for determination of total serum cholesterol. Clin Chem. 1982;28:5–8.
23. Tagliacozzi D, Mozzi AF, Casetta B, Bertucci P, Bernardini S, Di IC, Urbani A, Federici G. Quantitative analysis of bile acids in human plasma by liquid chromatography-electrospray tandem mass spectrometry: a simple and rapid one-step method. Clin Chem Lab Med. 2003;41:1633–41.
24. Bjorkhem I, Falk O. Assay of the major bile acids in serum by isotope dilution-mass spectrometry. Scand J Clin Lab Invest. 1983;43:163–70.
25. Dzeletovic S, Breuer O, Lund E, Diczfalusy U. Determination of cholesterol oxidation-products in human plasma by isotope-dilution mass-spectrometry. Anal Biochem. 1995;225:73–80.
26. Acimovic J, Lovgren-Sandblom A, Monostory K, Rozman D, Golicnik M, Lutjohann D, Bjorkhem I. Combined gas chromatographic/mass spectrometric analysis of cholesterol precursors and plant sterols in cultured cells. J Chromatogr B Anal Tech Biomed Life Sci. 2009;877:2081–6.
27. Lund E, Sisfontes L, Reihner E, Bjorkhem I. Determination of serum levels of unesterified lathosterol by isotope dilution-mass spectrometry. Scand J Clin Lab Invest. 1989;49:165–71.
28. Lovgren-Sandblom A, Heverin M, Larsson H, Lundstrom E, Wahren J, Diczfalusy U, Bjorkhem I. Novel LC-MS/MS method for assay of 7alpha-hydroxy-4-cholesten-3-one in human plasma. Evidence for a significant extrahepatic metabolism. J Chromatogr B Analyt Technol Biomed Life Sci. 2007;856:15–9.
29. Parini P, Johansson L, Broijersen A, Angelin B, Rudling M. Lipoprotein profiles in plasma and interstitial fluid analyzed with an automated gel-filtration system. Eur J Clin Invest. 2006;36:98–104.
30. van den Ingh TSGA, Krogdahl Å, Olli JJ, Hendriks HGCJ, Koninkx JGJF. Effects of soybean-containing diets on the proximal and distal intestine in Atlantic Salmon (*Salmo salar*) - A Morphological-Study. Aquaculture. 1991;94:297–305.
31. Baeverfjord G, Krogdahl Å. Development and regression of soybean meal induced enteritis in Atlantic salmon, *Salmo salar* L, distal intestine: A comparison with the intestines of fasted fish. J Fish Dis. 1996;19:375–87.
32. Gatlin DM, Barrows FT, Brown P, Dabrowski K, Gaylord TG, Hardy RW, Herman E, Hu GS, Krogdahl Å, Nelson R, Overturf K, Rust M, Sealey W, Skonberg D, Souza EJ, Stone D, Wilson R, Wurtele E. Expanding the utilization of sustainable plant products in aquafeeds: a review. Aquaculture Res. 2007;38:551–79.
33. Naylor RL, Hardy RW, Bureau DP, Chiu A, Elliott M, Farrell AP, Forster I, Gatlin DM, Goldburg RJ, Hua K, Nichols PD. Feeding aquaculture in an era of finite resources. PNAS. 2009;106:15103–10.
34. Nordrum S, Bakke-McKellep AM, Krogdahl Å, Buddington RK. Effects of soybean meal and salinity on intestinal transport of nutrients in Atlantic salmon (*Salmo salar* L.) and rainbow trout (*Oncorhynchus mykiss*). Comp Biochem Physiol B Biochem Mol Biol. 2000;125:317–35.
35. Lilleeng E, Froystad MK, Ostby GC, Valen EC, Krogdahl Å. Effects of diets containing soybean meal on trypsin mRNA expression and activity in Atlantic salmon (*Salmo salar* L). Comp Biochem Physiol A Mol Int Physiol. 2007;147:25–36.
36. Penn MH, Bendiksen EA, Campbell P, Krogdahl Å. High level of dietary pea protein concentrate induces enteropathy in Atlantic salmon (*Salmo salar* L.). Aquaculture. 2011;310:267–73.
37. Krogdahl Å, Penn M, Thorsen J, Refstie S, Bakke AM. Important antinutrients in plant feedstuffs for aquaculture: an update on recent findings regarding responses in salmonids. Aquaculture Res. 2010;41:333–44.
38. Stojancevic M, Stankov K, Mikov M. The impact of farnesoid X receptor activation on intestinal permeability in inflammatory bowel disease. Can J Gastroenterol. 2012;26:631–7.
39. Marjara IS, Chikwati EM, Valen EC, Krogdahl A, Bakke AM. Transcriptional regulation of IL-17A and other inflammatory markers during the development of soybean meal-induced enteropathy in the distal intestine of Atlantic salmon (*Salmo salar* L.). Cytokine. 2012;60:186–96.
40. Salze GP, Davis DA. Taurine: a critical nutrient for future fish feeds. Aquaculture. 2015;437:215–29.
41. Tocher DR, Bendiksen EA, Campbell PJ, Bell JG. The role of phospholipids in nutrition and metabolism of teleost fish. Aquaculture. 2008;280:21–34.
42. Kortner TM, Bjorkhem I, Krasnov A, Timmerhaus G, Krogdahl A. Dietary cholesterol supplementation to a plant-based diet suppresses the complete pathway of cholesterol synthesis and induces bile acid production in Atlantic salmon (*Salmo salar* L.). Br J Nutr. 2014;111:2089–103.

4

Genome-wide association study for hereditary ataxia in the Parson Russell Terrier and DNA-testing for ataxia-associated mutations in the Parson and Jack Russell Terrier

Alana Christina Gast[1], Julia Metzger[1], Andrea Tipold[2] and Ottmar Distl[1*]

Abstract

Background: Spinocerebellar ataxia also referred to as hereditary ataxia comprises different forms of progressive neurodegenerative diseases. A complex mode of inheritance was most likely in Parson Russell Terriers (PRT) and in Jack Russell Terriers (JRT). Recently, the missense mutation *KCNJ10*:c.627C > G was shown to be associated with the spinocerebellar ataxia (SCA) in JRT and related Russell group of terriers, whereas the missense mutation *CAPN1*:c.344G > A was associated with late onset ataxia (LOA) in PRT.

Results: We performed a genome-wide association study (GWAS) in PRT including 15 cases and 29 controls and found a statistically strong signal in the genomic region on dog chromosome 38 (CFA38) where *KCNJ10* is located. We tested the *CAPN1*:c.344G > A and *KCNJ10*:c.627C > G (Transcript XM_545752.4) mutations in a sample of 77 PRT and 9 JRT from Germany as well as further 179 controls from 20 different dog breeds. All cases and controls genotyped carried the wild-type for the *CAPN1*:c.344G > A mutation. Among the PRT, 17/77 (22.1 %) dogs were homozygous for the mutant *KCNJ10* allele and 22/77 (28.6 %) dogs were heterozygous. Three cases of PRT had the homozygous *KCNJ10* wild-type. In JRT, 1/3 cases did show the mutant *KCNJ10* allele homozygous. Thus, we sequenced the *KCNJ10* exons with their adjacent regions from 10 PRT and 3 JRT including the animals with imperfect co-segregation of the c.627C > G mutation. We identified a total of 45 genetic variants within *KCNJ10*. The most likely variant explaining the cases appeared a 1-bp-insertion in a C-stretch within exon 3 (*KCNJ10*:g.22141027insC). In silico analysis showed that this indel may influence the regulation of gene expression.

Conclusions: In the present study, 16/21 cases of hereditary ataxia perfectly co-segregated with the *KCNJ10*:c.627C > G mutation. The *CAPN1*:c.344G > A mutation could not be validated and seems to be a rare variant in the samples screened. Screening *KCNJ10* for further mutations did result in a genetic variant explaining 2 JRT cases but further 3 cases with a non-mutant homozygous c.627C > G genotype could not be resolved. Breeders have to be aware that DNA-testing for hereditary ataxia in PRT and JRT does not capture all cases of hereditary ataxia in these dog breeds. At least one further form of hereditary ataxia not yet resolved by a mutation may occur in PRT and JRT.

Keywords: Hereditary ataxia, Association, *KCNJ10*, *CAPN1*, Parson Russell Terrier, Jack Russell Terrier

* Correspondence: ottmar.distl@tiho-hannover.de
[1]Institute for Animal Breeding and Genetics, University of Veterinary Medicine Hannover, Bünteweg 17p, 30559 Hannover, Germany
Full list of author information is available at the end of the article

Background

In dogs, spinocerebellar ataxia (hereditary ataxia) is characterized by progressive incoordination of gait, loss of balance, hypermetric and spastic movements. This condition may be associated with changes of brainstem auditory evoked potentials, myokymia, neuromyotonia and muscle fasciculation or seizures [1–7].

Hereditary ataxia is classified according to different aspects like age of onset (neonatal, juvenile and adult) and location of the pathomorphological lesions (spinal cord and/or cerebellar cortex) [8]. In Parson (PRT) and Jack Russell Terriers (JRT) lesions were found in the spinal cord and in the brain [2]. In Fox Terriers, lesions were only present in the spinal cord [9], whereas a more recent study reported histopathological degenerative changes in the brainstem [10]. Histopathological examinations of the central nervous system in PRT and JRT demonstrated a bilateral symmetrical myelopathy, predominantly a neuronal axonopathy in the dorsal and ventral or ventromedial funiculi [1, 2]. Loss of axons and myelin and astrogliosis were primarily seen in the spinocerebellar tracts of the cervical cord but were also present in all parts of the brain [1, 2, 7].

A complex segregation analysis using regressive logistic models was performed to elucidate the mode of inheritance in PRT and JRT [2]. The data included 3 pedigrees with a total of 115 dogs, either JRT or PRT, and 27 affected with the typical clinical signs and 9/27 with a histopathological examination showing a bilateral symmetric myelopathy in the nervous system. A monogenic mode of inheritance could be clearly ruled out. Mixed models with a major gene effect and a polygenic model were most likely for these pedigrees. The analysis could not differentiate how many loci may segregate in these two dog breeds.

In JRT, PRT and related breeds, the missense mutation c.627C > G in the *KCNJ10* (*potassium inwardly-rectifying channel, subfamily J, member 10)* gene (Transcript XM_545752.4) was found to be strongly associated with spinocerebellar ataxia (SCA) [7, 11]. This *KCNJ10* variant was identified screening a whole-genome sequence of a single JRT with spinocerebellar ataxia and myokymia under the assumptions of an autosomal recessive inheritance and a mutation altering the protein structure. Data filtering included other 81 canids that had not shown SCA. Affected animals showed ataxia, myokymia and/or seizures beginning from 2–12 months of age. The spinal cord sections revealed a bilateral myelopathy. Brain magnetic resonance imaging showed no abnormalities and hearing loss was not evident [7].

A missense mutation in the *CAPN1* gene (c.344G > A) was associated with a late-onset spinocerebellar ataxia phenotype (LOA) in a cohort of PRT [12]. Signs of symmetric spinocerebellar ataxia had been noticed in affected dogs between 6 and 12 months of age. The *CAPN1* missense mutation c.344G > A was identified using a genome-wide association study (GWAS) followed by the massively parallel sequencing of affected and control PRT for the LOA-associated chromosomal interval.

The objectives of this study were to perform a genome-wide association study (GWAS) in PRT for hereditary ataxia using the canine Illumina high density bead chip and then to show whether the previously reported SCA- and LOA-associated *KCNJ10* and *CAPN1* genes in PRT and JRT are in windows of significantly associated genomic regions. In addition, we sequenced *KCNJ10* and validated the previously reported *KCNJ10* and *CAPN1* mutations in PRT and JRT and further control samples of other breeds of dog.

Methods

We collected EDTA-blood samples from 77 PRT and 9 JRT whereof 16 PRT and 3 JRT were clinically affected by SCA (Additional file 1). All 19 cases were presented at the clinic for Small Animals, University of Veterinary Medicine Hannover. Controls did not show any signs of ataxia, myokymia or seizures based on medical records of practitioners and clinical examinations at the clinic for Small Animals, Hannover. In addition, controls had to be >4 years of age. For 17 PRT a pedigree could be constructed. A subsample of the cases for the present study had been previously described elsewhere [2]. In brief, all clinically affected dogs showed symmetric generalized ataxia with hypermetric and spastic movements in all 4 legs at 2–9 months of age. Generalized seizures were observed in some cases. In all affected dogs clinical signs worsened and had to be euthanized at an age <3.5 years. All dogs had their origin in Germany. Out of the 16 clinically SCA-affected PRT cases, 14 were confirmed through a histopathological examination. In all examined 14 PRT, a bilateral symmetrical myelopathy was evident. Predominantly an axonopathy combined with myelin loss, in the dorsal and ventral or ventromedial funiculi was seen. Swelling of axons and dilatation of myelin sheaths with loss of myelin adjacent to a mild astrogliosis were observed primarily in the spinocerebellar tracts of the cervical cord but were also observed in all parts of the brain.

Genomic DNA was isolated using standard methods with RBC (Red Blood Cell) lysis buffer and SE (sodium EDTA) buffer. The DNA concentration of the samples was adjusted to 50 ng/µl using the Nanodrop ND-1000 (Peqlab Biotechnology, Erlangen, Germany) and quality control was performed by gel electrophoresis using 1 % agarose gels (peqGold Universal Agarose, Peqlab Biotechnologie).

We performed a GWAS in 44 PRT using the canine Illumina high density beadchip (Illumina, San Diego,

CA, USA) containing 173,662 single nucleotide polymorphisms (SNPs). The data set included 15 cases and 29 controls. Out of these 15 cases, 12 had a histopathological examination confirming the clinical diagnosis. Controls had to be unrelated with the cases at the parent level and >4 years of age. Among controls, 11 were male and 18 female. Cases included 7 males and 8 females. After quality control (genotyping rate per SNP and animal >0.90), filtering for minor allele frequency >0.05 and Hardy-Weinberg equilibrium (HWE) ($p < 0.000001$) using SAS/Genetics, version 9.4 (Statistical Analysis System, SAS-Institute, Cary, NE, USA), 128,863 SNPs were left for the analysis.

The GWAS was performed with a general linear model. The analysis was run using TASSEL, version 3.0.164 [13]. The GLM explained for sex effects and the SNP genotypes. In addition, we tested several extended models employing up to five principal components (PCAs) to show the robustness of the outcome of the GWAS. All these models yielded the same genome-wide associated SNPs as the GLM model. Thus, adding principal components for cryptic data structure did not change the results of the GLM model. A plot of the first two PCAs for cases and controls employed for the GWAS is shown in Additional file 2. We applied the Bonferroni correction to determine the threshold for genome-wide significance in order to avoid false-positive associations. The Bonferroni correction set the threshold for significance at $0.05/128{,}863 = 3.88e^{-7}$ for a P-value of 0.05. A sex-stratified case-control analysis was performed using SAS/Genetics, version 9.4 (SAS). Homozygosity mapping was done in sliding windows with a minimum of 4 consecutive homozygous SNPs within a range of 50 kb using PLINK, version 1.07 [14].

A polymerase chain reaction-restriction fragment length polymorphism (PCR-RFLP) for a sample of 77 PRT, 9 JRT from Germany and 179 controls from 20 different dog breeds was employed for genotyping the *CAPN1*:c.344G > A and *KCNJ10*:c.627C > G mutations. The design of primers was carried out using Primer 3 (http://bioinfo.ut.ee/primer3-0.4.0/) and the dog genome assembly CanFam3.1 (Additional file 3).

The gene model we used for *KCNJ10* was based on the transcript XM_005640901.1 of the dog genome assembly CanFam3.1 (Additional file 4). This transcript includes three exons whereof only two exons (exon 2 and 3) are translated into a protein with 414 amino acids (aa). A previous study [7] used the transcript XM_545752.4 as gene model (denoted XM_545752.3 in previous reports [7, 11]) with two exons encoding 379 aa. Exon 2 and 3 of *KCNJ10* and their adjacent genomic regions were sequenced in 10 PRT (cases PRT I-III and PRT IV-VIII and controls PRT IX and PRT X) and 3 JRT (cases JRT I-III) using an ABI 3500 Genetic Analyzer (Applied Biosystems by Life Technologies, Darmstadt, Germany) (Additional file 3). In total, 45 genetic variants were detected in these 13 dogs. Exon 1 could not be amplified because several prime pairs designed for this canine genomic region or primer pairs designed from other species including human, mouse and rat did not result in amplicons with the expected size nor the amplicons could be sequenced. The exon 1 region did not seem to be correctly annotated in the dog reference genome and thus, may prevent retrieval of possible genetic variants for *KCNJ10* exon 1 in whole genome sequence data.

In addition, we tried to amplify the gene *KCNJ9* (gene ID 100855823) annotated at 22,100,627–22,104,165 base pairs (bp) on dog chromosome (CFA) 38 (CanFam3.1). The record of this gene contained large gaps. We searched for canine expressed sequence tags (ESTs) using the canine coding sequence of *KCNJ9* and the basic local alignment tool (blast) of NCBI (https://blast.ncbi.nlm.nih.gov/Blast.cgi). The best hit with an E-value of $1e^{-77}$ and a total score of 293 (DN374672.1) of this search did not fit to the genomic region where *KCNJ9* was annotated in the dog genome reference assembly. The same was found for hits with larger E-values. Therefore, we were not able to build a gene model for *KCNJ9* or sequence this gene.

All *KCNJ10* genetic variants detected in the 10 PRT and 3 JRT were further evaluated by sequencing *KCNJ10* from one dog of 9 other breeds. These dogs had a normal phenotype in regard to SCA and included the following breeds: Akita, Bernese mountain dog, Dalmatian, German Drahthaar, German shepherd, Irish wolfhound, Shar Pei, Tibetan terrier and Briard. Analysis of sequencing results had been performed using Sequencher software, version 4.8 (Gene Codes, Ann Arbor, MI, USA). The evaluation study resulted in 16 private variants for PRT and JRT. We then filtered the 16 genetic variants for homozygous mutant genotypes in affected PRT and JRT. The single nucleotide variant (SNV) reported in a previous study [7] and only one other variant (*KCNJ10*:g.22141027insC) remained. Validation of this result was performed in further 17 PRT. We developed a test on a LI-COR 4300 DNA Analyzer (LI-COR Biosciences, Lincoln, NE, USA) using a 167-bp amplicon (Additional file 3). The forward primer was labelled with IRD700 at the 5′end. All samples of the 77 PRT and 9 JRT as well as 84 dogs from 40 other different breeds were used to generate the *KCNJ10*:g.22141027insC containing amplicon. The amplicons were size-fractionated using gel electrophoresis on an automated sequencer LI-COR 4300 DNA Analyzer on 6 % polyacrylamide denaturing gels. Allele sizes were scored against IRD700-labeled DNA ladders (Additional file 5). For bioinformatic analysis of the effects of the *KCNJ10*:g.22141027insC variant we used the complete fasta-sequence of *KCNJ10* and employed the Regulatory RNA Motifs and Elements

Finder (RegRNA) (http://regrna.mbc.nctu.edu.tw/html/about.html) [15] and the variant effect predictor (http://www.ensembl.org/Homo_sapiens/Tools/VEP?db=core).

Results

Genome-wide association study

The GWAS using 15 cases and 29 controls identified three genome-wide significantly associated SNPs on dog chromosome 38 (CFA38) (Additional file 6) and a quantile-quantile plot (Q-Q plot) for expected versus observed $-\log_{10}P$-values was calculated to control for population stratification (Additional file 7). All SNPs with $-\log_{10}$P-values >5 are located on CFA38 and were in HWE. The genomic inflation factor was equal to 1, indicative that data stratification had no effect on the outcomes of the GWAS. The significantly associated SNPs are located at 18.53, 25.21 and 25.31 Mb (CanFam2) and at 15.53, 22.19 and 22.30 Mb (CanFam3.1) on CFA38 with the strongest signal at 22.30 Mb ($P_{raw} = 5.14\times10^{-9}$). The *P*-values for the SNPs with the highest associations after Bonferroni-correction were at 0.031 (BICF2G63072533), 0.036 (BICF2P378938) and 6.6×10^{-4} (BICF2P478530) (Additional file 8). In the associated interval, 9/15 cases and one control shared a homozygous region over 147 consecutive SNPs spanning 1893 kb at 23,387,952–25,280,713 bp (CanFam2) and at 20,388,358–22,267,778 (CanFam3.1). Inclusion of further two cases resulted in an even shorter homozygous interval with a size of 124 kb. However, for all other cases, an extended homozygosity region could not be determined (Additional file 9). This may indicate that hereditary ataxia had its origin in several founders or recombinations broke down the homozygous identical-by-descent region caused by a common founder to a very small region not detectable via the beadchip data.

A potential candidate gene in the associated and homozygous interval is *KCNJ10* at 25,148,668–25,149,816 bp (CanFam2) and at 22,114,718–22,143,618 bp (CanFam3.1) [7, 11]. The two closest and significantly associated SNPs are 58,212 (BICF2P378938) and 149,816 (BICF2P478530) bp downstream to *KCNJ10*. An association was not evident for SNPs on CFA18 where *CAPN1* is located. The gene *KCNJ9* could not be verified using expressed sequence tags (ESTs) for searching this region. Other candidate genes could not be detected in the associated interval. Further members of the *KCNJ*-gene family were not considered because the GWAS did not indicate significant signals on locations outside CFA38.

Genotyping *CAPN1* and *KCNJ10* variants

CAPN1 genotyping results showed that all 77 PRT and 9 JRT were homozygous wild-type. Genotyping the *KCNJ10*:c.627C > G mutation revealed 38/77 PRT (49.4 %) with the wild-type, 22/77 (28.6 %) as heterozygous and 17/77 (22.1 %) as homozygous mutated. In 1/38 of the homozygous wild-type tested PRT, hereditary ataxia was clinically and histopathologically confirmed. Two other homozygous wild-type tested PRT were diagnosed to be affected after clinical examination and/or according to the report of the owner. Among JRT, only 1/9 dogs was homozygously affected and 7/9 heterozygous. Each one of the heterozygous and homozygous wild-type JRT were clinically affected (Table 1). In addition, 179 controls from 20 different dog breeds were genotyped for both mutations. All these dogs were homozygous wild-type for both mutations (Additional file 10).

Sequencing *KCNJ10*

In order to identify further mutations associated with hereditary ataxia explaining the cases with the homozygous *KCNJ10* C/C genotype, exon 2 and 3 of *KCNJ10* with their exon/intron or exon/UTR boundaries were sequenced in PRT and JRT. We included 3 affected PRT with the homozygous *KCNJ10* C/C genotype and all 3 affected JRT with the different *KCNJ10* genotypes. In addition, we sequenced 7 PRT (5 affected PRT and 2 unaffected) with the concordant *KCNJ10* genotype. A total of 45 genetic variants could be identified including 41 single nucleotide variants (SNVs) and 4 indels (3 insertions and 1 deletion) (Additional file 11) whereof

Table 1 Distribution of ataxia phenotypes by the *KCNJ10*:c.627C > G genotypes for Parson Russell (PRT) und Jack Russell Terriers (JRT)

Breed	Phenotype		*KCNJ10*:c.627C > G		
		n	C/C	C/G	G/G
PRT	A	12	1	0	11
	B	4	1	0	3
	C	2	1	0	1
	D	20	7	13	0
	E	3	1	2	0
	F	36	27	7	2
Subtotal		77	38	22	17
JRT	A	0	0	0	0
	B	3	1	1	1
	C	0	0	0	0
	D	0	0	0	0
	E	0	0	0	0
	F	6	0	6	0
Subtotal		9	1	7	1

A: hereditary ataxia clinically and histopathologically diagnosed, B: clinical signs of ataxia, C: clinical signs of ataxia, according to the medical records of the veterinary clinic and the report of the owner, D: unaffected dogs, E: unaffected dogs, but affected dogs in progeny or siblings, F: no information on health status; the phenotype group A contains 4 PRT shown in the pedigree (Pedigree numbers (P.n.) 14, 15, 16, 17, see Additional file 12), group D contains 7 PRT (P.n. 2, 6, 7, 8, 9, 10, 11, see Additional file 12) and group F includes 6 PRT (P.n. 1, 3, 4, 5, 12, 13, see Additional file 12)

most of them were located in the 3′UTR (CanFam3.1) (Additional file 4). Sequencing further 9 dogs of other breeds (Additional file 12) and filtering showed 16 variants private for PRT and JRT (Additional file 13). A further filtering for homozygous mutant genotypes in affected PRT and JRT resulted in a 1-bp-insertion (*KCNJ10:*g.22141027insC) prevalent in these animals. This 1-bp-insertion was located within a stretch of 7 consecutive C bases (Additional file 5). Bioinformatic analysis using RegRNA indicated the *KCNJ10:*g.22141027insC affecting regulation of gene expression via a regulatory RNA motif or miRNA target site. A regulatory RNA motif (5′-GGGAGGGG-3′) was identified 6 bp downstream to the *KCNJ10:*g.22141027insC. The motif of the miRNA (hsa-miR-1180) target site contains the *KCNJ10:*g.22141 027insC (5′-acACAACCCCCCCGACGCCGGGAg-3′). Genotyping a pedigree containing 17 PRT for both mutations, *KCNJ10:*g.22141027insC and *KCNJ10:*c.627C > G, showed segregation of both mutations with the affection status with exception of one animal (Additional file 14). Genotyping results of the *KCNJ10:*g.22141027insC are summarized in Table 2. Out of the 77 PRT, 34 (44.2 %) showed the wild-type, 26 (33.8 %) the heterozygous and 17 (22.1 %) the homozygous mutated genotype. In 2/26 of the heterozygous PRT, hereditary ataxia was clinically and histopathologically confirmed and 2/34 homozygous wild-type tested PRT were affected according to a clinical examination and/or according to the report of the owner. The genotyping results for the *KCNJ10:*g.22141027insC mutation of JRT showed two homozygous mutated genotypes among the affected individuals. A further affected individual had the wildtype genotype. Genotyping further 84 dogs of 40 other breed dogs revealed 59 (70.3 %) wild-type homozygous, 21 (25.0 %) heterozygous and 4 (4.8 %) homozygous mutated genotypes (Additional file 15).

Table 2 Distribution of ataxia phenotypes by the *KCNJ10:g.22141027insC* genotypes for Parson Russell (PRT) und Jack Russell Terriers (JRT)

Breed	Phenotype	*KCNJ10:*g.22141027insC			
		n	wt/wt	wt/mut	mut/mut
PRT	A	12	0	2	10
	B	4	1	0	3
	C	2	1	0	1
	D	20	7	12	1
	E	3	1	2	0
	F	36	24	10	2
Subtotal		77	34	26	17
JRT	A	0	0	0	0
	B	3	1	0	2
	C	0	0	0	0
	D	0	0	0	0
	E	0	0	0	0
	F	6	0	6	0
Subtotal		9	1	6	12

A: hereditary ataxia clinically and histopathologically diagnosed, B: clinical signs of ataxia, C: clinical signs of ataxia according to the medical records of the veterinary clinic and report of the owner, D: unaffected dogs, E: unaffected dogs, but affected dogs in progeny or siblings, F: no information on health status; the phenotype group A contains 4 PRT shown in the pedigree (Pedigree numbers (P.n.) 14, 15, 16, 17, see Additional file 12), group D contains 7 PRT (P.n. 2, 6, 7, 8, 9, 10, 11, see Additional file 12) and group F includes 6 PRT (P.n. 1, 3, 4, 5, 12, 13, see Additional file 12)

Discussion

The results of the GWAS indicate that the associated genomic region on CFA38 may harbour the most likely candidate genes for hereditary ataxia in the sample under study. Thus, our study corroborated the previous candidate gene search using whole genome sequence data [7]. We could not detect samples with the *CAPN1:*c.344G > A mutation. This may indicate that this mutation may be rare in the German PRT and JRT populations. In agreement with a previous study [7], one histopathologically confirmed case of hereditary ataxia and two clinically affected cases carried neither the *CAPN1:*c.344G > A allele nor the homozygous *KCNJ10:*c.627C > G genotype. This may indicate that at least one further mutation may be involved in hereditary ataxia of PRT and JRT. As the largest proportion of affected dogs were concordant with the segregation of the *KCNJ10:*c.627C > G alleles the remaining unexplained cases may harbour a rare mutation. However, breeders have to be aware that selective breeding based on genetic tests for the *KCNJ10:*c.627C > G and *CAPN1:*c.344G > A mutations cannot completely preclude affected dogs of the breeds PRT or JRT despite of homozygous wild-type genotypes of the parents.

The present sequence analysis tagged a 1-bp-insertion associated with hereditary ataxia in PRT and JRT. This mutation may have an effect on regulation of *KCNJ10* expression as indicated through bioinformatic results from RegRNA. However, the presence of this 1-bp-insertion in other breeds may require further research in phenotyping spinocerebellar ataxia associated with myokymia, seizures, or both. In conclusion, a few but not all cases of hereditary ataxia being heterozygous or homozygous for the wild-type allele of *KCNJ10* could be explained by the *KCNJ10:*g.22141027insC mutation.

Conclusions

Our data confirmed the presence of the *KCNJ10:*c.627C > G mutation in PRT and JRT affected with hereditary ataxia. However, some cases of hereditary ataxia could not be explained through the *KCNJ10:*c.627C > G nor the *CAPN1:*c.344G > A mutation. Genetic testing using the *KCNJ10:*c.627C > G and the *CAPN1:*c.344G > A mutations deems not to be sufficient to capture all cases of hereditary ataxia in PRT and JRT. This lets us assume that at least one additional form of hereditary ataxia may segregate in the breeds PRT and JRT. The *KCNJ10*:g.22141027insC mutation was evident in a few cases but could not explain all not yet resolved cases. Further efforts are necessary to collect cases of hereditary ataxia not explained by the presently known mutations to unravel the responsible mutations in these cases of hereditary ataxia.

Additional files

Additional file 1: Distribution of ataxia phenotypes for Parson Russell (PRT) and Jack Russell Terriers (JRT). (DOCX 15 kb)

Additional file 2: Plot of the first (PCA1) versus the second principal component (PCA2) by hereditary ataxia affected Parson Russell Terriers (affected) and controls (non-affected) used for the genome-wide association study (GWAS). The black dots indicate controls and the orange dots affected PRT. Number of single nucleotide polymorphisms (SNPs) that informed PCAs was at 128,863 SNPs. Variance of SNPs explained by PCA1 and PCA2 was at 0.19 and 0.17, respectively. (DOC 69 kb)

Additional file 3: Primer pair sequences, restriction enzymes, annealing temperature (AT) and amplicon size used for genotyping the mutations *CAPN1*:c.344G > A and *KCNJ10*:c.627C > G by PCR-RFLP are given. Primer pair sequences, annealing temperature (AT) and amplicon size of PCR for genotyping the mutation *KCNJ10*:g.22141027insC validated on a LI-COR 4300 DNA Analyzer as well as primer pair sequences and product-sizes for Sanger sequencing PCR-amplicons of exon 2 and 3 of *KCNJ10* are shown. (DOC 57 kb)

Additional file 4: Canine gene model of *KCNJ10* and detected variants. The gene model was built using the Ensemble annotation (assembly CanFam3.1). (A) represents transcript XM_005640901.1 and (B) represents XM_545752.4. Translated exons are shown as black boxes and untranslated exons are shown as open boxes. Exon numbers are given above the boxes. Continuous lines indicate introns. Sizes of exons and introns are given below the boxes and lines. Positions of start codon and stop codon are also present. Locations and motifs of variants identified in our study are listed above the exons. Both the single nucleotide variant (SNV) reported by Gilliam et al. [7] (*KCNJ10*:c.627C > G) and the variant validated in our study (*KCNJ10*:g.22141027insC) are framed by a black open box. (PDF 41 kb)

Additional file 5: (A) The genomic sequences of an unaffected and affected Parson Russell Terrier (PRT) are shown. The unaffected dog is homozygous for the wild-type allele. The sequence of the dog affected by hereditary ataxia shows a 1-base pair (bp) insertion in a seven-C stretch within exon 3 of the *KCNJ10* gene. The seven-C stretch with and without the inserted base C is framed by a red open box. The homozygous wild-type and the homozygous mutant variant in the forward sequence as well as the heterozygous variant in both the forward and reverse sequence are shown. (B) Fragment length analysis on a 6 % polyacrylamide gel for evaluating the 1-bp insertion in *KCNJ10* in hereditary ataxia affected Parson and Jack Russell Terriers. The homozygous wild-type (wt/wt) in two unaffected PRT are shown. The size of the normal PCR-product is 166 bp. The heterozygous genotype (wt/mut) in one unaffected and the homozygous genotype (mut/mut) for the mutant allele in two affected PRT are also present. (PDF 169 kb)

Additional file 6: Manhattan plot of $-\log_{10}P$-values of the genome-wide association study for hereditary ataxia in Parson Russell Terriers using a general model analysis. On the X-axis, the SNPs are given by dog chromosome number. The $-\log_{10}$P-values for each SNP genotype effect are plotted against the SNP position on each chromosome. Chromosomes are differentiated by colors. The color keys are given below the plot. The blue line indicates the threshold of the $-\log_{10}P$-values for genome-wide significance after Bonferroni correction. (PDF 138 kb)

Additional file 7: Q-Q-plot of expected $-\log_{10}P$-values versus observed-$\log_{10}P$-values from the general model analysis for hereditary ataxia in Parson Russell Terriers. Shown are all 128,863 SNPs included in the genome-wide association analysis with the grey line corresponding to the null hypothesis of no association. (PDF 56 kb)

Additional file 8: Summary of results for the genome-wide association study using a general model analysis and sex-stratified case-control analysis for hereditary ataxia in Parson Russell Terriers. The SNP-ID, the position on dog chromosome (CFA) in base pairs (bp) according to the dog genome assembly CanFam2, minor allele, minor allele frequency (MAF) for all, affected (MAF_A) and unaffected (MAF_U) dogs (controls), variance explained by the single SNP (V_{SNP}), $-\log_{10}P$-values ($-\log_{10}$P) and Bonferroni-corrected $-\log_{10}P$-values ($-\log_{10}P_{Bonf}$) of the general model analysis are given. Odds ratios (OR) with 95 % confidence intervals (CI) are from a sex-stratified case-control analysis for cases and controls. (DOC 42 kb)

Additional file 9: Overview on the results of extended homozygosity mapping in Parson Russell Terriers (PRT) genotyped on the canine Illumina high density beadchip. The IDs of PRT, *KCNJ10* c.627C > G genotype, the SNP-IDs and positions in base pairs (bp) for the start and end of the homozygosity region are given. The PRT-ID 2 indicates dogs which were used for sequencing in this study and PRT-ID 3 indicates the designation for PRT (P.n.) which are shown in the pedigree (see Additional file 12). *KCNJ10* is located at 25,148,668–25,149,816 on CFA38 (CanFam2). (DOC 51 kb)

Additional file 10: Distribution of genotyping results for the mutation *CAPN1*:c.344G > A and *KCNJ10*:c.627C > G in different dog breeds. Numbers of tested homozygous wild-type (wt/wt), heterozygous (wt/mut) and homozygous mutant (mut/mut) genotypes are given. (DOC 51 kb)

Additional file 11: Identification of variants in the gene *KCNJ10* in affected and unaffected Parson Russell Terriers (PRT) and Jack Russell Terriers (JRT). IDs of the variants, locations in the gene, accession numbers and the genotype for each variant are given. The single nucleotide variant reported by Gilliam et al. [7] (*KCNJ10*:c.627C > G) written in bold. Indel mutations are denoted as wt (wild-type) or mut (mutant). (DOC 108 kb)

Additional file 12: Sequencing results of nine dogs of different breeds for evaluation of the variants detected in Parson Russell Terriers (PRT) and Jack Russell Terriers (JRT). IDs of the variants and the genotype for each variant are given. The single nucleotide variant reported by Gilliam et al. [7] (*KCNJ10*:c.627C > G) written in bold. Indel mutations are denoted as wt (wildtype) or mut (mutant). Indel mutations are denoted as wt (wild-type) or mut (mutant). (DOC 97 kb)

Additional file 13: Variants in the gene *KCNJ10* which are private for Parson Russell Terriers (PRT) and Jack Russell Terriers (JRT). IDs of the variants, locations in the gene, accession numbers and the genotype for each variant are given. Both the single nucleotide variant reported by Gilliam et al. [7] (*KCNJ10*:c.627C > G) and *KCNJ10*:g.22141027insC identified as further putative variant written in bold. Indel mutations are denoted as wt (wild-type) or mut (mutant). (DOC 64 kb)

Additional file 14: The pedigree demonstrates the relationship of 17 Parson Russell Terriers (PRT) (pedigree number 1–17) selected from the sample of our study. Genotypes for both, the *KNCJ10*:g.22141027insC (first row) and *KCNJ10*:c.627C > G [7] (second row) variant are given for each of the 17 dogs. *KNCJ10*:g.22141027insC genotyping resulted in 5/17 wild-type (wt/wt), 9/17 heterozygous (wt/mut) and 3/17 homozygous mutant (mut/mut) PRT. *KCNJ10*:c.627C > G genotyping resulted in 9/17 wild-type (wt/wt), 5/17 heterozygous (wt/mut) and 3/17 homozygous mutant (mut/mut) PRT. (PDF 22 kb)

Additional file 15: Distribution of genotyping results for the mutation *KCNJ10*:g.22141027insC in different dog breeds. Numbers of tested homozygous wild-type (wt/wt), heterozygous (wt/mut) and homozygous mutant (mut/mut) genotypes are given. (DOC 57 kb)

Abbreviations

CFA: Dog chromosome; GWAS: Genome-wide association study; JRT: Jack Russell Terrier; *KCNJ10*: *Potassium inwardly-rectifying channel, subfamily J, member 10*; LOA: Late onset ataxia; PRT: Parson Russell Terrier; SCA: Spinocerebellar ataxia; SNP: Single nucleotide polymorphism; SNV: Single nucleotide variant

Acknowledgements
The authors thank the dog breeders for providing EDTA-blood samples, pedigree data and veterinary diagnoses for hereditary ataxia. All dog owners gave informed consent to participate in this study.

Funding
ACG obtained internal funds of the University of Veterinary Medicine Hannover. The funders had no role in the design of the study and collection, analysis, and interpretation of data and in writing the manuscript.

Authors' contributions
OD and AT conceived and designed the study. ACG, JM and OD performed the experiments and analysed the data. ACG, OD and AT coordinated the collection of samples. ACG, JM and OD drafted and finalized the manuscript. All authors read and approved the final manuscript.

Competing interests
The authors declare that they have no competing interests.

Consent for publication
Not applicable.

Author details
[1]Institute for Animal Breeding and Genetics, University of Veterinary Medicine Hannover, Bünteweg 17p, 30559 Hannover, Germany. [2]Department of Small Animal Medicine and Surgery, University of Veterinary Medicine Hannover, Bünteweg 9, 30559 Hannover, Germany.

References
1. Hartley WJ, Palmer AC. Ataxia in Jack Russell Terriers. Acta Neuropathol (Berl). 1973;26(1):71–4.
2. Wessmann A, Goedde T, Fischer A, Wohlsein P, Hamann H, Distl O, Tipold A. Hereditary ataxia in the Jack Russell Terrier–clinical and genetic investigations. J Vet Intern Med. 2004;18(4):515–21.
3. Van Ham L, Bhatti S, Polis I, Fatzer R, Braund K, Thoonen H. 'Continuous muscle fibre activity' in six dogs with episodic myokymia, stiffness and collapse. Vet Rec. 2004;155(24):769–74.
4. Vanhaesebrouck AE, Van Soens I, Poncelet L, Duchateau L, Bhatti S, Polis I, Diels S, Van Ham L. Clinical and electrophysiological characterization of myokymia and neuromyotonia in Jack Russell Terriers. J Vet Intern Med. 2010;24(4):882–9.
5. Vanhaesebrouck AE, Bhatti SF, Franklin RJ, Van Ham L. Myokymia and neuromyotonia in veterinary medicine: A comparison with peripheral nerve hyperexcitability syndrome in humans. Vet J. 2013;197(2):153–62.
6. Bhatti SF, Vanhaesebrouck AE, Van Soens I, Martlé VA, Polis IE, Rusbridge C, Van Ham LM. Myokymia and neuromyotonia in 37 Jack Russell terriers. Vet J. 2011;189(3):284–8.
7. Gilliam D, O'Brien DP, Coates JR, Johnson GS, Johnson GC, Mhlanga-Mutangadura T, Hansen L, Taylor JF, Schnabel RD. A homozygous KCNJ10 mutation in Jack Russell Terriers and related breeds with spinocerebellar ataxia with myokymia, seizures, or both. J Vet Intern Med. 2014;28(3):871–7.
8. Urkasemsin G, Olby NJ. Canine Hereditary Ataxia. Vet Clin North Am Small Anim Pract. 2014;44(6):1075–89.
9. Björck G, Mair W, Olsson SE, Sourander P. Hereditary ataxia in Fox Terriers. Acta Neuropathologica (Berl). 1962; Suppl 1:45–48.
10. Rohdin C, Lüdtke L, Wohlsein P, Jäderlund KH. New aspects of hereditary ataxia in smooth-haired fox terriers. Vet Rec. 2010;166(18):557–60. doi:10.1136/vr.b4821.
11. Rohdin C, Gilliam D, O'Leary CA, O'Brien DP, Coates JR, Johnson GS, Jäderlund KH. A KCNJ10 mutation previously identified in the Russell group of terriers also occurs in Smooth-Haired Fox Terriers with hereditary ataxia and in related breeds. Acta Vet Scand. 2015;57:26. doi:10.1186/s13028-015-0115-1.
12. Forman OP, DeRisio L, Mellersh CS. Missense mutation in CAPN1 is associated with spinocerebellar ataxia in the Parson Russell Terrier dog breed. PLoS One. 2013;8(5):e64627. doi:10.1371/journal.pone.0064627.
13. Bradbury PJ, Zhang Z, Kroon DE, Casstevens TM, Ramdoss Y, Buckler ES. TASSEL: software for association mapping of complex traits in diverse samples. Bioinformatics. 2007;23(19):2633–5.
14. Purcell S, Neale B, Todd-Brown K, Thomas L, Ferreira MA, Bender D, Maller J, Sklar P, de Bakker PI, Daly MJ, Sham PC. PLINK: a tool set for whole-genome association and population-based linkage analyses. Am J Hum Genet. 2007;81(3):559–75.
15. Huang HY, Chien CH, Jen KH, Huang HD. RegRNA: an integrated web server for identifying regulatory RNA motifs and elements. Nucleic Acids Res. 2006;34(Web Server issue):W429–434.

5

Fibrinogen deficiency in a dog

Franck Jolivet[1], Armelle Diquélou[1,2], Catherine Trumel[1], Simon Privat[1] and Olivier Dossin[1,2*]

Abstract

Background: Among coagulation disorders, primary fibrinogen deficiency is very rare in dogs. It is divided into hypofibrinogenemia, afibrinogenemia and dysfibrinogenemia. Afibrinogenemia has been described in three dogs. There are, however, no published case reports of primary hypofibrinogenemia in dogs.

Case presentation: A 1.5 year-old male German Pointer dog was evaluated for a locked-jaw syndrome associated with eye protrusion which appeared after a minor head trauma. Three months before the trauma, a persistent increase in coagulation times was detected by the referring veterinarian after a strong suspicion of snake envenomation. Apart for the primary complaint, physical examination was normal. A complete hemostatic profile revealed a moderately increased prothrombin time, activated partial thromboplastin times and a dramatically decreased fibrinogen concentration (0.34 g/L, reference interval [1.3–4.8 g/L]). Platelet count, plasma D-dimers and antithrombin, were all within the reference intervals and not consistent with a disseminated intravascular coagulation. Other possible causes of hypofibrinogenemia such as chronic hemorrhage and liver failure were excluded by laboratory work-up and imaging studies. Finally, antifibrinogen circulating anticoagulants were excluded using a dilution of citrated plasma from the pooled plasma of healthy dogs. These results supported a diagnosis of congenital fibrinogen deficiency and secondary retrobulbar hematoma and/or cellulitis. The dog's condition improved rapidly after symptomatic treatment with corticosteroids and antibiotics. At the 1 year follow-up, the dog was clinically normal but a persistent hypofibrinogenemia (≤ 0.8 g/L) remained.

Conclusions: Various clinical presentations may occur in canine primary hypofibrinogenemia which should be included in the list of coagulation disorders. Diagnosis should include fibrinogen determination by coagulometric and non-coagulometric methods to differentiate from dysfibrinogenemia. There is no specific treatment but care should be taken to prevent bleeding and trauma. Emergency management of bleeding episodes with cryoprecipitate is the treatment of choice.

Keywords: Fibrinogen deficiency, Hypofibrinogenemia, Dysfibrinogenemia, Bleeding disorders, Dog

Background

Congenital disorders of coagulation are rare in veterinary medicine, and consist mainly of hemophilia A and B [1]. Other clotting factor deficiencies have however been described and can be a diagnostic challenge. Among these deficiencies, hypofibrinogenemia has seldom been described in dogs.

Fibrinogen, the soluble precursor of fibrin, is a key coagulation factor involved in both primary and secondary hemostasis, promoting platelet aggregation and clot formation. Fibrinogen is the most abundant clotting factor, with usual blood concentrations ranging from 1.3 g/L to 4.8 g/L in adult dogs (reference interval (RI) from the veterinary clinical pathology laboratory of the Veterinary Teaching Hospital of the University of Toulouse (VTH UT)). In human and veterinary medicine, three congenital fibrinogen abnormalities have been described: afibrinogenemia (absence of fibrinogen), hypofibrinogenemia (quantitative deficiency) and dysfibrinogenemia (qualitative deficiency) [2–6].

Humans with congenital hypofibrinogenemia are usually asymptomatic but may bleed when the hemostatic

* Correspondence: o.dossin@envt.fr
[1]Department of Clinical Sciences, ENVT, University of Toulouse, 31076 Toulouse, France
[2]IRSD, INSERM 1220, INSERM, INRA, ENVT, UPS, University of Toulouse, 31024 Toulouse, France

system is strongly solicited, for example in such situations as trauma or surgery [2].

This report describes a 1.5 year-old German Pointer dog with a protrusion of the right third eyelid and a locked-jaw syndrome associated with extreme pain on mouth-opening due to a congenital hypofibrinogenemia.

Case presentation

A 1.5 year-old male German Pointer dog weighing 27 kg was referred to the VTH UT for a protrusion of the right third eyelid, and a locked-jaw syndrome associated with extreme pain when the dog tried to open his mouth. These signs had appeared 10 days earlier, after the dog was hit on the head by a ball. The dog had remained stable since then. History revealed a strong suspicion of snake envenomation 3 months earlier. At that time, the dog was presented in shock to a veterinarian with marks on the head suggestive of a snake bite. The laboratory workup revealed markedly increased prothrombin time (PT) and activated partial thromboplastin time (aPTT). The veterinarian started a symptomatic treatment [fluid-therapy (Ringer Lactate), corticosteroids (prednisolone, 1 mg/kg, IV, q 12 h), antibiotics (marbofloxacin, 4 mg/kg, IV, q 12 h) and K1 vitamin] and clinical signs improved within a few days. However, the PT and aPTT remained moderately increased after this suspected envenomation. One month later, a gingival wound appeared, requiring a surgical suture to stop the bleeding. On this occasion, PT and APPT were still markedly increased (PT >35 s, RI [12–19 s] and aPTT >200 s, RI [75–105 s]).

Upon admission at the VTH UT, physical examination showed an exophthalmia of the right eye associated with protrusion of third eyelid. The dog was reluctant to be touched on the head and opening the mouth elicited severe pain. Apart from this, clinical examination was unremarkable and a thorough ocular examination did not reveal any other abnormality. The ocular ultrasonography was consistent with a retrobulbar cellulitis with no image suggesting the presence of a foreign body. Because of the history of abnormal coagulation, the retrobulbar fine needle aspiration was postponed until the laboratory results were available.

An extensive laboratory profile, including complete hemostatic profile[1], was performed at the veterinary clinical pathology laboratory of the VTH UT. Severe hypofibrinogenemia (0.34 g/L, RI [1.30–4.80 g/L] assessed by Clauss'coagulometric method), increased PT (15.0 s, RI [7.10–9.00 s]) and aPTT (19.3 s, RI [12.8–17.2 s]) were observed. All other results including buccal mucosal bleeding time, complete blood count (CBC), D-dimers (DDi), and antithrombin (AT) were within reference intervals (Table 1). The fibrinogen/fibrin degradation products (FDPs) value was however in the grey zone (between 5 and 20 μg/mL, RI [< 5 μg/mL]).

Table 1 Complete hemostasis profile

Variable	Value	Reference Interval
Buccal Mucosal Bleeding Time	3 min10 s	3–5 min
Platelet count	175,000 /μL	64,000–613,000 /μL
PT	15.0 s	7.1–9.0 s
aPTT	19.3 s	12.8–17.2 s
Fibrinogen	0.34 g/L	1.30–4.80 g/L
FDPs	5–20 μg/mL	<5 μg/mL
DDi	0.51 mg/L	<0.56 mg/L
AT	115%	109–195%

The hypofibrinogenemia was observed on repeated coagulometric measurements as well as by physical measurement using the Millar heat-precipitation method based on the ability of fibrinogen to precipitate at 56 °C [7]. This method confirmed the severe hypofibrinogenemia with an almost undetectable fibrinogen precipitation band.

A screening for possible causes of hypofibrinogenemia was performed. The normal liver profile, including a normal bile acid test, excluded liver failure (Table 2). The absence of clinical signs of disease conditions that are associated with disseminated intra-vascular coagulation (DIC) together with the absence of any other laboratory signs of hemostasis system activation (normal platelet count, DDi and AT) was not consistent with DIC. Chronic bleeding was ruled out by clinical, diagnostic imaging and CBC findings. To rule out the hypothesis of circulating anticoagulant interfering with the fibrinogen determination, a 1/1 dilution of the dog's citrated plasma with pooled healthy dog plasma (PHDP) was performed. PHDP was prepared by pooling identically prepared plasma samples from 9 clinically healthy dogs. The fibrinogen concentration assessed by coagulometric method in the mixture was consistent with the expected calculated result (Table 3). This finding ruled

Table 2 Complete blood chemistry profile

Variable	Value	Reference Interval
Creatinine	75 μmol/L	44–133 μmol/L
Cholesterol	4.7 mmol/L	3.3–9.3 mmol/L
Triglycerides	0.4 mmol/L	0.2–1.3 mmol/L
Total Protein	76.1 g/L	48.0–66.0 g/L
Albumin	35.3 g/L	23.0–39.0 g/L
Alanine Aminotransferase	45 U/L	0.3–50 U/L
Alkaline Phosphatase	195 U/L	20–155 U/L
Gamma-glutamyltransferase	5 U/L	0.5–25 U/L
Total Bilirubin	1.8 μmol/L	1.7–12.0 μmol/L
Pre-Prandial Bile Acids	2.0 μmol/L	0–10.0 μmol/L
Post-Prandial Bile Acids	2.0 μmol/L	0–20.0 μmol/L

Table 3 Fibrinogen concentration after plasma dilution with PHDP

Sample	Fibrinogen concentration
PHDP	1.70 g/L
Patient	0.51 g/L
PHDP + Patient (1/1, V/V dilution)	1.13 g/L

Theoretical expected result for the dilution: 1.105 g/L
PHDP Pooled Healthy Dogs Plasma

out the presence of circulating anticoagulant with fibrinogen inhibitory properties. A congenital hypofibrinogenemia was hence diagnosed.

Retrobulbar fine needle aspiration was not performed due to the high risk of puncture-induced hemorrhage. In the hypothesis of a retrobulbar cellulitis, the following treatment was administered: antibiotics (gentamicin 6.6 mg/kg, IV, q 24 h for 6 days, and amoxicillin/clavulanic acid 20 mg/kg, IV, q 8 h for 6 days, then 12.5 mg/kg, PO, q 12 h for 6 weeks) and corticosteroid therapy (prednisolone 0.3 mg/kg, IV, q 24 h for 6 days then 0.3 mg/kg, PO, q 24 h for 3 weeks, and finally 0.3 mg/kg, PO, every other day, for 2 weeks).

After 2 days of treatment, the protrusion of the third eyelid and the pain associated with mouth opening decreased and resolved after 2 weeks. One month later, the dog was completely normal. Two months later, the dog was stable but fibrinogen remained persistently below the reference interval (Table 4) and the FDP value was negative (< 5 μg/mL). Six months after the initial presentation, no clinical relapse was observed but plasma fibrinogen value remained low.

There is no specific treatment for congenital hypofibrinogenemia, other than plasma transfusion during acute bleeding crisis. It was therefore strongly recommended to avoid strenuous exercise or hunting with the dog to prevent trauma.

Discussion

This case describes fibrinogen deficiency, an extremely rare congenital bleeding disorder in dogs [1, 8]. Very little data is published on the subject in veterinary medicine, with only three case reports on dogs with afibrinogenemia: a Bernese mountain dog [3], a Chihuahua [4], and a Bichon Frise [5]. In an international registry of animal hemostatic disorders, Dodds mentioned a case of dysfibrinogenemia in an inbred family of Borzois and a case of hypofibrinogenemia in a family of Saint Bernard dogs [6] but to our knowledge these cases have not been reported in detail in a peer-reviewed journal.

Table 4 Follow-up of fibrinogen concentrations

Test time	Fibrinogen concentration	RI
Admission	0.34 g/L	
1 month later	0.70 g/L	1.30–4.80 g/L
2 months later	0.51 g/L	

In human medicine, congenital fibrinogen deficiency represents 7% of rare congenital bleeding disorders, hemophilia-excluded [2, 9]. Three categories of fibrinogen deficiency have been described: afibrinogenemia when fibrinogen is not detectable; hypofibrinogenemia when the value is below the lower limit of the reference interval; and dysfibrinogenemia when the fibrinogen molecule is abnormal and dysfunctional. The only way to differentiate hypofibrinogenemia from dysfibrinogenemia in humans is a low fibrinogenemia assessed by coagulometry with a concurrent normal or subnormal fibrinogen concentration by an immunologic method. Unfortunately, such a method is not routinely available in veterinary medicine [10, 11]. Therefore dysfibrinogenemia was not completely excluded in our dog. However, because the fibrinogen concentration was similarly decreased with both coagulometric method and heat precipitation method, we concluded it was hypofibrinogenemia.

The clinical presentation of ocular signs in this case is unusual. Ocular ultrasonography was suggestive of a retrobulbar cellulitis with effusion. To confirm this diagnosis, cytological and bacteriological analysis of a fine needle aspiration of retrobulbar space is needed. In this case, the first hypothesis was a hematoma because the ocular problems started after the dog was hit on the head and the patient had a background history of sustained increase of coagulation times and abnormal bleeding following a benign gingival wound. However, the nature of the retrobulbar ultrasonographic abnormality could not be confirmed by fine needle aspiration due to the risk of bleeding. Given the extreme pain associated with jaw opening, a primary hematoma with secondary inflammation/infection was a possible hypothesis. The dog was therefore treated with antibiotic and anti-inflammatory drugs. The rapid clinical improvement after onset of the treatment in a dog, whose signs had been stable for the previous 10 days was consistent with this hypothesis.

When hypofibrinogenemia is detected, the first clinical step is to exclude all possibility of a preanalytic error and to confirm the fibrinogen value using another method such as Millar's method. If the decreased concentration is confirmed, all other causes of decreased fibrinogen production or increased fibrinogen consumption need to be explored before considering a diagnosis of congenital hypofibrinogenemia. Liver function must be assessed because fibrinogen is produced by the liver. In our case, normal clinical examination and bile acid test excluded decreased hepatic fibrinogen synthesis. The second step is to rule out increased and sustained fibrinogen consumption by activation of the coagulation cascade, namely DIC or chronic bleeding, by laboratory work-up and diagnostic imaging. No systemic disease, bleeding or inflammatory site, other than the ocular bulging, was suspected in our dog. No signs of chronic blood loss were detected on CBC, and normal platelet count, AT and DDi concentrations were inconsistent with DIC.

In our patient, the only hemostatic abnormality other than hypofibrinogenemia was FDPs in the grey zone. FDPs reflect the action of the fibrinolytic enzyme, plasmin, on fibrin and fibrinogen whereas DDi appear only when fibrin is degraded by plasmin [12]. Decreased FDPs clearance due to a failing liver or kidney was excluded by the laboratory results. The FDPs value results could indicate primary hyperfibrinolysis (*ie* spontaneous activation of plasmin not triggered by coagulation activation). However, primary hyperfibrinolysis had not previously been described in dogs and was considered very unlikely in our case for other reasons including the absence of primary diseases causing hyperfibrinolysis in humans, such as liver cirrhosis [13] or bronchiectasis [14]. Moreover, if the severe hypofibrinogenemia in this dog had been caused by hyperfibrinogenolysis, FDPs would have been very high and not only slightly increased. Finally, the dog's fibrinogen concentration remained low at the 1 and 2 month follow-ups which was not compatible with a primary hyperfibrinogenolysis that is not a persistent condition. Therefore, we hypothesized that the slight increase of the FDPs could be the consequence of the suspected retrobulbar hematoma.

Furthermore, the unusual context of this case's clinical scenario made it difficult to determine whether the disorder was congenital or acquired. The onset of the condition, discovered by the veterinarian in association with a strong suspicion of snake bite, was initially confusing. It concerned an adult dog, with no previous coagulation profile evaluation or surgical history, making it impossible to determine if the coagulation disorders were present prior to this episode. According to the owner, the dog had been perfectly healthy which is consistent with the few cases of hypofibrinogenemia described in the veterinary literature [1, 8].

Because the PT and aPTT values were consistently above the reference intervals after the presumed envenomation, the hypothesis of circulating anticoagulants, such as antibodies that would have developed after envenomation and would be directed against fibrinogen, or would impair the coagulation reactions involved in the transformation of fibrinogen into fibrin, had to be investigated. The dilution method with a PHDP is a simple method used to explore circulating anticoagulants. It is easily performed in-house when coagulation times are sufficiently increased (at least 1.5 times the upper limit of RI), only requiring the measurement of PT or aPTT in PHDP, the citrated plasma of the affected animal and a 1/1 (vol/vol) mixture of the two. If PT or aPTT are not normalized in the mixture, it strongly suggests a circulating anticoagulant/antibody against a coagulation factor [15]. In our case, we chose to measure the fibrinogen concentration ([Fibrinogen]) using a coagulometric method rather than coagulation times. Because the fibrinogen concentration in the mixture was close to [PHDP Fibrinogen]/2 + [affected dog's Fibrinogen]/2, we ruled out the presence of a circulating anticoagulant in the plasma of the affected dog. A possible limitation to this approach would be that serial dilutions might have been more sensitive to detect a circulating antibody if the optimal concentrations had not been obtained at the 1/1 dilution. However, in the only case report of circulating antibody against fibrinogen described in the dog [5], the fibrinogen concentration of the 1/1 mixture was more than 50% below the expected theoretical concentration. A circulating anticoagulant was therefore considered unlikely in our case. Once all the hypotheses had been excluded, the final diagnosis was consistent with a congenital fibrinogen deficiency.

Testing the parents and the siblings to assess coagulation abnormalities would have been interesting to investigate the disorder in the whole family and document a possible genetic/hereditary background. Unfortunately, this was not possible in our case.

Cryoprecipitate is the treatment of choice for fibrinogen deficiencies because it supplies high concentrations of fibrinogen in a low volume. Fresh frozen plasma is an alternative product when cryoprecipitate is unavailable. For patients with active hemorrhage and decreased PCV, a blood transfusion is also indicated. The target fibrinogen value is 1.0 g/L [16]. The half-life of fibrinogen is 4.2 days and relatively long compared to most coagulation factors [17]. Therefore, fewer transfusions are often sufficient to temporarily support haemostasis in such patients.

Conclusions

This case is the first complete report of congenital hypofibrinogenemia in a dog. Moreover, it is an original presentation of bleeding disorders suggesting that clinicians should consider bleeding disorders in differential diagnosis of locked jaw syndrome or eye protrusion.

Endnotes

[1]Sta-Compact, Diagnostica Stago, France.

Abbreviations

aPTT: Activated partial thromboplastin time; AT: Antithrombin; CBC: Complete blood count; DDi: D-dimers; DIC: Disseminated intra-vascular coagulation; FDPs: Fibrinogen/fibrin degradation products; PCV: Packed cell volume; PHDP: Pooled healthy dog plasma; PT: Prothrombin time; RI: Reference interval; VTH UT: Veterinary Teaching Hospital of the University of Toulouse

Acknowledgements
We would like to acknowledge Royal Canin for supporting the position of F. Jolivet as an ECVIM Internal Medicine resident, Michelle Ingelbach for final reviewing and editing of the manuscript and the primary veterinarian for referring the case.

Funding
Not applicable.

Authors' contributions
FJ and OD dealt with the case, drafted the manuscript and FJ, AD, CT, SP and OD have read, and participated in reviewing the manuscript and approved the final manuscript.

Authors' information
Franck Jolivet, DVM; Armelle Diquélou, DVM, PhD; Catherine Trumel, DVM, PhD, Dipl.ECVCP; Simon Privat, DVM; Olivier Dossin, DVM, PhD, Dipl. ECVIM-CA.

Competing interests
The authors declare that they have no competing interests.

Consent for publication
The owner of the dog gave his consent for publication.

References
1. Barr JW, McMichael M. Inherited disorders of hemostasis in dogs and cats. Top Companion Anim Med. 2012;27:53–8.
2. Moen JL, Lord ST. Afibrinogenemias and Dysfibrinogenemias. In: Colman RW, Marder VJ, Clowes AW, et al., editors. Hemostasis and Thrombosis. Basic Principles and Clinical Practice. 5th ed. Philadelphia: Lippincott Williams and Wilkins; 2006. p. 939–52.
3. Kammermann B, Gmür J, Stünzl H. Afibrinogenemia in dogs. Zentralbl Veterinarmed A. 1971;18:192–205.
4. Chambers G. Treatment of afibrinogenemia in a Chihuahua. J Am Anim Hosp Assoc. 2013;49:70–4.
5. Wilkerson MJ, Johnson GS, Stockham S, Riley L. Afibrinogenemia and a circulating antibody against fibrinogen in a Bichon Frise dog. Vet Clin Pathol. 2005;34:148–55.
6. Doods WJ. Spontaneous (naturally occurring) disease models: hereditary. In: Doods WJ. Second International Registry of Animal Models of Thrombosis and Hemorrhagic Diseases. Washington DC: National Academy Press; 1981. pp. R3-R25.
7. Millar HR, Simpson JG, Stalker AL. An evaluation of the heat precipitation method for plasma fibrinogen estimation. J Clin Pathol. 1971;24:827–30.
8. Brooks M. A review of canine inherited bleeding disorders: biochemical and molecular strategies for disease characterization and carrier detection. J Hered. 1999;90:112–8.
9. Peyvandi F. Epidemiology and treatment of congenital fibrinogen deficiency. Thromb Res. 2012;130(Suppl 2):S7–11.
10. Münster AM, Olsen AK, Bladbjerg EM. Usefulness of human coagulation and fibrinolysis assays in domestic pigs. Comp Med. 2002;52:39–43.
11. Ravanat C, Freund M, Dol F, Cadroy Y, Roussi J, Incardona F, et al. Cross-reactivity of human molecular markers for detection of prethrombotic states in various animal species. Blood Coagul Fibrinolysis. 1995;6:446–55.
12. Marder VJ, Francis CW. Physiologic regulation of fibrinolysis. In: Colman RW, Marder VJ, Clowes AW, et al., editors. Hemostasis and Thrombosis. Basic Principles and Clinical Practice. 5th ed. Philadelphia: Lippincott Williams and Wilkins; 2006. p. 427–36.
13. Nair GB, Ljin M, Muslimani A. A cirrhotic patient with spontaneous intramuscular hematoma due to primary hyperfibrinolysis. Clin Adv Hematol Oncol. 2011;9:249–52.
14. Wei D, Huang G, Su J, Cheng Y. Bronchiectasis combined with primary hyperfibrinolysis : report of two cases. Nan Fang Yi Ke Da Xue Xue Bao. 2012;32:1528–9.
15. Ortel TL. Antiphospholipid syndrome: laboratory testing and diagnostic strategies. Am J Hematol. 2012;87:S75–81.
16. O'Shaughnessy DF, Atterbury C, Bolton Maggs P, Murphy M, Thomas D, Yates S, et al. Guidelines for the use of fresh-frozen plasma, cryoprecipitate and cryosupernatant. Br J Haematol. 2004;126:11–28.
17. Madden RE, Gould RG. The turnover rate of fibrinogen in the dog. J Biol Chem. 1952;196:641–50.

6

Mucopolysaccharidosis VI in cats–clarification regarding genetic testing

Leslie A. Lyons[1*], Robert A. Grahn[2], Francesca Genova[3], Michela Beccaglia[4], John J. Hopwood[5] and Maria Longeri[3]

Abstract

The release of new DNA-based diagnostic tools has increased tremendously in companion animals. Over 70 different DNA variants are now known for the cat, including DNA variants in disease-associated genes and genes causing aesthetically interesting traits. The impact genetic tests have on animal breeding and health management is significant because of the ability to control the breeding of domestic cats, especially breed cats. If used properly, genetic testing can prevent the production of diseased animals, causing the reduction of the frequency of the causal variant in the population, and, potentially, the eventual eradication of the disease. However, testing of some identified DNA variants may be unwarranted and cause undo strife within the cat breeding community and unnecessary reduction of gene pools and availability of breeding animals. Testing for mucopolysaccharidosis Type VI (MPS VI) in cats, specifically the genetic testing of the L476P (c.1427T>C) and the D520N (c.1558G>A) variants in *arylsulfatase B (ARSB)*, has come under scrutiny. No health problems are associated with the D520N (c.1558G>A) variant, however, breeders that obtain positive results for this variant are speculating as to possible correlation with health concerns. Birman cats already have a markedly reduced gene pool and have a high frequency of the MPS VI D520N variant. Further reduction of the gene pool by eliminating cats that are heterozygous or homozygous for only the MPS VI D520N variant could lead to more inbreeding depression effects on the breed population. Herein is debated the genetic testing of the MPS VI D520N variant in cats. Surveys from different laboratories suggest the L476P (c.1427T>C) disease-associated variant should be monitored in the cat breed populations, particularly breeds with Siamese derivations and outcrosses. However, the D520N has no evidence of association with disease in cats and testing is not recommended in the absence of L476P genotyping. Selection against the D520N is not warranted in cat populations. More rigorous guidelines may be required to support the genetic testing of DNA variants in all animal species.

Keywords: *ARSB*, DNA, Feline, *Felis silvestris catus*, Genetic testing, *N-acetylgalactosamine-4-sulfatase*, MPS VI

Background

Genetic testing represents one of the most important hot topics in the field of veterinary small animal practice [1, 2]. The discovery and release of DNA-based diagnostics has tremendously increased, and the impact of these tests on animal breeding and health and population management is significant. All DNA tests need extensive "vetting" by the research community to document sensitivity, specificity and correlation with disease since the downstream consequences of publishing ambiguous or benign genetic variants have the potential to dramatically impact the genetic health of a population.

One recent example of a controversial DNA test in cats was the A31P and A74T variants in *myosin-binding protein C3* (*MYBPC3*) for hypertrophic cardiomyopathy (HCM) [3]. The A31P variant has a strong correlation with disease – as an indicator of risk, with a late-onset Mendelian autosomal dominant transmission, in Maine Coon cats. However, an A74T variant was presented in an abstract and suggested as causative for the same disease, which elicited a strong debate in the veterinary community [4]. Genetic testing was initiated by several commercial laboratories in worldwide cat breed populations. However, data strongly indicated that the A74T was a common polymorphism in a large number of breeds, and not significantly correlated to HCM [5]. Therefore, the A74T DNA variant testing was subsequently removed from many commercial laboratory offerings and no breeding decisions should be influenced by the presence or absence of this variant in a domestic cat.

A similar situation has recently developed for the genetic testing of mucopolysaccharidosis Type VI (MPS VI), an *arylsulfatase B* (*ARSB*) variant in cat breeds [6–9]. The published phenotypes and implications of the L476P (c.1427 T > C) variant in *ARSB* that causes a

* Correspondence: lyonsla@missouri.edu
[1]Department of Veterinary Medicine and Surgery, College of Veterinary Medicine, University of Missouri – Columbia, Columbia, MO 65211, USA
Full list of author information is available at the end of the article

severe form of MPS VI have been recognized for many years [10]. However, a second variant of *ARSB* was identified within the same experimental feline colony [11, 12]. Several laboratories now offer this MPS VI D520N "mild" DNA test to the cat breeding community. Unlike HCM, veterinarians and cat owners are less familiar with MPS VI, both in regards to clinical presentation and disease course.

Unarmed with the proper knowledge and poor availability of genetic counselling, breeders have become alarmed since many cats have been genotyped as carriers or homozygous for the D520N *ARSB* variant. A wave of genotyping in Birmans for the D520N variant has escalated the concern with breeders, who are now attributing pyometra, pregnancy loss, infertility and other health problems as a result of the variant (Personal communication – several authors). Hence, the impetus for this positional paper and a perfect example of the questions the scientific, veterinarian and breeder community will frequently address in the future. The questions are: does this mutation cause a "real disease", a "dysfunction" and is it worthy of negative selection and elimination from breeding programs? Does this variant predict a strong association with disease – as a risk indicator? A quick and massive selection for any genetic traits can lead to a drastic reduction of the genetic variability in the breed and the potential emergence of other problems, potentially more devastating, such as the severe form of MPS VI.

The authors consider the *ARSB* D520N variant not causative of a dysfunction or health concern unless present in combination with the *ARSB* L476P variant. Selection against cats with the D520N variant is only warranted if also testing for L476P. However, the L476P variant has not been demonstrated to be present in cat breed and domestic cat populations that have been tested to date. Presented is an evaluation of current genotyping data that supports this position.

What is mucopolysaccharidosis Type VI (MPS VI)?

The lysosomal storage diseases (LSD) form a diverse group of conditions linked by the common pathological feature of abnormal accumulation of metabolites within cells (for review) [13]. LSD results from a deficiency of an enzyme of one of the lysosomal catabolic pathways. The lysosomes provide a suitable environment for enzyme-catalyzed hydrolysis, keeping other cellular structures protected from the harmful effects of unconfined degradative enzymes. The LSD group is organized into subgroup classifications comprised of more than 30 different diseases based of the metabolic pathways affected and the type of storage identified. Humans with MPS have at least seven different disease entities that include skeletal, cardiovascular, neurological and ocular abnormalities and these same conditions are found in MPS cats [6–8, 14–18].

MPS VI in humans

In humans, MPS VI, or Maroteaux - Lamy syndrome (OMIM:253200), is a rare autosomal recessive LSD [19]. MPS VI is caused by homozygous or compound heterozygous mutation in *ARSB* (OMIM:611542) [20]. The disease has been estimated to affect 1:200,000–1,500,000 people worldwide [21]. Pathogenic variants of *ARSB* result in reduced or absent activity of the enzyme arylsulfatase B. The reduced activity leads to high urinary excretion and intralysosomal accumulation of large amounts of partially degraded glycosaminoglycans (GAG - previously also known as a "mucopolysaccharide" dermatan sulfate) as well as chondroitin sulfate, N-acetylgalatosamine and N—acetylgalatosiamine-4,6-disulfate [22, 23]. GAG accumulation results in cell injury with a multi-systemic clinical picture of bone abnormalities, collectively referred to as dysostosis multiplex (disorder of the development of bone, in particular, the ossification), which affects growth, gait, and appearance.

Depending on the age of onset and progression of symptoms, patients with MPS VI have been classified into severe, intermediate, and "attenuated" forms [24]. The severe form of MPS VI is characterized by very early onset and severe progression of symptoms with various skeletal abnormalities (severe dysostosis), including dwarfism, facial dysmorphisms, and joint deformities that affect mobility. Individuals with MPS VI may develop a narrowing of the spinal canal (spinal stenosis) in the neck, which can compress and damage the spinal cord. Death generally occurs during childhood or adolescence.

The attenuated MPS VI form is characterized by very late onset with affected individuals living nearly normal life expectancies. Patients have been described with corneal clouding and joint stiffness [25], or mild dysostosis [26]. The intermediate form shows the middle of the spectrum of phenotypes, however, no fixed criteria for separating these descriptive categories are defined.

Since 1991, nearly 100 genetic mutations had been identified in *ARSB* in patients with MPS VI [20, 27–30] and are cataloged in a database (http://mps6-database.org) [31]. All types of variants can cause all severities of MPS VI and compound heterozygotes can also affect the severity of disease [28].

MPS VI in cats

Cowell et al., (1976) [32] reported the first case of an inherited disorder of mucopolysaccharide metabolism in the cat. Suzie, a 21-month-old blue point Siamese cat born of a mother-son mating, presented as "decidedly small" and "reluctant to walk". Suzie's head was "smaller than normal with an overall shortened and broadened appearance". The maxilla was remarkably broadened and

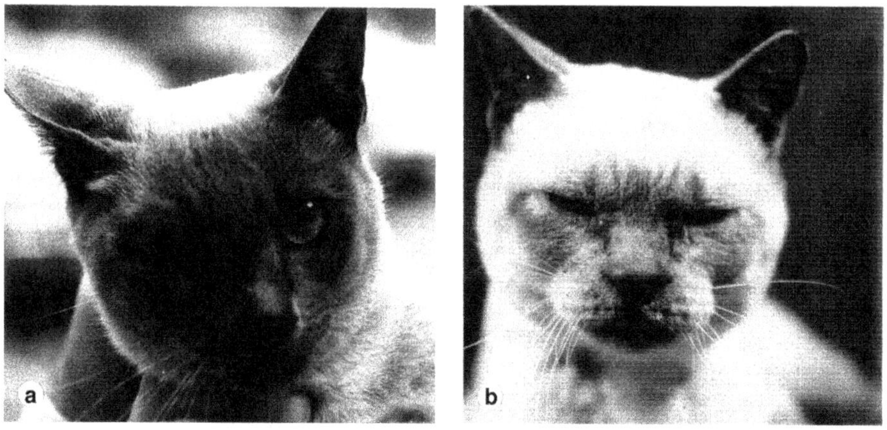

Fig. 1 a Phenotypically normal Siamese dam of the affected cat in **b. b** Siamese affected cat with *ARSB* variant causing severe MPS VI disease. Notice the broad maxillary area, slightly flattened face and half-closed eyes. (Reproduced with permission from Cowell et al., 1976.) [32]

decreased in length' (Fig. 1). The cat had bilateral pain at flection and extension of the joins with radiographic skeletal striking deformities, multifocal neurologic deficits, corneal clouding, retinal atrophy and significantly high concentration of mucopolysaccharide in the urine. A Siamese – Siamese x domestic shorthair cross experimental colony was established and more complete descriptions of pathologic and enzymologic findings were recorded (Fig. 2) [17, 33]. MPS VI has since been diagnosed in Siamese, [34–36] and domestic longhair [37] cats from different locations and all were reported as similarly affected (OMIA 000666-9685) [38]. In cats, autosomal recessive mutation consists of an amino acid substitution of a wild type leucine to a proline (L476P) in the arylsulfatase B enzyme, due to a thymine to cytosine transition (c. 1427 T > C) in *ARSB* [10].

A missense mutation (c.1558G > A), inherited independently from L476P and causing an amino acid substitution of the wild type aspartic acid to an asparagine at codon 520 (D520N) was identified in the same colony (Fig. 2) [11, 12]. The phenotype of the D520N variant in combination with the L476P variant was dubbed MPS VI "mild". Skin fibroblasts from adult D520N/L476P compound heterozygous cats expressed approximately 3.1 % of normal levels of ARSB activity and D520N homozygous cats contained approximately 4.6 %. L476P homozygous fibroblasts contained very low levels of ARSB activity at 0.46 %. All 18 colony cats that were D520N homozygotes were evaluated radiographically up to 5 years of age. This small increase in residual *ARSB* activity is sufficient to prevent the occurrence of degenerative joint disease in D520N homozygous cats. However, L476P/D520N compound heterozygous cats can develop severe joint disease as they age [11]. One cat exhibited an atypical joint disease in the shoulder. Therefore, in the clinical situation, these animals would most likely be indistinguishable from normal Siamese cats, although more clinically observable joint lesions could potentially develop

```
          ***  ** **  *    ********  *******  * ****  ***** **  * * ****** ** ***** ** *** ****  ****
   CAT WT CTGCGATACCCTCATCAGACCCACCGACCAAGACCCTCTGGCTCTTTGATATTGATCAGGACCCAGAAGAAAGACATGACCTGTCAAGAGA
CAT L476P ..........................................C................................................
      DOG ...T...C.....T..G....................G.................C.............................G.....
    HUMAN ...A.....................A...............................G......T....................C.....
    HORSE ....A..T...C.......................T.A...........C.......G......................G..........
      COW ...T............G........AG......................C.....C........C..G.....G.................
    MOUSE ...A......TC..GTG........A........T........T........CA..........T...........C...G....C.....

          ***** ** **** ******  **** ** ** **     * ** **  *     ********** ** ******  *** ** *  ***
   CAT WT TCCCGCCTCCAGTTCTACCACAAACATTCAGTGCCTGTGCATTTCCCGGCACAGGACCCCCGCTGTGACCCCAAGGGCACTGGGGCCTGGG
CAT D520N ......................................................A....................................
      DOG ........G.................C..G.........T.C........G.............................C..........
    HUMAN ........A...........T.....C.....C..C...T.C.....T....................T.......C........TG....
    HORSE .....T..G.................C..G.....C...T.C.................................A...............
      COW .....T..G...........G.....C..C.........T.C..T........A..............T.......C..............
    MOUSE ........G....A......TG.......T......TCT..C.....AC.CTT............C..T......A.......T.TG...A
```

Fig. 2 Alignment of *ARSB* DNA sequence fragments across mammals. Presented are the wildtype sequences for the domestic cat and other species and the cat sequences with variants at the nucleotide indicated with a box. The mutation sites are the L476P (C**T**C to C**C**C) and the D520N mutation (**G**AC to **A**AC). Note each mutation is on the wildtype sequence background and not compound heterozygotes. Both sites are conserved across mammals. Alignment produced by ClustalX software. The asterisks indicate conservation of the wildtype nucleotide across all species

in older animals since the cats were followed only for 5 years [39].

A population screening for both L476P and D520N was conducted on Siamese cats worldwide [39]. The prevalence was investigated in 101 clinically normal cats from North America, South America, Europe and Australia. In this general Siamese population, the D520N allelic frequency was 11.4 % (Table 1), but L476P was absent, suggesting either low frequency or higher prevalence within breeding lines excluded by the sampling. The authors noticed that "the high prevalence in the general population of the D520N, which might correspond to an expected D520N/D520N genotype frequency of 1.2 % in the sample, is "consistent with an extensive presence of carriers, to the extent two D520N/D520N homozygous were detected", suggesting Hardy-Weinberg equilibrium.

Commercial MPS VI screening

Commercial screening has been offered for MPS VI "mild", the D520N (c.1558G > A) variant. All data were generated as fee for service and not based on experimentation. Over 2200 cats have been genotyped and the variant was identified in 13 different breeds (Table 2), including, Abyssinian, Birman, British Shorthair, German Longhair, Oriental Shorthair, Ragdoll, Russian Blue, Russian White, Selkirk Rex, Siamese, and Tonkinese. Most of these breeds have South East Asian origins and the low occurrence in Western European breeds, such as British Shorthair, Ragdoll and Selkirk Rex is likely due to cross breeding. Interestingly, cats with South East Asian origins, such as Korat and Singapura, and cats bred from Abyssinians, such as Ocicats, were not found to have the variant in the populations tested.

Both the *ARSB* cat variants are variants on the Illumina 63 K iSelect Infinium DNA array for the cat. In a survey of approximately 2602 archival cat samples from various disease and phenotypic projects that were unrelated to MPS studies, only four domestic cats were identified as carriers for the severe variant, including a domestic shorthair, a Siamese, an Ocicat, and a Chartreux. This low rate could be within the genotyping error rate of the array. However, 435 were carriers and 103 were homozygous (3.5 %) for the D520N "mild" variant. A majority of the homozygous and heterozygous cats were Birmans, as well as many African and European wildcats – suggesting the variant segregates in the wildcat population and may be a common ancestral allele.

Table 1 Prevalence of feline *ARSB* variants in Siamese cats from the general Siamese population

Origins	No. Alleles tested	L476P	D520N	(Percent)
Bristol, England	10	0/10	0/10	
Dublin, Ireland	24	0/24	3/24[a]	(12.5 %)
Argentina	4	0/4	2/4[b]	(50 %)
The Netherlands	8	0/8	1/8	(12.5 %)
Melbourne, Australia	132	0/132	14/132[c]	(10.6 %)
Pennsylvania	24	0/24	3/24[c]	(12.5 %)
Total	202	0	23	(11.4)

(reproduced with permission from Crawley et al, 2003) [39]
[a]Two animals possibly related
[b]Possibly littermates
[c]One cat was a D520N homozygote

Table 2 Allele frequency of MPS VI variants in cat breeds

BREED	N	Frequency L476P Severe	D520N "Mild"
Abyssinian	114	0.00	0.179
Birman	150	0.00	0.313
Birman[a]	231	0.00	0.359
Birman (Italy)[b]	51	0.00	0.284
British Shorthair	244	0.00	0.006
Burmese	2	0.00	0.250
German Longhair[a]	3	0.00	0.333
Oriental Shorthair	5	0.00	0.200
Ragdoll	530	0.00	0.066
Ragdoll[a]	95	0.00	0.131
Russian Blue	44	0.00	0.239
Russian White	4	0.00	0.125
Selkirk Rex	16	0.00	0.063
Siamese	24	0.00	0.104
Somali	65	0.00	0.146
Tonkinese	1	0.00	0.500
39 additional breeds	678	0.00	0.000

[a]Indicates requested test
[b]Cats tested at Vetogene in Milan, Italy. All other cats were tested at the Veterinary Genetics Laboratory in Davis, California, USA

Conclusion

Genetics is an extremely powerful tool for animal health care and management because mating of cats can be controlled. Using genetic testing, cats can be bred in a manner to prevent illnesses, eliminating problems before they exist and even eradicating a disease from the population. However, genetics must be used wisely, not causing unwarranted strife and concern or causing elimination of individuals from a breeding pool that could make valuable contributions. Thus, researchers have the responsibility to vigorously define DNA variants that cause health problems in cats.

In humans, customized newborn screening programs that are tailored to the ethnicity of the population are active worldwide, screening for dozens of disease causing variants [40]. These DNA variants cause health problems where the negative health outcomes can be thwarted if early intervention can be applied. Concurrent with the screening programs, the fields of medical genetics and genetic counselling developed. Over 70 different genetic variants have been identified in cats that confer coat colors, fur types, morphological attributes, blood type and diseases [2]. However, formal medical genetic counselling programs do not exist for companion animals, thus the researchers and DNA testing laboratories must fulfill this role for the owners of cats with genetic diseases.

An uncontrolled selection against D520N is an example of how genetic testing can be used unwisely. The reduction of the already quite low genetic variability in some pedigreed breeds, such as Birmans, [41–43] which also have a high frequency of the D520N variant, can reduce genetic diversity and perhaps facilitate the proliferation of more detrimental mutations. Thinking this mutation must do "something", breeders tend to find any health condition, especially common problems due to overcrowding and stress, and make an unscientific and highly biased association with disease, including concerns that are not associated with *ARSB* variants.

Summary

The relevance of a genetic trait in terms of pain and impediment to function should be considered when publishing a DNA variant that may ultimately be requested as a genetic test both by veterinary practitioners and breeders. Severe genetic dysfunctions need to be tested, monitored and eventually eradicated. Conversely, elimination of genetic polymorphisms weakly or not associated to undefined or mild phenotypic forms endanger the genetic pool of at risk breeds.

Only the MPS VI L476P (c.1427 T > C) variant in *ARSB* causes severe disease in cats. Because the variant was found in the DNA array survey of unbiased cat breed sampling, perhaps this disease-associated variant should be monitored in the cat breed populations, particularly breeds with Siamese derivations and outcrosses. However, the *ARSB* D520N (c.1558G > A) has no evidence of association with disease and the authors recommend breeders discontinue testing for this variant, unless in combination with the L476 variant. Testing for D520N should be considered in heterozygous L476P cats, however, the L476P variant itself is extremely rare in the general cat population and should not be tested unless a MPS disease is suspected. Selection against the D520N variant is not warranted in cat populations. Researchers and commercial genetic testing laboratories need to carefully examine the published literature and perhaps openly discuss issues with genetic testing at forums such as the International Society of Animal Genetics (ISAG; http://www.isag.us/) and with the appropriate researchers with vested interests in the given disease or trait. Veterinarians and breeders are encouraged to be proactive and support research with samples, clinical records and funds to decipher the causes of health concerns in their cats.

Abbreviations

ARSB, N-acetylgalactosamine-4-sulfatase; GAG, glycosaminoglycan; HCM, hypertrophic cardiomyopathy; MPS VI, mucopolysaccharidosis type VI; *MYBPC3, myosin-binding protein C3;* OMIM, Online Mendelian Inheritance in Man

Acknowledgements

Vetogene and P.Valiati for technical assistance. This work was supported in part by funding from the National Center for Research Resources R24 RR016094 and is currently supported by the Office of Research Infrastructure Programs/OD R24OD010928 (LAL) and the University of California – Davis, Veterinary Genetics Laboratory (LAL, RAG).

Authors' contributions

LAL, RAG and FG provided data and analysis for the manuscript. All authors edited and approved of the manuscript.

Competing interests

The Authors declare that there is no conflict of interest. Financial interests: RAG, ML are staff at commercial genetic testing laboratories that have income from cat DNA testing. LAL receives support from the Veterinary Genetic Laboratory for cat genetic research.

Author details

[1]Department of Veterinary Medicine and Surgery, College of Veterinary Medicine, University of Missouri – Columbia, Columbia, MO 65211, USA. [2]Veterinary Genetics Laboratory, School of Veterinary Medicine, University of California - Davis, Davis, CA, USA. [3]Department of Veterinary Medicine, University of Milan, Milan, Italy. [4]Ambulatorio Veterinario, Lissone, Monza e Brianza, Italy. [5]Lysosomal Diseases Research Unit, South Australian Health and Medical Research Institute, Adelaide, Australia.

References

1. Jones BR, Little S, Lyons LA, Malik R, Nicholas F, O'Brien DP, Pedersen NC. Understanding genetics: why should vets care? J Feline Med Surg. 2015;17(3):201–2.
2. Lyons LA. DNA mutations of the cat: the good, the bad and the ugly. J Feline Med Surg. 2015;17(3):203–19.
3. Meurs KM, Sanchez X, David RM, Bowles NE, Towbin JA, Reiser PJ, Kittleson JA, Munro MJ, Dryburgh K, Macdonald KA et al. A cardiac *myosin binding protein C* mutation in the Maine Coon cat with familial hypertrophic cardiomyopathy. Hum Mol Genet. 2005;14(23):3587–93.
4. Kittleson MD, Meurs K, Munro M. Re: Association of A31P and A74T polymorphisms in the myosin binding protein C3 gene and hypertrophic cardiomyopathy in Maine Coon and other breed cats. J Vet Intern Med. 2010;24(6):1242–3. author reply 1244.
5. Longeri M, Ferrari P, Knafelz P, Mezzelani A, Marabotti A, Milanesi L, Pertica G, Polli M, Brambilla PG, Kittleson M et al. *Myosin-binding protein C* DNA variants in domestic cats (A31P, A74T, R820W) and their association with hypertrophic cardiomyopathy. J Vet Intern Med. 2013;27(2):275–85.
6. Abreu S, Hayden J, Berthold P, Shapiro IM, Decker S, Patterson D, Haskins M. Growth plate pathology in feline mucopolysaccharidosis VI. Calcif Tissue Int. 1995;57(3):185–90.
7. Aguirre G, Stramm L, Haskins M. Feline mucopolysaccharidosis VI: General ocular and pigment epithelial pathology. Invest Ophthalmol Vis Sci. 1983;24(8):991–1007.

8. Sheridan O, Wortman J, Harvey C, Hayden J, Haskins M. Craniofacial abnormalities in animal models of mucopolysaccharidoses I, VI, and VII. J Craniofac Genet Dev Biol. 1994;14(1):7–15.
9. Vine DT, McGovern MM, Haskins ME, Desnick RJ. Feline mucopolysaccharidosis VI: purification and characterization of the resident arylsulfatase B activity. Am J Hum Genet. 1981;33(6):916–27.
10. Yogalingam G, Litjens T, Bielicki J, Crawley AC, Muller V, Anson DS, Hopwood JJ. Feline mucopolysaccharidosis type VI. Characterization of recombinant *N-acetylgalactosamine 4-sulfatase* and identification of a mutation causing the disease. J Biol Chem. 1996;271(44):27259–65.
11. Crawley AC, Yogalingam G, Muller VJ, Hopwood JJ. Two mutations within a feline mucopolysaccharidosis type VI colony cause three different clinical phenotypes. J Clin Invest. 1998;101(1):109–19.
12. Yogalingam G, Hopwood JJ, Crawley A, Anson DS. Mild feline mucopolysaccharidosis type VI. Identification of an *N-acetylgalactosamine-4-sulfatase* mutation causing instability and increased specific activity. J Biol Chem. 1998;273(22):13421–9.
13. Parenti G, Andria G, Ballabio A. Lysosomal storage diseases: from pathophysiology to therapy. Annu Rev Med. 2015;66:471–86.
14. Haskins ME, Otis EJ, Hayden JE, Jezyk PF, Stramm L. Hepatic storage of glycosaminoglycans in feline and canine models of mucopolysaccharidoses I, VI, and VII. Vet Pathol. 1992;29(2):112–9.
15. Walkley SU, Thrall MA, Haskins ME, Mitchell TW, Wenger DA, Brown DE, Dial S, Seim H. Abnormal neuronal metabolism and storage in mucopolysaccharidosis type VI (Maroteaux-Lamy) disease. Neuropathol Appl Neurobiol. 2005;31(5):536–44.
16. Sleeper MM, Kusiak CM, Shofer FS, O'Donnell P, Bryan C, Ponder KP, Haskins ME. Clinical characterization of cardiovascular abnormalities associated with feline mucopolysaccharidosis I and VI. J Inherit Metab Dis. 2008;31(3):424–31.
17. Haskins ME, Aguirre GD, Jezyk PF, Patterson DF. The pathology of the feline model of mucopolysaccharidosis VI. Am J Pathol. 1980;101(3):657–74.
18. Haskins ME, Jezyk PF, Desnick RJ, Patterson DF. Feline models of mucopolysaccharidosis. Birth Defects Orig Artic Ser. 1980;16(1):219–24.
19. Litjens T, Baker EG, Beckmann KR, Morris CP, Hopwood JJ, Callen DF. Chromosomal localization of *ARSB*, the gene for human *N-acetylgalactosamine-4-sulphatase*. Hum Genet. 1989;82(1):67–8.
20. Wicker G, Prill V, Brooks D, Gibson G, Hopwood J, von Figura K, Peters C. Mucopolysaccharidosis VI (Maroteaux-Lamy syndrome). An intermediate clinical phenotype caused by substitution of valine for glycine at position 137 of *arylsulfatase B*. J Biol Chem. 1991;266(32):21386–91.
21. Valayannopoulos V, Nicely H, Harmatz P, Turbeville S. Mucopolysaccharidosis VI. Orphanet J Rare Dis. 2010;5:5.
22. Hopwood JJ, Elliott H. Urinary excretion of sulphated N-acetylhexosamines in patients with various mucopolysaccharidoses. Biochem J. 1985;229(3):579–86.
23. Byers S, Rozaklis T, Brumfield LK, Ranieri E, Hopwood JJ. Glycosaminoglycan accumulation and excretion in the mucopolysaccharidoses: characterization and basis of a diagnostic test for MPS. Mol Genet Metab. 1998;65(4):282–90.
24. Neufeld EF, Muenzer J. The mucopolysaccharidoses. In: Scriver CR, Beaudet AL, Sly WS, Valle D, editors. The Metabolic and Molecular Bases of Inherited Disease. 7th ed. New York: McGraw-Hill; 2001. p. 2465–94.
25. Quigley HA, Kenyon KR. Ultrastructural and histochemical studies of a newly recognized form of systemic mucopolysaccharidosis. (Maroteaux-Lamy syndrome, mild phenotype). Am J Ophthalmol. 1974;77(6):809–18.
26. Jin WD, Jackson CE, Desnick RJ, Schuchman EH. Mucopolysaccharidosis type VI: identification of three mutations in the *arylsulfatase B* gene of patients with the severe and mild phenotypes provides molecular evidence for genetic heterogeneity. Am J Hum Genet. 1992;50(4):795–800.
27. Villani GR, Balzano N, Vitale D, Saviano M, Pavone V, Di Natale P. Maroteaux-lamy syndrome: five novel mutations and their structural localization. Biochim Biophys Acta. 1999;1453(2):185–92.
28. Litjens T, Hopwood JJ. Mucopolysaccharidosis type VI: Structural and clinical implications of mutations in *N-acetylgalactosamine-4-sulfatase*. Hum Mutat. 2001;18(4):282–95.
29. Garrido E, Chabas A, Coll MJ, Blanco M, Dominguez C, Grinberg D, Vilageliu L, Cormand B. Identification of the molecular defects in Spanish and Argentinian mucopolysaccharidosis VI (Maroteaux-Lamy syndrome) patients, including 9 novel mutations. Mol Genet Metab. 2007;92(1–2):122–30.
30. Karageorgos L, Brooks DA, Pollard A, Melville EL, Hein LK, Clements PR, Ketteridge D, Swiedler SJ, Beck M, Giugliani R et al. Mutational analysis of 105 mucopolysaccharidosis type VI patients. Hum Mutat. 2007;28(9):897–903.
31. Saito S, Ohno K, Sekijima M, Suzuki T, Sakuraba H. Database of the clinical phenotypes, genotypes and mutant arylsulfatase B structures in mucopolysaccharidosis type VI. J Hum Genet. 2012;57(4):280–2.
32. Cowell KR, Jezyk PF, Haskins ME, Patterson DF. Mucopolysaccharidosis in a cat. J Am Vet Med Assoc. 1976;169(3):334–9.
33. Haskins ME, Jezyk PF, Patterson DF. Mucopolysaccharide storage disease in three families of cats with arylsulfatase B deficiency: leukocyte studies and carrier identification. Pediatr Res. 1979;13(11):1203–10.
34. Breton L, Guerin P, Morin M. A case of Mucopolysaccharidosis VI in a cat. J Am Anim Hosp Assoc. 1983;19:891–6.
35. Macrì B, Marino F, Mazzullo G, Trusso A, De Maria R, Amedeo S, Divari SMC. Mucopolysaccharidosis VI in a Siamese/Short-Haired European Cat. J Vet Med Assoc. 2002;49:438–42.
36. Di Natale P, Annella T, Daniele A, Spagnuolo G, Cerundolo R, de Caprariis D, AE G. Animal models for lysosomal storage diseases: a new case of feline mucopolysaccharidosis VI. J Inherit Metab Dis. 1992;15(1):17–24.
37. Beekman GK. Mucopolysaccharidosis VI in a kitten: a case report and discussion of feline Maroteaux-Lamy syndrome. Feline Pract. 1993;21:7–11.
38. Online Mendelian Inheritance in Animals, OMIA. [http://omia.angis.org.au/home/].
39. Crawley AC, Muntz FH, Haskins ME, Jones BR, Hopwood JJ. Prevalence of mucopolysaccharidosis type VI mutations in Siamese cats. J Vet Intern Med. 2003;17(4):495–8.
40. Hoffmann GF, Lindner M, Loeber JG. 50 years of newborn screening. J Inherit Metab Dis. 2014;37(2):163–4.
41. Alhaddad H, Khan R, Grahn RA, Gandolfi B, Mullikin JC, Cole SA, Gruffydd-Jones TJ, Haggstrom J, Lohi H, Longeri M et al. Extent of linkage disequilibrium in the domestic cat, *Felis silvestris catus*, and its breeds. PLoS One. 2013;8(1):e53537.
42. Kurushima JD, Lipinski MJ, Gandolfi B, Froenicke L, Grahn JC, Grahn RA, Lyons LA. Variation of cats under domestication: genetic assignment of domestic cats to breeds and worldwide random-bred populations. Anim Genet. 2013;44(3):311–24.
43. Lipinski MJ, Froenicke L, Baysac KC, Billings NC, Leutenegger CM, Levy AM, Longeri M, Niini T, Ozpinar H, Slater MR et al. The ascent of cat breeds: genetic evaluations of breeds and worldwide random-bred populations. Genomics. 2008;91(1):12–21.

7

Evaluation of an open source method for calculating physical activity in dogs from harness and collar based sensors

C. Westgarth[1*] and C. Ladha[2]

Abstract

Background: The ability to make objective measurements of physical activity in dogs has both clinical and research applications. Accelerometers offer a non-intrusive and convenient solution. Of the commercialy available sensors, measurements are commonly given in manufacturer bespoke units and calculated with closed source approaches. Furthermore, the validation studies that exist for such devices are mounting location dependant, not transferable between brands or not suitable for handling modern raw accelerometry type data.

Methods: This paper describes a validation study of $n = 5$ where 4 sensors were placed on each dog; 2 on a harness and 2 on a collar. Each position held two sensors from different manufacturers; Actigraph (which has previously been validated for use on the collar) and VetSens (which provides un-filtered accelerometry data). The aims of the study was to firstly evaluate the performance of an open-design method of converting raw accelerometry data into units that have previously been validated. Secondly, comparison was made between sensors mounted at each location for determining physical activity state.

Results: Once the raw actigraphy data had been processed with the open-design method, results from a 7 day measurement revealed no significant difference in physical activity estimates via a cutpoint approach between the sensor manufacturers. A second finding was a low inter-site variability between the ventral collar and dorsal harness locations (Pearsons $r^2 = 0.96$).

Conclusions: Using the open-design methodology, raw, un-filtered data from the VetSens sensors can be compared or pooled with data gathered from Actigraph sensors. The results also provide strong evidence that ventral collar and dorsal harness sites may be used interchangeably. This enables studies to be designed with a larger inclusion criteria (encompassing dogs that are not well suited for wearing an instrumented collar) and ensures high levels of welfare while maintaining measurement validity.

Keywords: Dogs, Physical activity, Accelerometer, Harness, Collar, Exercise, Sensor

Background

In the past decade, accelerometers have gained popularity as tools for measuring dogs' physical activity. They offer low cost, objective measurements and the size of modern sensors does little to hinder everyday movements and behaviour of the subject; they can be worn continuously as concluded in [1]. Amongst other applications, accelerometers have found use in measuring dysfunction or disease [2–4], making unsupervised behaviour observations [5, 6] and forming part of dog-owner communication systems [7].

The majority of commercially available physical activity sensors contain an accelerometer chip. Fundamentally accelerometers measure movement, or more exactly, they afford a sensitive platform to capture any force exerted on them. This makes them particularly good at detecting both cyclic motions (e.g walking) as well as orientation changes, such as posture transitions. In its raw form, the output of any accelerometer contains a timestamped stream of data containing

* Correspondence: Carri.westgarth@liverpool.ac.uk
[1]Institute of Infection and Global Health and Institute of Veterinary Science, University of Liverpool, Leahurst Campus, Chester High Road, Neston, Cheshire CH64 7TE, UK
Full list of author information is available at the end of the article

information related to the forces on each of its 3-axis. Internally, this stream may be sampled up-to several hundred times per second, although a study on human data demonstrated sample rates above 50 Hz provided little benefit (even for complex machine learning activities working in the frequency domain [8]). Even when stationary, accelerometers are sensitive to the reaction forces of gravity. This property allows them to be used effectively used as inclinometers and subsequently good detectors of posture transition and sleep as shown in [9].

When making physical activity measurements the aim is to use the accelerometer chip to detect movements and have the sensor record them for retrospective analysis. For example, in locomotion, the signal measured via the sensor is mostly an attenuated derivative of the reaction force of the thoracic limbs striking the floor. Due to attenuation through skeletal and soft-tissue structures, sensor location may affect the signal. Modelling these attenuations is a complex task is out of scope of this paper. However, from fundamental principles [10] a power spectral analysis will reveal that body accelerations of lower frequencies contain higher energy and will propagate more effectively through bone and soft tissue.

The majority of movements related to physical activity are the result of gross motor functions (e.g. locomotion or posture transitions).For such measurements, it is common to summarise the raw output stream into manageable time-slices of data called epochs (methodology described in [11]). This technique is common practice in human studies and is now also widely adopted for canine measurements [2, 4, 12]. The concept is that a single epoch summary measure contains enough information to make inferences to a coarse physical activity state (over its time period). It is common to give states names such as sedentary, light, moderate or vigorous and each state is associated with a threshold (often termed cutpoint). Depending on the topic of interest, hourly or daily estimates of time in each state can be estimated. Within the field of canine physical activity measurement using accelerometers, current topics of debate are: suitable epoch duration ([4, 12, 13] use 1, 10 and 15 s respectively); best placement location for different types of measurement [12]; and attachment protocol where the current consensus is to use a separate collar for sensor and leash [14, 15].

Although the concept of making summary epoch measures is common, the practicalities of combining a time-slice of 3-axis accelerometer data (which could be hundreds of samples) into a single epoch is complex. Each manufacturer has their own algorithm which will often contain filters to remove non-wear, filter mechanical vibrations and minimise the effect of un-wanted orientation changes (e.g. collar rotations). Subsequently, it is problematic to validate a set of cutpoint thresholds that can be used across device brands. For example, studies such as [16] have used the GT3X (Actigraph Corp, USA) sensor and suggested values which are not directly compatible with [1] which use the Actical (Philips Respironics, Netherlands) sensor. In human studies, an attempt has been made to harmonise across sensor designs by publication of an open methodology for calculating epoch summaries [17]. Using a shaker table resonating at frequencies resembling human movement, this method has been demonstrated to very closely replicate Actigraph Count measures; a unit bespoke to that manufacturer.

For research using animals to be ethical it should minimise discomfort or distress and allow natural behaviour. The latter is particularly important when the purpose of the research is to capture typical behaviour/movement. For the majority of dogs, the collar offers a convenient attachment site for the accelerometer and many studies have reported using it [1, 2, 4, 13, 18]. However, for some breeds (e.g. very small) or a dog with a sensitive throat/neck, the burden of an additional collar (as recommended in [14, 15]) may lead to discomfort and poor quality measurements. In such cases a harness may offer more comfort. As an attachment site, a harness has its own set of idiosyncrasies. Studies such as [6, 7] have reported good compliance with dogs carrying sensors on this site and thus the question arises if measurements made from a collar can be directly compared to those from a harness. Having multiple mounting options and the ability to interchange attachment location within a cohort has the benefit that a wider range of dogs can be recruited without compromising welfare. The ability to use a harness for physical activity measurements also supports the experimentation of combining other sensors (which would be too burdening to be worn on a collar). For example, in humans the addition of GPS data to physical activity has been previously shown to provide context on how environment relates to exercise [19].

The uncertainty as to whether cutpoint values derived for the collar are applicable to the harness originates from the underlying mode of sensor operation; accelerometers are a sensitive platform for measuring forces. For example, a sensor mounted dorsally (e.g. on a harness), has sagittal signal components that reference the angular force between the cervical spine and the crest of the scapula. In contrast, a sensor mounted ventrally (say on a collar) has similar components that reference the rotation of the sternal notch around the dorsal crest of the scapulohumeral joint. While on a skeletal level the forces involved are of the same order of magnitude (if they were not the joint would become unstable), the accelerometer must detect these forces through several layers of fat, muscle and fur. In addition, if the collar is to remain comfortable, it is highly likely that it may move or rotate. Previous work [12] has demonstrated that the attenuation of these signals is sufficient to make estimating walking speed difficult from any other location than a tightly fitting harness.

The first aim of this study is to validate if the open-method for calculating epoch summaries functions on data from dogs. Having a consistent methodology that functions across sensor brands allows for data pooling, prevents brand lock-in and safeguards against scenarios where manufacturers change data processing methodologies without notifying users [20]. Our hypothesis for this part of the study is that the signals originating from a dog and human are sufficiently similar in the frequency domain that the methods developed for humans can be transferred without modification and our two sensors will give similar results.

The second aim of this study is to determine if epoch summary measures obtained from a collar can be compared to those similarly from a harness. The ability to do so will provide flexibility in study design and ensure a consistent level of welfare is maintained through the choice of either a second collar or harness to carry sensors. Our hypothesis is that the coarse nature of the cutpoint methodology will mask effects of mounting specific signal attenuation found to be problematic in approaches such as [12] and thus the findings from each location will be similar.

Methods

Experiment design

For this study, $n = 5$ dogs were recruited from a convenience sample belonging to Veterinary School staff members. The sample purposefully included a range of breeds, sizes and ages in order to maximise variability in the captured signal characteristics (see Table 1). The cohort size was chosen to provide sufficient variety in order to test equivalency across a range of movements and is similar to that of a previous validation study [12] (this study had a cohort of $n = 6$). All dogs were deemed healthy by their owners and assessment by the last author. The study was approved by the University of Liverpool Veterinary Ethics Committee.

All dogs were selected to wear both an instrumented collar and an instrumented harness. Some had previously worn a harness and for others it was new. Both the collar and harness were fitted with a GT3X (Actigraph Corp, USA) and a VetSens sensor (VetSens UK); a total of four sensors per dog. The Actigraph sensor was chosen as it is a sensor previously validated for canine physical activity measurements and a set of validated cutpoints have been reported [16]. The VetSens sensor was chosen as it compatible with OpenMovement [21] open-source software, provides access to raw unfiltered accelerometer measurements and has had its raw output data verified for equivalency on a shaker table experiment [22]. The sensors were all configured with the same workstation which provided a synchronisation mechanism (to the system time). All the sensors were configured to record continuously for a period of 7 days. The Actigraph sensors automatically measured in Actigraph Count units (the proprietary manufacturer unit) of 60 s epoch duration. The VetSens sensors were set to measure in raw mode with F_s = 100 Hz and sensitivity of ±8 g as recommended for capture of canine activity [5].

The two sensors at each site were physically strapped together using non-stretch tape. The first pair of sensors were attached around the dog neck using a shortened elastic belt and clips supplied with the Actigraph GT3X so that they fit snugly but comfortably to the dog neck (in accordance with recommendations set out in [15]). A dorsal collar position was initially attempted but we found that rotation to the ventral position frequently occurred and efforts to prevent this were abandoned during the capture period. The second pair of sensors were mounted onto a Perfect Fit (Dog Games, UK) three-piece fleece-lined harness using a specially designed pouch integral to the top piece (See Fig. 1).

Data processing

For convenience and due to their previous validation research, cutpoints suggested by [16] were used as a basis for comparison between sensors. As these figures are specified in manufacturer proprietary units (Actigraph Counts) a prior conversion step was made to the VetSens data such that it was compatible. This conversion step has been openly described and validated in humans

Table 1 Participant information and sensor agreement per dog

Dog	Age (Years)	Breed	Height (cm)	R^2 VetSens C + H	R^2 Actigraph C + H	R^2 Harness Ac + Vs	R^2 Collar Ac + Vs
A	13	Spaniel cross	48	0.98	0.96	0.97	0.28
B	4	Pug x Chihuahua x Pomeranian	27	0.98	0.97	0.93	0.96
C	6	Patterdale cross	37	0.97	0.97	0.94	0.97
D	0.5	Miniature American Shepherd	36	0.96	0.98	0.95	0.92
E	5	Poodle x Golden retriever	57	0.98	0.97	0.96	0.97

Ac Actigraph, *Vs* VetSens, *C* collar, *H* harness

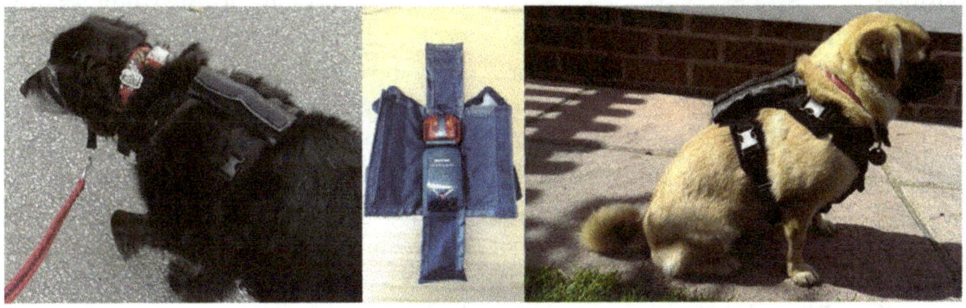

Fig. 1 Harness components; a generic compartment housing all sensing equipment and a multisize strap system suitable for different size dogs

[17]. In summary, a 3rd order band-pass Butterworth filter (f_c 0.25–2.5 Hz) is applied to remove DC offset and high frequency noise; such as would be expected from mechanical noise or vibration. The axis are then combined as their Euclidean distance vector into a measure that is reported equivalent in scale to the Actigraph Count.

Measurements from both collar and harness, from each sensor, on each dog, were subsequently summarised into epochs of 60 s. This value was chosen for convenience of processing; it is of similar design to many other studies [1, 23, 24], and the length is sufficient to minimise any synchronisation issues between sensors. Individual epoch summary measures were then first compared across sensor types (within the same location) and then secondly across sites (but within the same sensor type).

Statistical processing

The resulting data from the two sensors from each location was directly compared; Actigraph-Collar vs VetSens-Collar and Actigraph-Harness vs VetSens-Harness. Correlations were made on time-synchronised epochs of Counts, within each dog, and a mean overall Pearson's correlation squared (r^2) value was calculated.

To estimate disagreement between harness-collar for each sensor, a normalised difference is taken against the number of 60 s epochs in 24 h,

$$disagreement = (|A_{collar} - A_{harness}|)/(24*60)$$

where A = activity expressed in counts per min and disagreement is in percentage of a 24-h period.

Results

Sensor equivalency tests

All sensors recorded as configured and a total of 10,080 60s epoch measurements were collected from each sensor (total of 403,200 min over all sensors and dogs). Figure 2 depicts counts from all dogs over a 24 h period and highlights sensor type to illustrate difference. Seven day data from each Actigraph-VetSens sensor pair, on both sites, over all dogs were compared to yield a mean Pearson's r^2 = 0.97 and r^2 = 0.96 for collar and harness location respectively; see Fig. 2. (i). Results per dog are presented in Table 1.

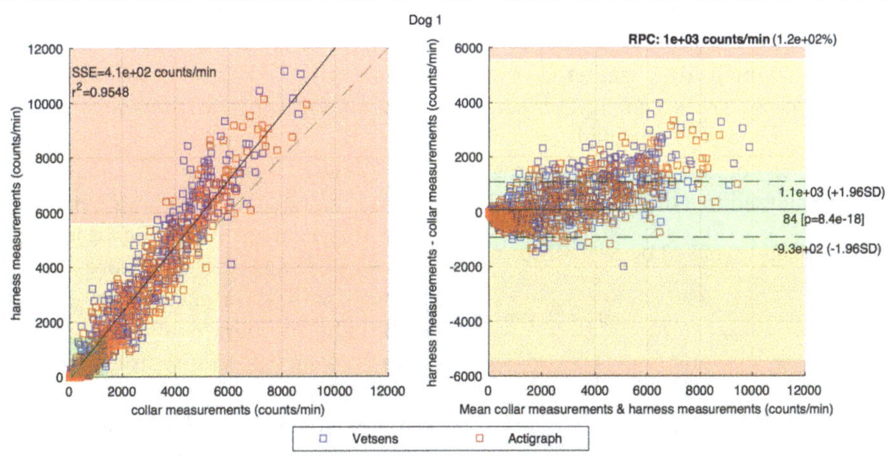

Fig. 2 Comparison between harness and collar positions for Vetsens and Actigraph sensors on 1 dog for 24 h. Green, Orange and Red areas mark Sed, Light-Mod and Vig activity levels as defined in [8]

Collar vs harness position

Applying the cutpoint thresholds from [16] gives results in Table 2. These results represent mean daily averages for all dogs over the 7-day collection period. Reassuringly, the proportion of time spent in Sedentary, Light-Moderate and Vigorous were in line with previous findings for adult dogs [2] (this study reports a 88:10:2 percentage daily time split between Sed:Light-Mod:Vig states). For the VetSens sensor, disagreement between measurements at the harness and collar is 1.2%, 1.5% and 0.3% for Sed, Light-Moderate and Vigorous respectively. For the Actigraph sensor the disagreement between sites is marginally higher at 2.2%, 0.5% 0.4% for Sed, Light-Moderate and Vigorous respectively.

Acceptability of the method

With the exception of one (dog C), all dogs tolerated wearing the instrumented harness; for this dog it was removed after 5 days as it was thought it may be becoming uncomfortable. This finding may be incidental as there had not been issues over the first 5 days of the dog wearing it. For the other dogs no adverse effects were reported other than noticing that the dogs were possibly slightly less settled and relaxed in the evenings than they normally would be without the harness. For the very small dog (B), the sensors on the collar were observed to be more intrusive than the harness.

Discussion

The first aim of this study was to test whether raw data output from the VetSens sensor can be processed using an open-design method to be equivalent to a closed-source equivalent (Actigraph). The results from the intra-site sensor comparisons (VetSens vs Actigraph at the collar and harness locations) was in line with the levels of agreement reported in [15]. Although not perfect, this high degree of correlation provides confidence in replicating the manufacturers bespoke epoch summary units (Actigraph Counts); data gathered from VetSens and Actigraph sensor types can be compared like-for-like basis using previously validated cutpoint sets. Furthermore, data may be pooled with heterogeneous sensor types and analysed together.

Table 2 Mean number of minutes captured by each sensor in each activity state per day

Sensor	Position	S (mins)	LM (mins)	V (mins)
Vetsens	Collar	1154	259	27
	Harness	1171	238	31
Actigraph	Collar	1157	228	37
	Harness	1189	220	31

Activity states determined as per Morrison 2013. N = 5 dogs. (S = Sedentary, LM = Light-Moderate, V = Vigorous)

The second aim of this study was to evaluate if accelerometer measurements made at the collar could directly be compared to those made at a harness on an epoch-by-epoch basis. Before our experiments, we hypothesised that the epoch summary method would be not be sensitive to the subtle differences in how signal components propagate through the bone and soft-tissue between collar or harness locations. The results from the inter-site comparison (collar vs harness) revealed a high level of agreement between the sites, supporting our hypothesis. Were this level of disagreement translated into a time (0.3% of the day in minutes equates to ~4mins), it would be an order of magnitude below what is considered a reasonable time to spend exercising (~40mins). This result gives confidence in the interchangeability between sites using this technique. Furthermore, this result was consistent across all sizes of dog in our cohort. Our findings are in contrast to previous work [12] that suggested non-compatibility, however the purpose of that study was to determine walking speed (rather than physical activity intensity) and used a much shorter epoch duration (1 s) with only 3 min of recorded data per participant (n = 6).

A review into some of the disagreements pointed towards possible root causes of collar rotation or looseness; the harness has the advantage of being unable to rotate. This stresses the importance of consistent and proper mounting protocol and a separate collar for attaching the leash whilst walking. A review of time-synchronised raw signal components from each site was also done and revealed significantly different signal characteristics; predominantly phase and frequency. This leads us to hypothesize that while the relatively coarse approach of constructing epoch summary measures to estimate physical activity will transfer between sites, methods making use of more complex signal features or time-frequency components (such as those in [5, 6]) would not transfer well.

The number of dogs used in this study was relatively small and thus could be considered a limitation; no meaningful inter-dog comparisons could be made for confounding factors such as age, breed, size, weight. However, the scope of this study was limited to equivalency evaluation and correlations were made on an intra-dog basis. The dogs recruited were specifically chosen to provide variability in both physical activity intensity as well as time in spent in each light, moderate and vigorous physical activity states. None of the sampled dogs appeared as an outlier and a long duration was collected to provide optimal chance of all natural behaviour types to be displayed with multiple occurrences (7 continuous days of data on 5 dogs equates to over 400,000 epochs correlation points).

Conclusions

An open-design methodology for gathering canine physical activity data was evaluated for replication of closed source epoch measurements in manufacturer-specific units. Strong correlation demonstrates its effectiveness and provides the confidence to move towards consistent and validated methodologies of handling raw-data streams; a format sensor manufacturers are trending towards. The open-method also may allow pooling of previously gathered raw accelerometer data across different sensor platforms.

The study also demonstrated equivalency between data gathered from a sensor mounted a harness and a sensor mounted on a collar. Put simply, for the sensors types in this study, cutpoint thresholds validated for the collar can be confidently applied to epoch measurements gathered at the harness. This finding enables studies to be designed with more flexible inclusion criteria enabling measurement of dogs better suited to wearing a harness or use of a harness for reasons such as carrying additional sensors. Being able to interchange collar and harness within a cohort also ensures that consistent levels of welfare can be sought while retaining measurement validity.

Acknowledgements

The authors would like to thank John Grainger and Dog Games Ltd. for the development and supply of bespoke harnesses.

Funding

This research was funded by a Medical Research Council Population Health Scientist Fellowship (Grant ref.: G1002402) held by CW. The funders played no role in study design or conclusions.

Authors' contributions

CW designed the study and collected the data. CL analysed the data and drafted the manuscript. Both revised and approved the final manuscript.

Consent for publication

CW approves the images of her dogs in Fig. 1.

Competing interests

Author CW has no competing interests. CL is engaged in development of the VetSens product.

Author details

[1]Institute of Infection and Global Health and Institute of Veterinary Science, University of Liverpool, Leahurst Campus, Chester High Road, Neston, Cheshire CH64 7TE, UK. [2]Institute of Neuroscience, Henry Wellcome Building, The Medical School, Newcastle University, Newcastle upon Tyne NE2 4HH, UK.

References

1. Dow CC, Michel KEK, Love M, Brown DC. Evaluation of optimal sampling interval for activity monitoring in companion dogs. Am J Vet Res. 2009;70: 444-48. Available from: http://avmajournals.avma.org/doi/abs/10.2460/ajvr.70.4.444. [cited 2016 Jun 2].
2. Michel KEK, Brown DCD. Determination and application of cut points for accelerometer-based activity counts of activities with differing intensity in pet dogs. Am J Vet Res. 2011;72:866–70.
3. Ladha C, O'Sullivan J, Belshaw Z, Asher L. GaitKeeper: A System for Measuring Canine Gait. Sensors [Internet]. Multidisciplinary Digital Publishing Institute; 2017 [cited 2017 Jun 28];17:309. Available from: http://www.mdpi.com/1424-8220/17/2/309
4. Morrison R, Reilly JJ, Penpraze V, Pendlebury E, Yam PS. A 6-month observational study of changes in objectively measured physical activity during weight loss in dogs. J Small Anim Pract. 2014;55:566–70.
5. Ladha C, Hammerla N, Hughes E, Olivier P, Ploetz T. Dog's life: Wearable Activity Recognition for Dogs. Proc. 2013 ACM Int. Jt. Conf. Pervasive ubiquitous Comput. - UbiComp '13 [Internet]. 2013;415. Available from: http://dl.acm.org/citation.cfm?id=2493432.2493519
6. Gerencsér L, Vásárhelyi G, Nagy M, Vicsek T, Miklósi A. Identification of Behaviour in Freely Moving Dogs (*Canis familiaris*) Using Inertial Sensors. de Polavieja GG, editor. PLoS One [Internet]. The Japanese Society of Veterinary Science; 2013 [cited 2017 Sep 4];8:e77814. Available from: http://dx.plos.org/10.1371/journal.pone.0077814
7. Jackson MM, Kshirsagar Y, Starner T, Zeagler C, Valentin G, Martin A, et al. FIDO - facilitating interactions for dogs with occupations. Proc. 17th Annu. Int. Symp. Int. Symp. wearable Comput. - ISWC '13 [Internet]. New York, New York, USA: ACM Press; 2013 [cited 2017 Sep 4]. p. 81. Available from: http://dl.acm.org/citation.cfm?doid=2493988.2494334
8. Khan A, Hammerla N, Mellor S, Plötz T. Optimising sampling rates for accelerometer-based human activity recognition. Pattern Recognit. Lett. 2016; 70(4):444-48.
9. Clarke N, Fraser D. Automated monitoring of resting in dogs. Appl Anim Behav Sci. 2016;174:99–102.
10. Stoica P, Moses R. Spectral Analysis of Signals. Spectr. Elem. Method Struct. Dyn. [Internet]. Prentice Hall; 2009 [cited 2017 Sep 5]. p. 11–38. Available from: http://doi.wiley.com/10.1002/9780470823767.ch2
11. Trost SG, Mciver KL, Pate RR. Conducting accelerometer-based activity assessments in field-based research. Med Sci Sports Exerc. 2005;37:531–43.
12. Preston T, Baltzer W, Trost S. Accelerometer validity and placement for detection of changes in physical activity in dogs under controlled conditions on a treadmill. Res Vet Sci. 2012;93:412–6.
13. Wrigglesworth DJ, Mort ES, Upton SL, Miller AT. Accuracy of the use of triaxial accelerometry for measuring daily activity as a predictor of daily maintenance energy requirement in healthy adult Labrador retrievers. Am J Vet Res. 2011;72:1151–5.
14. Olsen A, Evans R, Duerr F. Evaluation of accelerometer inter-device variability and collar placement in dogs. Vet. Evid. [Internet]. 2016 [cited 2016 Jun 2];1:1–9. Available from: https://www.veterinaryevidence.org/index.php/ve/article/view/40
15. Martin KW, Olsen AM, Duncan CG, Duerr FM. The method of attachment influences accelerometer-based activity data in dogs. BMC Vet. Res. [Internet]. 2016;13:48. Available from: http://bmcvetres.biomedcentral.com/articles/10.1186/s12917-017-0971-1
16. Morrison R, Penpraze V, Beber A, Reilly JJ, Yam PS. Associations between obesity and physical activity in dogs: a preliminary investigation. J Small Anim Pract. 2013;54:570–4.
17. Van Hees VT, Pias M, Taherian S, Ekelund U, Brage S. A method to compare new and traditional accelerometry data in physical activity monitoring. 2010 IEEE Int. Symp. 'A World Wireless, Mob. Multimed. Networks', WoWMoM 2010 - Digit. Proc. 2010.
18. Buckley CMF, Colyer A, Skrzywanek M, Jodkowska K, Kurski G, Gawor J, et al. Use of pedometers to measure the relationship of dog walking to body condition score in obese and non-obese dogs. Br. J. Nutr. [Internet]. 2011; 106:S11–4. Available from: http://www.ncbi.nlm.nih.gov/pubmed/22005441
19. Evenson KR, Wen F, Hillier A, Cohen DA. Assessing the contribution of parks to physical activity using global positioning system and accelerometry. Med. Sci. Sports Exerc. [Internet]. NIH Public Access; 2013 [cited 2017 Sep 5];45: 1981–7. Available from: http://www.ncbi.nlm.nih.gov/pubmed/23531716
20. Brønd JC, Arvidsson D. Sampling frequency affects the processing of Actigraph raw acceleration data to activity counts. J. Appl. Physiol. [Internet].

2016 [cited 2017 Aug 24];120:362–9. Available from: http://www.ncbi.nlm.nih.gov/pubmed/26635347

21. Ladha C, Jackson D, Ladha K, Olivier P. Open Movement: An open source sensor platform. github Repos. 2013. p. www.openmovement.co.uk.
22. C Ladha, K Ladha, D Jackson PO. Shaker table validation of OpenMovement AX3 accelerometer. ICAMPAM. 3rd Int. Conf. Ambul. Monit. Phys. Act. Mov. Amherst; 2013. p. 69–70.
23. Michel KE, Brown DC. Association of signalment parameters with activity of pet dogs. J Nutr Sci. 2014;3:e28.
24. Hansen BD, Lascelles DX, Keene BW, Adams AK, Thomson AE. Evaluation of an accelerometer for at-home monitoring of spontaneous activity in dogs. Am J Vet Res. 2007;68:468–75.

8

In vitro physiological and antibacterial characterization of ZnO nanoparticle composites in simulated porcine gastric and enteric fluids

Marina S.R. Barreto[1], Cristina T. Andrade[1], Luiz Cláudio R. P. da Silva[2], Lúcio M. Cabral[2], Vânia M. Flosi Paschoalin[3] and Eduardo M. Del Aguila[3*]

Abstract

Background: Diarrhea in piglets is one of the main causes of animal death after weaning; zinc oxide (ZnO) has been used in high doses for the control of this sickness. The aim of this study was to determine the physicochemical properties of ZnO nanoparticles synthesized and immobilized on a chitosan/alginate (CH/SA) complex and investigate the antimicrobial activity and in vitro release profile of zinc (Zn^{2+}) from these new compounds. The ZnO nanoparticles composites were prepared and combined with CH/SA or CH/SA and sodium tripolyphosphate (TPP). The structure and morphology of the composites were analyzed by characterization methods such as X-ray diffraction, FTIR spectroscopy, thermogravimetric analysis, atomic absorption spectrophotometry and scanning electron microscopy.

Results: The crystallite size of ZnO nano was 17 nm and the novel ZnO composites were effective in protecting ZnO in simulated gastric fluid, where Zn^{2+} reached a concentration six-fold higher than the levels obtained with the unprotected commercial-zinc oxide. In addition, the novel composites suggest effective antimicrobial activity against *Escherichia coli* and *Staphylococcus aureus*.

Conclusions: The results described herein suggest that the novel nano composites may work as an alternative product for pig feeding as verified by the in vitro assays, and may also contribute to lower the zinc released in the environment by fecal excretion in animals waste.

Keywords: Chitosan/alginate coatings, ZnO nanoparticles, Biological properties, Piglets

Background

For decades, farms have used pharmacological concentrations of zinc oxide (ZnO) to combat post-weaning diarrhea [1, 2]. Different modes of action for the antibacterial activity of ZnO have been proposed, one of them being the partial dissolution of the ZnO particles in the enteric region and the release of Zn^{2+} [3]. When ZnO is formulated to reduce this undesirable dissociation in the stomach, less ZnO may be added to the diet [4]. This is important, since much of the ZnO given to the piglets is excreted with their waste, causing accumulation of this metal in the environment [5, 6]. The incorporation of ZnO nanoparticles in polymer matrices can facilitate their gradual and sustained release [7].

Chitosan (CH) and alginate (SA) are two of the most commonly studied biopolymers, particularly for drug delivery [8]. CH is the partially deacetylated derivative of chitin, composed of repeating units of β-(1,4)-2-amino-2-deoxy-D-glucose and β-(1,4)-2-acetamido-2-deoxy-D-glucose [9]. SA is extracted from brown seaweeds and contains carboxylic acid groups [8], presents linear chains with blocks of 1–4–linked α-L-gluronic (G-block), β-D-mannuronic acid (M-block) residues, and blocks of alternated G and M residues [10].

* Correspondence: emda@iq.ufrj.br
[3]Instituto de Química, Universidade Federal do Rio de Janeiro, Av. Athos da Silveira, Ramos 149, Bloco A, sala 545, Rio de Janeiro 21941-909, Brazil
Full list of author information is available at the end of the article

In the present study, CH and SA, with and without the addition of sodium tripolyphosphate, were combined to encapsulate nanostructured ZnO particles aiming for the control of their enteric release. To protect ZnO from the gastric acid environment, the composite structures were designed to maintain acid-soluble chitosan in the internal phase of the complex. The physical, chemical and rheological characteristics of the resulting products were analyzed by infrared spectroscopy, X-ray diffraction, atomic absorption spectrophotometry, thermogravimetry and scanning electron microscopy. The antibacterial properties of the composites were tested against *Escherichia coli* and *Staphylococcus aureus* and the MICs were calculated. The in vitro release profile of Zn^{2+} from the composites in both gastric and enteric simulated fluids was also investigated.

Methods

Reagents and solvents

The commercial zinc oxide (ZnO) sample (D_{XRD} = 0.22 µm) was supplied by Brasóxidos Indústria Química Ltda. (Sertãozinho-Mauá, SP, Brazil). Chitosan (CH) (75%–85% DA), sodium alginate (SA), sodium tripolyphosphate (TPP) (85% PA) and zinc acetate dehydrate (99% PA) were purchased from Sigma-Aldrich Co. (St. Louis, MO, USA). Acetic acid (99.7% PA), sodium hydroxide (99% PA), hydrochloric acid (37% PA), hydrated potassium phosphate (P.A.) and sodium chloride were purchased from Vetec Química Ltd. (Rio de Janeiro, RJ, Brazil).

Preparation of biopolymer solutions, zinc oxide dispersion and microcapsules

The CH solution at 2% (m/v) concentration was prepared by adding 2 g CH slowly to 100 mL of acetic acid 1% (*v*/v), under magnetic stirring. This solution was heated for 30 min and maintained for 12 h under stirring at room temperature. The SA aqueous solution at 2% (m/v) was prepared using 2 g of SA in 100 mL water with magnetic stirring for 12 h. The TPP solution at 3% (m/v) was prepared in 100 mL ultrapure Milli-Q water (18.2 MΩ·cm at 25 °C).

A zinc acetate dihydrate 0.2 M solution (13.2 g in 500 mL water) was prepared with Milli-Q water under magnetic stirring and at room temperature in a two-necked 1000 mL flask adapted to a heating mantle and a reflux condenser. The reaction mixture was refluxed for 30 min. After cooling, a 5 M NaOH solution was added dropwise, until achieving pH 11 [11], after which refluxing was continued for 3 h. The reaction product was decanted and the supernatant solution discarded. After successive washings with Milli-Q water, the product was oven-dried at 100 °C for 24 h, characterized and used for the preparation of the microcapsules.

Commercial ZnO (250 mg) was dispersed in water (Millipore, model Direct-Q3, São Paulo, SP, Brazil) at 4 g/100 mL composition, at 10.000 rpm with a Ultra-Turrax dispersing IKA T25 equipment (IKA®, São Paulo, Brazil) for 40 min, oven-dried at 100 °C for 24 h and characterized.

ZnO nanoparticles were added to 20 mL of acetic acid 1% solution in a 50 mL beaker, and manually dispersed until no more granules were observed. Subsequently, this dispersion was homogenized in a Turrax at 10,000 rpm for 30 min and 15 mL of the CH 2% solution was added, dropwise, with the aid of a Pasteur pipette, at a Turrax stirring speed of 5000 rpm. Then, 30 mL of the SA 2% solution was added, dropwise, still under stirring at 5000 rpm, resulting in ZnO nanoparticles and both CH and SA (ZnO/CA) and ZnO microparticles with CH, SA and TPP (ZnO/CAT), in which 15 mL of a TPP solution 3% in Milli-Q water were also added to the reaction mixture. The resulting mixtures were subjected to ultrasonic radiation for 15 min (40% amplitude, 1 s/1 s intervals, in ice baths) (750 W Sonics & Materials Inc., Newtown, CT, USA) and dried at 60 °C for further characterization.

Physicochemical and morphological characterizations

The XRD curve for the samples was obtained on a Miniflex diffractometer (Rigaku Corporation, Osaka, Japan) operating at a CuK_α wavelength of 1.542 Å. The samples were exposed to the X-ray beam with the X-ray generator running at 30 kV and 15 mA. Scattered radiation was detected at ambient temperature in the angular region (2θ) of 2–80° at a rate of 3°/min and a step size of 0.05°. The diffractogram was smoothed (Savitsky-Golay, polynome = 2, points = 7) and the baseline was corrected. Scherrer's equation (Eq. (1)) was used to estimate the average size of the ZnO crystallites.

$$D_{XRD} = K\lambda/\beta\cos\theta \tag{1}$$

where D is the average crystallite diameter in Å, K = 0.9 is the shape factor, λ = 1.5418 Å is the wavelength of the CuK_α radiation and θ is the angle of Bragg diffraction. The β value was determined by Eq. (2)

$$\beta^2 = \left(B^2 - b^2\right)^{1/2} \tag{2}$$

where B is the full width at half maximum (FWHM) of the (101) reflection of ZnO and b is the FWHM of the (101) reflection of the quartz standard, which was taken directly from the software provided with the equipment.

The ZnO, ZnO/CAT and ZnO/CA samples were characterized by FTIR spectroscopy on a Perkin Elmer spectrophotometer, Frontier model (Waltham, MA, USA) using KBr disks, with accumulation of 20 scans and 2 cm^{-1} resolution. The KBr used to prepare transparent disks was permanently maintained in an oven at 50 °C. Samples were thoroughly dried and carefully weighed (2 mg) before grinding with 100 mg of KBr.

Rheological measurements were performed at 25 °C using a controlled AR2000 stress rheometer (TA Instruments Inc., New Castle, DE, USA), fitted with a cone-and-plate geometry (2° cone angle, 40 mm diameter, 54 μm gap). The strain sweep was measured first as the evolution of the complex modulus at 6.28 rad s^{-1} for the determination of the linear viscoelastic region. Subsequently, the frequency sweep (mechanical spectra) was measured from 10^{-1} to 10^{2} rad s^{-1} (at a strain value of 1%), within the viscoelastic region.

Thermogravimetric analysis (TGA) was performed under a controlled N_2 atmosphere using a Q500 thermoanalyzer equipment from TA Instruments (New Castle, DE, USA). The measurements were performed at a heating rate of 10 °C/min from room temperature to 700 °C.

Zinc contents were determined according to the standard AOAC method (2005) using a Varian AA280 atomic absorption spectrometer (Les Ulis, France). Each sample was heated at 550 °C and the ash boiled with 10 mL of 20% HCl in a beaker and then filtered into a 100 mL standard flask. All samples were analyzed in triplicate.

Scanning electron microscopy (SEM) was used to visualize the samples with a FEI Quanta™ 400 (Hillsboro, OR, USA) scanning electron microscope, at the acceleration voltage of 20 kV. The samples were vacuum-coated with gold before measurements.

The particle size distribution (PSD) of the samples was determined by laser diffraction, using the Masterisizer 2000 Malvern equipment (Malvern Instruments, Malvern, UK). The samples were dispersed in water on a Hydro 2000SM apparatus until the laser obscuration index reached 10–12%. The PSD values for the samples were determined in triplicate and were expressed as equivalent volume diameters at 10% ($d_{10\%}$), 50% ($d_{50\%}$) and 90% ($d_{90\%}$) of the cumulative volume, as the average of the diameter values ($D_{4,\ 3}$) and Span. The Span values indicated the particle polydispersity, and were calculated according to Eq. (3).

$$\text{Span} = d_{90\%} - d_{10\%}/d_{50\%} \tag{3}$$

Bioactivity of ZnO complexes

Two solutions were prepared: simulated gastric juice solution (SGS) with 2 g of NaCl in 7 mL of HCl, with pH adjusted to 2.5, and simulated enteric juice solution (SES) using 6.8 g of KH_2PO_4 in 250 mL distilled water, adding 77 mL of 0.2 N NaOH at pH 6.8 and distilled water to complete the volume of 1 L for each [12].

The assays were performed in triplicate, in 250 mL beaker, using 175 mL of SGS or SES with 10 mg of each composite. This was added to 25 mL of the same solution into previously hydrated dialysis membranes (MEMBRA-CEL® dialysis tubing, MWCO 7000, 34 mm, 14 × 100 CLR). The systems were kept at 39 °C under gently magnetic stirring and the solutions (SGS or SES) and 15 mL aliquots were collected in different time intervals (0, 15, 30 and 45 min) and the solutions were replenished with the same volume. Aliquots were stored and submitted to AAS analysis to determine the amount of Zn^{2+} released each time in the simulated media.

The minimum bacteriostatic concentration (MBC) evaluation of commercial ZnO, ZnO nano, ZnO/CAT and ZnO/CA samples was performed by the well diffusion method and by liquid growth-inhibition assay against *Escherichia coli* DH5α (strain 00379 INCQS-Fiocruz) and *Staphylococcus aureus* ATCC 6538 (INCQS-Fiocruz), Gram negative and Gram positive bacteria, respectively. The same assay was performed to investigate the antimicrobial activity of CH used in the formulation of the samples. The strains were grown in LB medium pH 7.0 (Luria-Bertani BD™) in an orbital shaker at 200 rpm, at 37 °C, for 24 h. The cellular density was adjusted in a saline solution (0.8% of NaCl) where the turbidity equivalent to McFarland 0.5 standard (1.5×10^{8} CFU/mL) was used as an inoculum in the presence of the composites at increasing concentrations, at 37 °C for 18 h at 200 rpm. Subsequently, cells were serially diluted in saline solution (0.8% of NaCl), plated on solid LB, and incubated at 37 °C for 18 h. Colony-forming units were counted. The MBC was taken as the concentration at which 100% growth inhibition was observed.

Results

The crystallite size of nano and commercial ZnO (D_{XRD} = 17 nm and 0.22 μm, respectively) was calculated from Scherrer's formula applied to the most intense reflection (101), as observed in the diffractogram displayed in Fig. 1a. It was observed that the reflections obtained for nano ZnO (trace II) were less crystalline with wider bases, characteristic of nanoparticles. Figure 1c shows that ZnO nanoparticles reduced the crystallinity when comparing to chitosan (CH) (Fig. 1b, trace II), as reflections were weaker and wide, as observed in a previous study [13]. Three strong reflections could be noticed, displayed in Fig. 1a between the angles of 2θ = 30° and 40°, corresponding to ZnO, but the diffraction corresponding to ZnO/CAT and ZnO/CA samples were very small, revealing the intense reduction in the orientation of crystallinity (Fig. 1c). It should also be noted that the ZnO/CAT samples encapsulated 10.2% of zinc and had a higher crystallinity than the ZnO/CA samples, with 12.6% Zn.

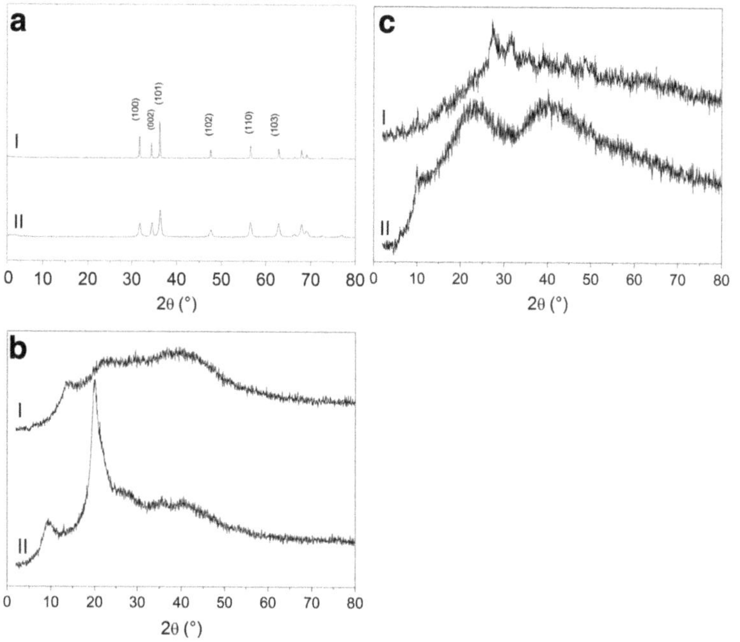

Fig. 1 X-ray diffractogram in the 2θ region of 2.0° to 80° for the (**a**) I- Commercial ZnO, II- ZnO nano synthesized sample, (**b**) I- sodium alginate and II- chitosan, (**c**) I- ZnO/CAT and II- ZnO/CA

The FTIR spectrum for SA (Fig. 2a, trace I) shows intense absorption bands with maximums at 3402, 2920, 1613, 1419 and 1032 cm^{-1}. These bands were attributed to stretching vibrations of O-H, C-H bonds, asymmetrical and symmetrical stretching vibrations of the carboxylate groups and, finally, to C-O-C bonds from the polysaccharide structure. For the CH samples, the broad absorption with maximum at 3401 cm^{-1} was assigned to -OH and -NH_2 stretching vibrations (Fig. 2a, trace II). The absorptions at 1657 cm^{-1} and 1594 cm^{-1}were attributed, respectively, to the amide I (C = O stretching) and amide II (C–N stretching and C–N–H bending vibrations) from amide functional groups in the solid state. In this region (1650–1580 cm^{-1}), the absorption attributed to the N-H bending (scissoring) vibration would be expected to appear. The strong absorption at 1094 cm^{-1} was attributed to the C-O-C bond from the polysaccharide structure.

Figure 2b displays the spectra for nano ZnO (trace I), the product obtained by encapsulating ZnO in the CH/SA complex (ZnO/CA, trace IV) and by encapsulating ZnO in the CH/SA complex reinforced with TPP (ZnO/CAT, trace III). For ZnO/CA (trace IV), the absorption at 471 cm^{-1}, which also appeared in the ZnO nano (trace I), in commercial ZnO (trace II) and in ZnO/CAT spectra, were attributed to the Zn-O stretching vibration. This result pointed to the incorporation of ZnO to the CH/SA and CH/SA/TPP complexes.

The dynamic rheological results are displayed in Fig. 3 with the mechanical spectra for the SA/CH (CA) and SA/CH/TPP (CAT) complexes shown in Fig. 3a. The elastic behavior (G' > G"), observed for both products, along the range of studied frequencies, revealed the formation of a tridimensional network.

Surface morphologies by SEM analysis of the nano and commercial ZnO, ZnO/CAT and ZnO/CA are displayed in Fig. 4. The surface morphology of pure ZnO nanoparticles (Fig. 4a) showed a fine powder with strong aggregation, characteristic of nanomaterials. In the ZnO/CAT micrograph, microparticles can also be observed as influencing the crosslinking of the biopolymer and the surface structure of the material (Fig. 4b).

The presence of 78% Zn^{2+} in the new pure synthesized ZnO nano and 99% in the commercial ZnO was observed, while the ZnO/CAT and ZnO/CA composites showed 10.2 and 12.6%, Zn^{2+}, respectively by atomic absorption spectrophotometry (AAS). The particle size of each composite is displayed in Table 1 and Fig. 5. In all measurements, the ZnO/CAT samples were shown to be a smaller particle than the ZnO/CA samples. When the mean values were evaluated, a value of 114.32 μm of ZnO/CAT against 162.48 μm ZnO/CA was observed. However, the poly dispersion index expressed in Span value for this sample was higher (1.80 μm), revealing a less homogeneous distribution of particles in comparison with the ZnO/CA, that had a smaller span value (1.24 μm) (Fig. 5).

The amount of inorganic residues (after heating to 700 °C) can be observed in the TGA curve, that indicated mineral matter content of 40%, approximately, for ZnO/CA, and 55% for ZnO/CAT (Fig. 6). The largest

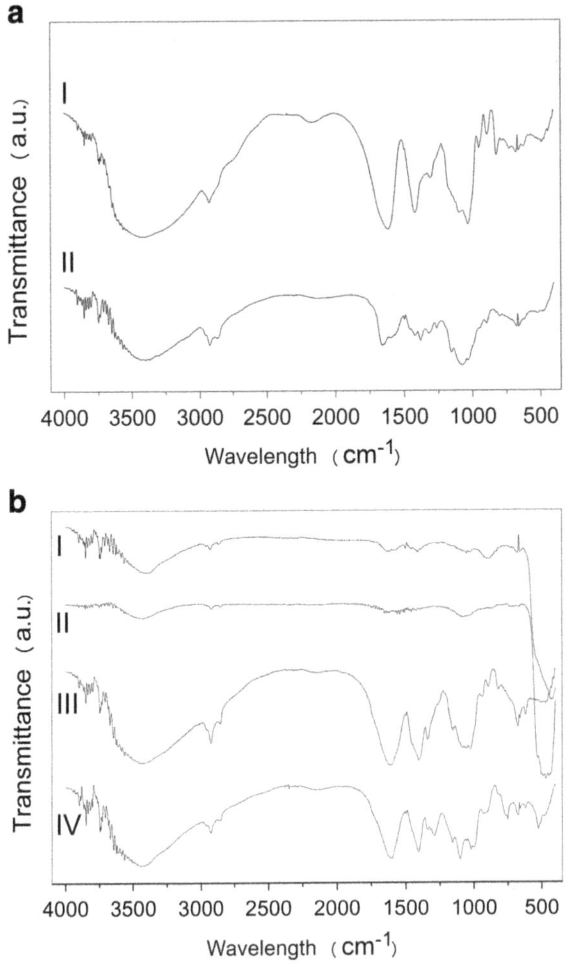

Fig. 2 Infrared spectra obtained for (**a**) sodium alginate (trace I) and chitosan (trace II); (**b**) ZnO nano (trace I), commercial ZnO (trace II), ZnO/CAT (trace III) and ZnO/CA (trace IV)

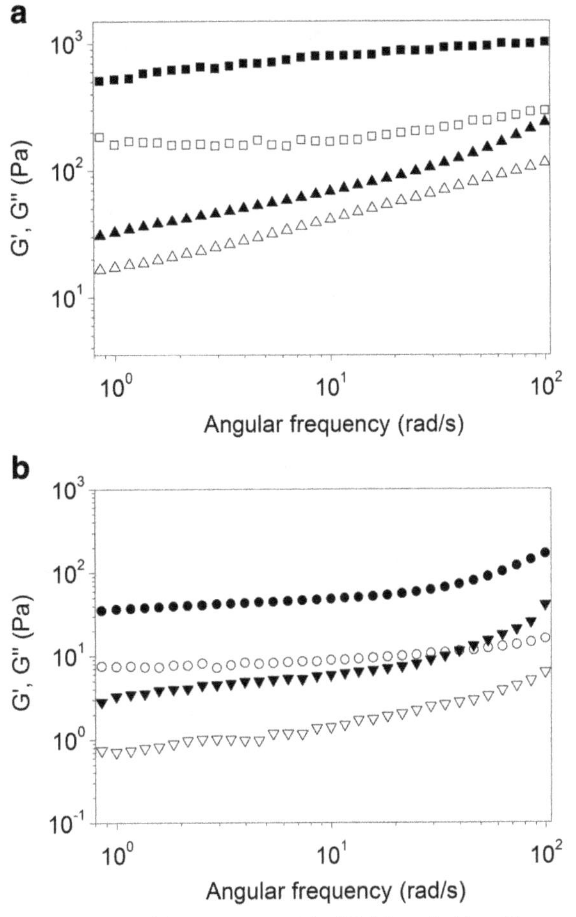

Fig. 3 Variation of the storage modulus (G′, full symbols) and loss modulus (G″, open symbols) values as a function of frequency. **a** microparticles without ZnO, CAT (squares), CA (triangles); **b** microparticles with ZnO, ZnO/CAT (circles) and ZnO/CA (triangles)

residue observed in the ZnO/CAT sample is due to phosphorus (P) from the TPP and Zn^{2+} present in ZnO. However, the results of the AAS Zn^{2+} quantification indicated that the ZnO/CAT samples have lower Zn^{2+} concentration (10.2%) compared to the ZnO/CA samples (12.6%). The in vitro release assay demonstrated that the ZnO samples complexed with CH, SA and TPP (ZnO/CAT) and no TPP (ZnO/CA) were effective in protecting Zn^{2+} in simulated gastric medium, as displayed in Fig. 7a. In SGF, at time zero, nano and commercial ZnO samples had the lowest release of Zn^{2+} between the 4 tested samples, however, the first 15 min revealed an increase of 11.2%, from 2.4 to 13.6% (commercial ZnO) and 7.4%, from 2.8 to 10.25% (ZnO nano). The release of ZnO/CA and release of the ZnO/CAT sample remained constant (4.5% and 6.2%) during the same period. From 15 min onwards, release by the ZnO nano and commercial sample increased and became more intense, reaching 40.4% and 27%, respectively, at 45 min. It was verified that despite the nano ZnO contain less Zn^{2+} in its formulation (78%) when compared to the commercial ZnO (99%), it released 1.5 times more at 45 min. This behavior was not observed in the protected samples, ZnO/CAT and ZnO/CA. Both samples had a low and constant release taxa as shown in Fig. 7a, 8.0 (5.3%) to 10.7 (6.9%) times lower than that observed in the ZnO nano sample. Figure 7b indicates that, at the beginning of the test using SES, nano ZnO released less Zn^{2+} (0.1%) than the ZnO/CAT (2.3%) and ZnO/CA (2.3%) samples and remained as such until the end time point (120 min) of the experiment, when a release of 4.2% and 4.5% was recorded, respectively. While commercial ZnO showed an initial release of 1.64% Zn^{2+} and a gradual increase of 2.62% tea at 120 min.

The antimicrobial activity of nano and commercial ZnO was tested. ZnO/CA sample exhibited the lowest MBC for both tested bacteria (*E. coli* and *S. aureus*) (Tables 2 and 3), where 1 mg/mL of ZnO/CA sample (126 μg/mL Zn^{2+} incorporated) provoked a total

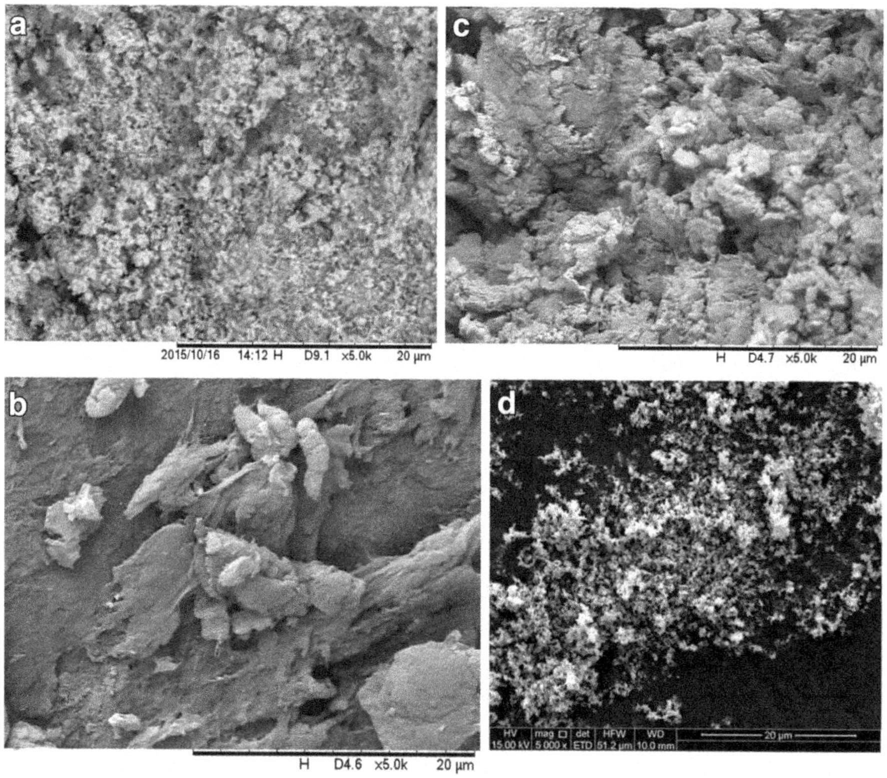

Fig. 4 SEM micrographs of the morphology of microparticles. **a** ZnO nano, **b** ZnO with CH, SA and TPP sample (ZnO/CAT), **c** ZnO with CH and SA sample (ZnO/CA) and **d** commercial ZnO

inhibition of *E. coli* and *S. aureus* growths. The ZnO/CAT sample inhibited *E. coli* growth at 2.25 mg/mL (229.5 µg/mL Zn^{2+} incorporated) and *S. aureus* at 2 mg/mL (204 µg/mL Zn^{2+} incorporated). When compared to the activities using the pure ZnO, *E. coli* growth was inhibited by 350 µg/mL (273 µg/mL Zn^{2+} incorporated) and *S. aureus* growth by 250 µg/mL (195 µg/mL Zn^{2+} incorporated), showing that the incorporated Zn^{2+} concentration is lower in the chitosan and alginate composites. On the other hand, the commercial ZnO showed the worst antimicrobial activity compared to other compounds, with a MBC of 500 µg/mL (495 µg/mL Zn^{2+} incorporated) and 650 µg/mL (643.5 µg/mL Zn^{2+} incorporated). These results can be explained by the larger particle size of commercial ZnO (0.22 µm), while the nano ZnO (contained in samples ZnO/CAT and ZnO/CA) presented a lower particle diameter (17 nm). Another study [13] has also described the TPP effect, including the decrease of particle size when crosslinker concentrations were increased, which allows to enhance ZnO protection in the simulated gastric fluid.

Table 1 Diameters of the ZnO/CAT and ZnO/CA microparticles

Sample	$d_{10\%}$ (µm)	$d_{50\%}$ (µm)	$d_{90\%}$ (µm)	$d_{4,3}$ (µm)	Span (µm)
ZnO/CAT	18.59	109.63	216.46	114.32	1.80
ZnO/CA	47.92	169.11	257.16	162.48	1.24

Discussion

The addition of TPP (Fig. 1c) to the formulation interfered in the acquired reflections, where the ZnO/CA samples showed higher amounts of amorphous structures, a sodium alginate (SA) characteristic, as observed

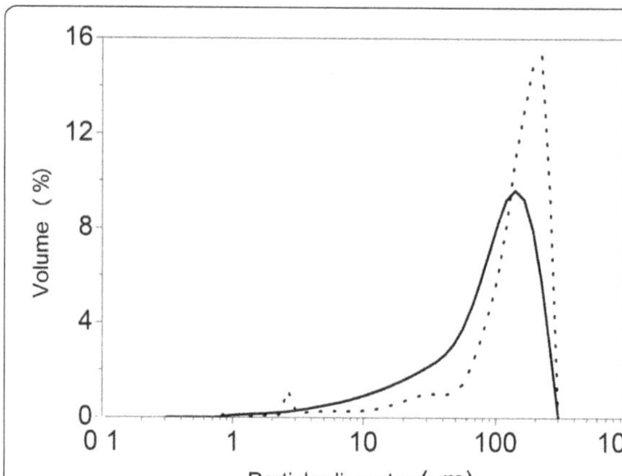

Fig. 5 Size distribution for ZnO/CA (*dotted* line) and ZnO/CAT sample (*continuous* line) microparticles

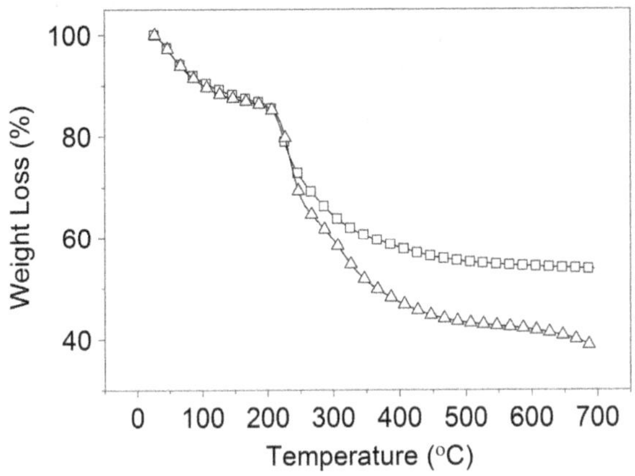

Fig. 6 TGA curves for ZnO/CAT and ZnO/CA samples at a heating rate of 10 °C/min

Table 2 Antimicrobial activity of commercial ZnO, ZnO nano, ZnO/CAT and ZnO/CA against *Escherichia coli*

Samples	Sample concentration (μg/mL)	Concentration of incorporated Zn^{2+} (μg/mL)[a]	*E. coli* inhibition (%)
Commercial ZnO	200	198	12.7 ± 0.7
	500	495	100 ± 0.00
ZnO nano	250	195	26.7 ± 2.0
	300	234	45.0 ± 0.6
	350	273	100 ± 0.0
ZnO/CAT	1700	173	6.8 ± 0.3
	2000	204	56.0 ± 0.6
	2250	229.5	100 ± 0.0
ZnO/CA	500	63	4.6 ± 0.9
	750	94.5	44.0 ± 1.1
	1000	126	100 ± 0.0

[a]Average concentration of incorporated Zn^{2+} as determined by atomic absorption spectrophotometry: commercial ZnO, 99%; ZnO nano, 78 mass%; ZnO/CAT, 10.2 mass%; ZnO/CA, 12.6 mass%

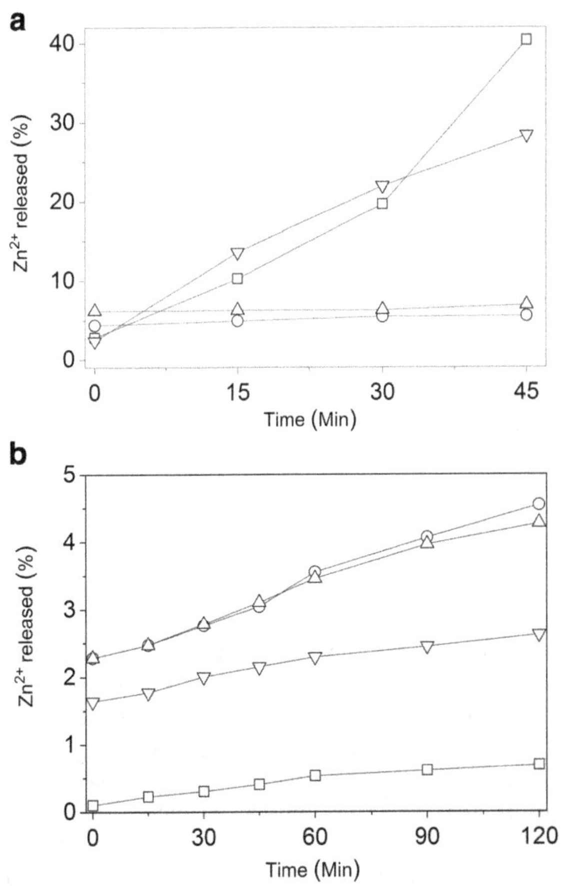

Fig. 7 In vitro Zn^{2+} release profile from ZnO commercial, ZnO nano, ZnO/CAT and ZnO/CA in gastric (SGF) (**a**) and enteric (SEF) (**b**) simulated fluids —▽— ZnO commercial, —□— ZnO, —○— ZnO/CAT, —△— ZnO/CA

in Fig. 1b, line I, corroborating data from a previous study [14].

The band shift attributed to the asymmetrical stretching vibrations of the carboxylate group, acquired by FTIR, reported the composite formation, where a linkage occurs between the SA carboxylate groups and the CH amine groups, but only a slight shift (from 1613 cm^{-1} for SA to 1612 cm^{-1} from the ZnO/CA composite) was observed (the band is broader and more intense). Interestingly, a much more expressive shift to lower

Table 3 Antimicrobial activity of commercial ZnO, ZnO nano, ZnO/CAT and ZnO/CA against *Staphylococcus aureus*

Samples	Sample concentration (μg/mL)	Concentration of incorporated Zn^{2+} (μg/mL)[a]	*S. aureus* inhibition (%)
Commercial ZnO	200	198	45.6 ± 1.3
	500	495	63.5 ± 1.4
	650	643,5	100 ± 0.00
ZnO nano	150	117	22.7 ± 1.1
	200	156	58.3 ± 1.0
	250	195	100 ± 0.0
ZnO/CAT	1000	102	4.6 ± 0.6
	1250	127.5	16.6 ± 0.9
	2000	204	100 ± 0.0
ZnO/CA	500	63	6.3 ± 0.2
	750	94.5	43.8 ± 0.2
	1000	126	100 ± 0.0

[a]Average concentration of incorporated Zn^{2+} as determined by atomic absorption spectrophotometry: commercial ZnO, 99%, ZnO nano, 78 mass%; ZnO/CAT, 10.2 mass%; ZnO/CA, 12.6 mass%

wavenumbers (from 1613 cm^{-1} and 1419 $cm^{-1}$for SA to 1600 cm^{-1}, and 1407 cm^{-1} for ZnO/CAT composite, respectively) of both bands was observed in the ZnO/CAT spectra (Fig. 2b, trace III). This clearly demonstrates the TPP contribution in increasing interactions in this composite.

Moreover, the spectra obtained for these products corroborated the FTIR data, reinforcing the role of TPP in increasing physical interactions between the gel components. The CAT matrix forms a stronger gel than CA (without TPP). On the other hand, the addition of ZnO (Fig. 3b) seems to disturb the gel structure. ZnO/CAT showed G' and G" values superior to those for ZnO/CA.

The ZnO/CAT complex showed a smooth and fine surface, corroborating a previous report by [15], which may be due to interfacial interactions between the CH chains and nano ZnO, which could possibly act as intermolecular crosslinks. Therefore, ZnO nano can contract and restrict the mobility of CH chains, and subsequently change the expansion of the surface morphology. On the other hand, when observing Fig. 4c, a rougher and crowded surface was observed, probably due to the lack of TPP. This reveals the influence of the addition of TPP on ZnO/CAT morphology (Fig. 4b), in addition to ZnO linking with CH. The addition of TPP decreased the particle size, probably due to crosslinking of polymeric chains, resulting in greater particle compression.

The high performance of the ZnO/CAT sample in SGF can be explained by the addition of TPP, the crosslinking agent, used in the preparation of CH due to its rapid gelling ability [16], where TPP reduces the gel pore size and effectively traps Zn^{2+} in the interstices of the support matrix [16, 17]. In simulated enteric juice, the ZnO/CAT and ZnO/CA complexes released more Zn^{2+} than ZnO nano and commercial samples, as expected. The ZnO delivery systems developed in this study allow for high concentrations of Zn^{2+} in the enteric environment, which are necessary to achieve the antimicrobial effect. The partial dissolution of ZnO particles releases zinc ions (Zn^{2+}), which contributes to the antimicrobial activity of the oxide [3] against the enteric microbiota of weanling pigs.

The Zn^{2+} dissociation from the ZnO composites is due to the formation of strong electrostatic but reversible bonds, even without the use of any covalent crosslinking agent [18]. Furthermore, the SA layer could have prevented the gastric degradation of CH, because the positive charges from CH reduced solubility at low pH. However, at around neutral pH, a higher amount of negative charges sequester positive CH charges, resulting in dissolution of the CH/SA complex and increase in the release of Zn^{2+} in the middle enteric region [19]. ZnO/CA and ZnO/CAT showed good release of Zn^{2+} in SEF, triggered by the change in the pH.

The lower concentrations of ZnO/CA are probably due to the absence of TPP, thus allowing closer contact between Zn^{2+} and the target microorganisms, where ZnO/CA showed a complete inhibition of *E. coli* growth at lower concentrations than ZnO/CAT (126 μg/mL Zn^{2+} incorporated against 229.5 μg/mL). For *S. aureus,* ZnO/CA prevented the growth complete at a lower incorporated concentration of Zn^{2+} (126 μg/mL), compared to the 204 μg/mL of ZnO/CAT. The CH/SA complex network, even in the absence of TPP, showed greater efficacy when compared to pure ZnO nano, which is effective in inhibiting *E. coli* and *S. aureus* at concentrations of 273 μg/mL and 195 μg/mL, respectively.

A comprehensive mechanism for the antimicrobial effect of nano-ZnO particles is still under debate. In an aqueous environment, the ZnO NPs aggregate to micrometer-sized particles and do not interact effectively with microorganisms. Thus, the antimicrobial activity has been mainly attributable to the dissolved zinc species [20–24]. The dissolution of ZnO nanoparticles and Zn^{2+} release seem to be able to generate radical oxygen species (ROS), consequently, activating a cytotoxic cascade of events that include intracellular calcium flux, mitochondrial depolarization, and plasma membrane leakage [25–28].

In the conditions of the present study, *S. aureus* was shown to be more sensitive to both the ZnO nano and ZnO/CAT samples in comparison to *E. coli.* The difference in antibacterial activity against both microorganisms can be related to differences in the chemical and structural composition of the cell membranes, particularly of the cell wall [29, 30] and to the preparation of the composites. *S. aureus* tends to develop defenses against oxidative stress by releasing products such as superoxide dismutase, catalase and thioredoxin reductase [31–33]. In our study, we can suggest that the new particles of ZnO were able to assemble at cellular membrane and damage it, despite the greater defense of *S. aureus* to the toxicity of ZnO.

Some ZnO particles can attach to the bacterial membrane surface, damaging it, and this mechanical damage has been postulated as a probable mechanism of antimicrobial inhibition [31]. According to the literature, ZnO nano bacteriostatic effectiveness can be ascribed to the disorganization of the membrane, increasing its permeability and resulting in the internalization of the nanoparticles. One possible explanation is that the antibacterial activity exhibited by ZnO composites is based on the abrasive texture of the ZnO surface. This abrasive texture, due to surface defects, fixes ZnO to the protein molecules from microorganism membranes, promotes internalization and consequent cell metabolism inhibition, killing the bacteria [34].

Several factors can interfere with the daily feed intake by animals, such as diet composition, the quality of raw materials and the sanitary conditions of farms [35, 36]. According to the health challenge of each farm and immune conditions of piglets, different concentrations of ZnO in their diets can be adopted, which usually range between 3000 and 5000 ppm (mg/kg). Considering an average daily intake of 400 g of feed by animal, established according to their growth phase (weaning- 21 days) [37–39], containing 4000 ppm (mg/kg) of the commercial ZnO, it should be expected the release of approximately 31.7 mg of Zn in the piglet gut, an amount 6 fold less than that, which corresponds to the MBC against *E. coli*, 198 mg Zn/0.4 kg of feed, and 8 fold less than MBC for *S. aureus* – 257.4 mg Zn/0.4 kg of feed. Released Zn2+ seems to be under the effective MBC threshold, particularly because considerations about the water intake and gut secretion should be done in order to calculate Zn2+ concentration in the gut.

The ZnO/CAT composites obtained in this study, at the same concentration of ZnO, led to a release of 7.4 mg of Zn, a value 12-fold lower than the MBC for *E. coli* (91.8 mg Zn^{2+}) and 11-fold lower than for *S. aureus* (81.6 mg). However, ZnO/CA, released 8.6 mg Zn^{2+}, which is 5.8-fold lower for the MBC for both evaluated bacteria (50.4 mg). Besides, the coating of ZnO showed a gut empowering effect due to the reduction in the release of Zn^{2+} in simulated porcine gastric fluid. This feature can reduce the amount of ZnO composites to be administered to weaned piglets.

These experiments revealed a remarkable advantage of the synthetized products compared to commercial ZnO, since the concentration of Zn in pig intestine released from those compounds should be higher. The intake dosage of 9.9 g of commercial Zn should be enough to ensure the release of 198 mg in the middle intestine, corresponding to the MBC value for *E. coli*. In the same way, the intake of 12.9 g of Zn might release 257.4 mg corresponding to ZnO MBC for *S. aureus*. These values are approximately 5 times higher than necessary (2 g) of ZnO/CAT to obtain a release of 91.2 mg that are enough to inhibit *E. coli* and 7 times greater than the intake (1.8 g) necessary to release 81. 6 mg Zn from ZnO/CAT and inhibit *S. aureus* in the gastrointestinal environment. The same would be true for ZnO/CA in a more pronounced way, because in order to release 50.5 mg of Zn (MIC of ZnO/CA to both bacteria) it would be necessary for each piglet to ingest at least 1.2 g of Zn, value 8 and 11 times lower than that observed for commercial ZnO inhibit *E. coli* and *S. aureus*, respectively. Although, the intake of ZnO composites can alter the gut microbiota composition, reducing the bacterial diversity and effecting even the probiotic bacteria, the overall supplementation effect of wearing piglets is positive since it can prevent attachment of pathogenic bacteria to the intestinal villi avoiding wearing unspecific diarrhea.

Conclusion

We have successfully synthesized new ZnO nanoparticles - ZnO/CA and ZnO/CAT, using CH/SA and an ultrasound-assisted methodology. The novel composites showed an optimum in vitro release profile of Zn^{2+} in simulated enteric fluids assays and expressive antimicrobial activities against *E. coli* and *S. aureus*. The physicochemical analysis and in vitro assays indicate that ZnO microparticles are a promising designed product to be applied for piglet livestock. The data from this study suggest that the ZnO nanoparticle composites may be effective in diets fed to weanling pigs, and may have the potential to significantly reduce fecal Zn excretion. Experiments with weanling pigs fed diets containing ZnO nanoparticle composites should be conducted to address the clinical evaluation of ZnO composites in piglets fed in controlled conditions.

Abbreviations

CH: Chitosan; MBC: Minimal bactericide concentration; SA: Alginate; SA, ZnO/CA: ZnO plus both CH; SEM: Scanning electron microscopy; SES: Simulated enteric juice solution; SGS: Simulated gastric juice solution;
TGA: Thermogravimetric analysis; TPP: Sodium tripolyphosphate; TPP, ZnO/CAT: ZnO plus CH, SA; ZnO: Zinc oxide

Acknowledgements

Not applicable.

Authors' contribution

MSRB performed the laboratory investigation. CTA, EMDA and VFP led the manuscript preparation. LCRPS performed the intestinal assays. MSRB, CTA, LMC, VFP, EMDA contributed to the interrogation of results and manuscript preparation. All authors read and approved the final manuscript.

Funding

This work was partially supported by the Fundação Carlos Chagas Filho de Amparo à Pesquisa do Estado do Rio de Janeiro (FAPERJ, Rio de Janeiro, Brazil), Conselho Nacional de Desenvolvimento Científico e Tecnológico (CNPq, Brasília, Brazil) and Coordenação de Aperfeiçoamento de Pessoal de Nível Superior (CAPES, Brasília, Brazil).

Competing interests

The author(s) declare that they have no competing interests.

Consent for publication

All authors have read and approved the manuscript for submission and publication.

Requesting animal ethics

Not applicable.

Author details
[1]Instituto de Macromoléculas Professora Eloisa Mano, Universidade Federal do Rio de Janeiro, Centro de Tecnologia, Bloco J, Rio de Janeiro, RJ 21941-598, Brazil. [2]Universidade Federal do Rio de Janeiro, Faculdade de Farmácia, Av. Carlos Chagas Filho, 373, CCS, Bloco L, sala 24, Rio de Janeiro, RJ 21941-902, Brazil. [3]Instituto de Química, Universidade Federal do Rio de Janeiro, Av. Athos da Silveira, Ramos 149, Bloco A, sala 545, Rio de Janeiro 21941-909, Brazil.

References

1. Carlson MS, Boren CA, Wu C, Huntington CE, Bollinger DW, Veum TL. Evaluation of various inclusion rates of organic zinc either as a polysaccharide or proteinate complex on the growth performance, plasma, and excretion of nursery pigs. J Anim Sci. 2004;82:1359–66.
2. Heo JM, Opapeju FO, Pluske JR, Kim JC, Hampson DJ, Nyachoti CM. Gastrointestinal health and function in weaned pigs: a review of feeding strategies to control post-weaning diarrhea without using in-feed antimicrobial compounds. J Anim Physiol Anim Nutr. 2013;97:207–37.
3. Pasquet J, Chevalier Y, Pelletier J, Couval E, Bouvier D, Bolzinger M-A. The contribution of zinc ions to the antimicrobial activity of zinc oxide. Colloids Surf A Physicochem Eng Asp. 2014;457:263–74.
4. Shen J, Chen Y, Wang Z, Zhou A, He M, Mao L, et al. Coated zinc oxide improves intestinal immunity function and regulates microbiota composition in weaned piglets. Br J Nutr. 2014;111:2123–34.
5. Hahn JD, Baker DH. Growth and plasma zinc responses of young pigs fed pharmacologic levels of zinc. J Anim Sci. 1993;71:3020–4.
6. Hill GM, Mahan DC, Carter SD, Cromwell GL, Ewan RC, Harrold RL, et al. Effect of pharmacological concentrations of zinc oxide with or without the inclusion of an antibacterial agent on nursery pig performance. J Anim Sci. 2001;79:934–41.
7. Juby KA, Dwivedi C, Kumar M, Kota S, Misa HS, Bajaj PN. Silver nanoparticle-loaded PVA/gum acacia hydrogel: synthesis, characterization and antibacterial study. Carbohydr Polym. 2012;89:906–13.
8. George M, Abraham TE. Polyionic hydrocolloids for the intestinal delivery of protein drugs: alginate and chitosan – a review. J Control Release. 2006;114:1–14.
9. Muzzarelli RAA. Chitins and chitosans as immune adjuvants and non-allergenic drug carriers. Mar Drugs. 2010;8:292–312.
10. Yang J-S, Xie Y-J, He W. Research progress on chemical modification of alginate: a review. Carbohydr Polym. 2011;84:33–9.
11. Chand P, Gaur A, Kumar A. Structural and optical properties of ZnO nanoparticles synthesized at different pH values. J Alloys Compd. 2012;539:174–8.
12. United States Pharmacopeial Staff. USP35-NF30 pharmaceutical compounding- sterile preparations 2012. USP® US. Pharmacopeia the standard of quality. Corporight© 2011. The United States Pharmacopeial Convention.
13. Gan Q, Wang T, Cochrane C, McCarron P. Modulation of surface charge, particle size and morphological properties of chitosan–TPP nanoparticles intended for gene delivery. Colloids Surf B Biointerfaces. 2005;44:65–73.
14. Jayasuriya AC, Aryaei A, Jayatissa AH. ZnO nanoparticles induced effects on nanomechanical behavior and cell viability of chitosan films. Mater Sci Eng C Mater Biol Appl. 2013;33:3688–96.
15. Monteiro OAC, Airoldi C. Some studies of crosslinking chitosan–glutaraldehyde interaction in a homogeneous system. Int J Biol Macromol. 1999;26:119–28.
16. Berger J, Reist M, Mayer JM, Felt O, Peppas NA, Gurney R. Structure and interactions in covalently and ionically crosslinked chitosan hydrogels for biomedical applications. Eur. J. Pharm. Biopharm. 2004;57;19:34.
17. Li N, Bai R. A novel amine-shielded surface cross-linking of chitosan hydrogel beads for enhanced metal adsorption performance. Ind Eng Chem Res. 2005;44:6692.
18. Luo Y, Wang Q. Recent development of chitosan-based polyelectrolyte complexes with natural polysaccharides for drug delivery. Int J Biol Macromol. 2014;64:353–67.
19. Hongliang D, Mengrui L, Xiaoye Y, Guangxi Z. The design of pH-sensitive chitosan-based formulations for gastrointestinal delivery. Drug Discov Today. 2015;20:1004–11.
20. Broom LJ, Miller HM, Kerr KG, Knapp JS. Effects of zinc oxide and *Enterococcus faecium* SF68 dietary supplementation on the performance, intestinal microbiota and immune status of weaned piglets. Res Vet Sci. 2006;80:45–54.
21. Liedtke J, Vahjen W. In vitro antibacterial activity of zinc oxide on a broadrange of reference strains of intestinal origin. Vet Microbiol. 2012;160:251–5.
22. Wang C, Liu L-L, Zhang A-T, Xie P, Lu J-J, Zou X-T. Antibacterial effects of zinc oxide nnanoparticles on *Escherichia coli* K88. Afr J Biotechnol. 2012;11:10248–54.
23. Xie Y, He Y, Irwin PL, Jin T, Shi X. Antibacterial activity and mechanism of action of zinc oxide nanoparticles against *Campylobacter jejuni*. Appl Environ Microbiol. 2011;77:2325–31.
24. Zhang L, Ding Y, Povey M, York D. ZnO nanofluids – a potential antibacterial agent. Progress in Nat Sci. 2008;18:939–44.
25. Wu W, Xiao H, Peng TC, Jiang CZ. Controllable synthesis and optical properties of connected zinc oxide nanoparticles. Chem Asian Jl. 2010;5:315–21.
26. George S, Xia T, Rallo R, Zhao Y, Ji Z, Lin S, et al. Use of a high-throughput screening approach coupled with in vivo zebrafish embryo screening to develop hazard ranking for engineered nanomaterials. ACS Nano. 2011;5:1805–17.
27. Applerot G, Perkas N, Amirian G, Girshevitz O, Gedanken A. Coating of glass with ZnO via ultrasonic irradiation and study of its antibacterial properties. Appl Surf Sci. 2009;2565:53–8.
28. George S, Pokhrel S, Xia T, Gilbert B, Ji Z, Schowalter M, et al. Use of a rapid cytotoxicity screening approach to engineer a safer zinc oxide nanoparticle through iron doping. ACS Nano. 2010;4:15–29.
29. Jones N, Ray B, Koodali RT, Manna AC. Antibacterial activity of ZnO nanoparticle suspensions on a broad spectrum of microorganisms. FEMS Microbiol Lett. 2008;279:71–6.
30. Shantikumar N, Abhilash S, Divya W, Deepthy M, Seema N, Satish KM. Antibacterial activity of zinc oxide nanoparticles. J Med Microbiol. 2008;24:465–71.
31. Anna LC, Mahmuda S, Bakhoria SKM, Sirelkhatima A, Mohamadb D, Hasanc H, et al. Antibacterial responses of zinc oxide structures against *Staphylococcus aureus*, *Pseudomonas aeruginosa* and *Streptococcus* pyogenes. Ceram Int. 2014;40:2993–3001.
32. Raghupathi KR, Manna RT, Koodali AC. Size-dependent bacterial growth inhibition and mechanism of antibacterial activity of zinc oxide nanoparticles. Langmuir. 2011;27:4020–8.
33. Ballal A, Manna AC. Control of thioredoxin reductase gene (*trxB*) transcription by SarA in *Staphylococcus aureus*. Int J Bacteriol. 1990;192:336–45.
34. Vani C, Sergin GK, Annamalai A. A study on the effect of zinc oxide nanoparticles in *Staphylococcus aureus*. Int J Pharma Bio Sci. 2011;2:326–35.
35. Dybkjær L, Jacobsen AP, Tøgersen FA, Poulsen HD. Eating and drinking activity of newly weaned piglets: effects of individual characteristics, social mixing, and addition of extra zinc to the feed. J Anim Sci. 2006;84:702–11.
36. Peet-Schwering CMC van der, Kemp B, Plagge JG, Vereijken PFG, Herzog LA den , Spoolder HAM and Verstegen MWA. Performance and individual feed intake characteristics of group-housed sows fed a non-starch polysaccharides diet ad libitum during gestation over three parities. J Anim Sci 2004;82;1246–1257.
37. Chai W, Zakrzewski SS, Günzel D, Pieper R, Wang Z, Twardziok S, et al. High-dose dietary zinc oxide mitigates infection with transmissible gastroenteritis virus in piglets. BMC Vet Res. 2014;10:75–85.
38. Tse MLP, Costa LB, Braz DB, Garcia AN, Berenchtein B, Miyada VS. Leitões recém-desmamados alimentados com dietas contendo proteína láctea e zinco suplementar. R Bras Zootec. 2010;39:2006–16.
39. Zhu L, Wang G, Dong B, Peng CC, Tian YY, Gong LM. Effects of sweetener neotame on diet preference, performance and hematological and biochemical parameters of weaned piglets. Anim Feed Sci Technol. 2016;214:86–94.

Isolation and identification of culturable fungi from the genitals and semen of healthy giant pandas (*Ailuropoda melanoleuca*)

Xiaoping Ma[1,2†], Changcheng Li[2†], Jiafa Hou[1*] and Yu Gu[3*]

Abstract

Background: In order to better understand the possible role of fungi in giant panda reproduction and overall health, it is important to provide a baseline for the normal fungal composition in the reproductive system. Using morphology and internal transcribed spacer (ITS) sequence analysis, we systematically isolated and identified fungal species from the vagina, foreskin, and semen of 21 (11 males and 10 females) healthy giant pandas to understand the normal fungal flora of the genital tracts.

Results: A total of 76 fungal strains were obtained, representing 42 genera and 60 species. Among them 47 fungal strains were obtained from vaginal samples, 24 from foreskins, and 5 from semen samples. Several fungal strains were isolated from more than one sample. More fungal species were isolated from females from males. The predominant genera were *Aspergillus*, *Trichosporon*, and *Penicillium*, followed by *Candida*, *Cladosporium*, *Sordariomycetes*, and *Diaporthe*. The average number of strains in the female vagina was significantly higher than in the foreskin and semen of male.

Conclusions: A total of 60 fungal species (belonging to 42 genera) were identified in the giant panda's genital tract. Some of the species were commonly shared in both males and females. These findings provide novel information on the fungal community in the reproductive tracts of giant pandas.

Keywords: Culturable fungi, Giant panda (*Ailuropoda melanoleuca*), Vagina, Foreskin, Semen

Background

The giant panda is one of the rarest endangered animals [1]. In recent years, breeding giant pandas in captivity has become necessary for conservation and improving their reproductive rate. Although the captive giant panda population has increased, its genetic diversity is far lower than that of the wild population [2], and some captive female giant pandas are unable to carry cubs to term or are subject to secondary infertility.

* Correspondence: jiafahou@163.com; guyu632@sicau.edu.cn
†Equal contributors
[1]College of Veterinary Medicine, Nanjing Agricultural University, Nanjing 210095, China
[3]College of Life Sciences, Sichuan Agricultural University, Ya'an 625014, China
Full list of author information is available at the end of the article

Microorganisms are responsible for diseases that can directly or indirectly affect reproductive success in animals. Fungi are one of the most important microorganisms that are known to cause abortion in cattle [3] and horses [4].

Fungal infections are becoming more frequent in humans due to the widespread use of antibiotics and immunosuppressors [5]. In 1929, a study confirmed the existence of fungi in the human vagina [6]. *Torulopsis* and *Candida* spp. were later identified from vaginal samples [7].

Studies have confirmed the presence of fungi in the reproductive organs of animals [8–10]. To date, few studies have been performed on microorganisms of the genitourinary tract of the giant panda [11], and fungal infections have been identified as a potential threat to giant panda fertility [12]. Low breeding rates strongly affect the population of giant pandas. There is a close relationship between sterility and vaginal dysbiosis, which is characterized by the imbalance of vaginal microflora due to various disorders and conditions. This highlights the importance of an improved understanding of the normal vaginal flora of giant pandas.

In this study, we investigated the fungal compositions in the vaginas, foreskins, and semen of 21 healthy giant pandas living in a semi-captive, semi-closed breeding environment. Our goal is to provide a baseline information on the normal fungal flora in the reproductive system to better understand the possible roles of fungi in the reproduction and overall health of giant pandas.

Methods

Animals

The giant pandas used in this study lived in a semi-captive, semi-closed breeding environment at the Chengdu Research Base of Giant Panda Breeding (Sichuan, China). The pandas were fed bamboo shoots and steamed corn bread. They were allowed to drink water *ad libitum.*

Samples were collected from 10 female during estrus and 11 male pandas. Details of the samples are listed in Table 1. None of the animals had previous genital infections noted in their files, and detailed physical examinations found no evidence of vaginitis or balanoposthitis. Pandas with a recent history of disease or animals treated with antifungal drugs during the last 6 months were excluded from this study.

Sampling procedure

Samples were collected during estrus when the female pandas were ready for artificial insemination from February to May of 2013. All personnel involved in sampling wore sterile protective clothing, hats, masks, and latex gloves. Ketamine was used for anesthesia in giant pandas, and isoflurane was administered via anesthetic machine to maintain anesthesia. Samples were collected from either the bottoms of vaginas (cervical orifice) or foreskins with sterilized cotton swabs when the pandas were supine after anesthesia. The vulvas, foreskins, and surrounding areas were rinsed three times with sterilized, warm physiological saline solution, then wiped with a disposable sterile towel. Samples were collected using guarded swabs by inserting a sterile cervical canal into the cervical. Sterile cotton swabs were then inserted to the vagina

Table 1 List of samples taken from giant pandas

Name	Sex	Sample	Age	Sample date	Note
A	female	vaginal secretion	11 yr. 5mo.	2013.4	Pre-procreated
B	female	vaginal secretion	5 yr.	2013.3	First artificial breeding
C	female	vaginal secretion	5 yr. 7mo.	2013.2	First artificial breeding
D	female	vaginal secretion	12 yr.	2013.4	First artificial breeding
E	female	vaginal secretion	6 yr. 9mo.	2013.5	First artificial breeding
F	female	vaginal secretion	7 yr. 8mo.	2013.3	First artificial breeding
G	female	vaginal secretion	5 yr. 7mo.	2013.4	First artificial breeding
H	female	vaginal secretion	–	2013.3	First artificial breeding
I	female	vaginal secretion	18 yr. 8mo.	2013.2	Not pregnant for 5 years
J	female	vaginal secretion	10 yr. 7mo.	2013.4	Not pregnant for 2 years
K	male	prepuce inclusions	10 yr. 3mo.	2013.3	
L	male	prepuce inclusions	14 yr. 7mo.	2013.4	
M	male	prepuce inclusions	10 yr. 7mo.	2013.5	
N	male	prepuce inclusions	10 yr. 7mo.	2013.4	
O	male	prepuce inclusions and semen	10 yr. 6mo.	2013.4	
P	male	semen	8 yr. 6mo.	2013.5	
Q	male	prepuce inclusions	7-10 yr	2013.3	
R	male	prepuce inclusions	8 yr	2013.4	
S	male	prepuce inclusions	7 yr.8mo	2013.2	
T	male	prepuce inclusions	8 yr.	2013.4	
U	male	prepuce inclusions and semen	8 yr. 7mo	2013.4	

Note: Because panda H was captured in the wild, its age is not known

bottoms (cervical orifice) through the cervical canal to collect the cervix outflow. The semen from three male giant pandas was collected through electroejaculation after general anesthesia, with sterilized cotton swabs using a sterilized special semen collection cup. Special care was taken to ensure that the swab did not come into contact with other parts of the body. All samples were quickly placed in sterilized plastic sample bags, transported into laboratory on ice within 2 h, and then immediately inoculated under a BSL-2 safety cabinet. A total of 23 samples were subjected to fungal analysis (Table 1).

Fungal culture and identification

Fungal culture

Samples were streak inoculated aerobically onto Sabouraud dextrose agar (MOLTOX, Inc., Boone, NC) containing 2% (*v/v*) sterile olive oil, malt extract agar, or yeast extract peptone dextrose agar. All media were supplemented with antibiotics (Chloramphenicol 0.005% (m/v)).

Cultural examination was carried out in a BSL-2 safety cabinet of a bioclean room. Sterilized sealing film was used to cover each plate. Blank plates were used as control to ensure no microorganisms were from aerial contamination. Each sample was plated in 3 culture plates with 3 control plates. All culture dishes were inoculated and stored at 25 °C for 7–30 days before being considered negative. As soon as a new fungal colony appeared, the colony was picked and planted in another dish containing the same medium for cultivation.

Morphology identification

Fungal morphology was determined according to previous procedures [13].

Genetic analysis

Genomic DNA of the isolates was individually extracted using a Yeast DNA Kit (Tiangen Biotech Co., Ltd., Beijing, China) and stored at −20 °C before further analysis.

Fungal DNA amplification was performed using the primer set of an ITS located between ITS1 to ITS4 that was specific for a ribosomal DNA gene: forward, 5′-TCC GTAGGTGAACCTGCG-3′; reverse, 5′-TCCTCCGCT TATTGATATGC-3′. PCR amplification was performed in a 50-μl reaction mixture containing 19 μl 2 × Taq Master Mix (Tiangen Biotech Co., Ltd., Beijing, China), 2 μl primers, 25 μl ddH2O, and 2 μl of fungal genomic DNA. The thermocycling conditions were as follows: 5 min at 94 °C (initial denaturation), 30 cycles of 45 s at 94 °C, 45 s at 58 °C, 72 °C extension for 60 s, cycle number 40, and a final extension of 7 min at 72 °C. The PCR products (8 μl) were examined using 1.0% agarose gel electrophoresis containing 0.5 mg/ml of ethidium bromide. A 300–600 bp fragment of the rDNA was produced. The PCR products were subjected to DNA sequencing performed by Invitrogen (Shanghai Invitrogen Biotechnology Company, Shanghai, China).

Partial gene sequences of the isolates were submitted to GenBank Accession and the numbers are listed in Table 2. A sequence similarity search was performed using BLAST (https://www.ncbi.nlm.nih.gov/nuccore/). Isolates were identified on the selection of the most similar sequences using BLAST. The phylogenetic tree was constructed by Mega 6.0 software with neighbor-joining method.

Statistical analysis

Data were analysized by IBM SPSS 20.0 software for Windows. The independent-samples test of nonparametric tests or one-way ANOVA were used. Differences showing *p*-values less than 0.05 were considered statistically significant.

Results

Morphological identification

In this study, a total of 23 samples from vaginas, foreskins, and semen were collected from 21 healthy giant pandas (Table 1). Fungi were isolated from 22 samples, and only one sample (foreskin inclusions of panda U, Table 1) was found free of any fungus. The fungi were identified either as multicellular filaments (mycetes) or single-celled yeasts. Mycetes were isolated from 9 of the 10 vaginal samples, 7 of the 10 foreskin inclusions, and 3 of the 3 semen samples. Yeasts were isolated from 5 of the 10 vaginal samples, 6 of the 10 foreskin inclusions, and none of the semen samples (Table 2).

Morphological identification revealed 82 total isolates, including 51, 26, and 5 from the vagina, foreskin, and semen samples, respectively.

Genetic identification

The 82 fungal isolates were sequenced and analyzed by NCBI Blast. The nucleotide sequence and blast results showed that several isolates had nearly the same base sequence; therefore, these were identified as the same strain. Finally, 76 fungi strains were obtained, and a phylogenetic tree was constructed (Fig. 1). Forty-seven strains were identified from the 51 isolates in vaginal samples, 24 strains from the 26 isolates in foreskin samples, and 5 strains from the 5 isolates in semen samples (Table 2, Fig. 1).

Table 2 Fungal strains identified in vaginal secretion, foreskin inclusion, and semen of giant pandas

Name	Gender	Strain No. in sample	Sample type	Fungal taxon	GenBank accession number
A	Female	1	VS	*Candida catenulate*	KF973198
H	Female	3	VS	*Pseudozyma aphidis*	KF973199
				Arthrinium sacchari	KF973200
				Trichoderma sp.LCC02–03	KJ531959
J	Female	3	VS	*Diaporthe melonis*	KF986543
				Myrmecridium schulzeri	KF986544
				Lecythophora sp.LCC06	KF986545
D	Female	5	VS	*Cladosporium cladosporioides*	KF986546
				Chaetomium globosum	KF986547
				Aspergillus niger	KF986548
				Sordariomycetes sp.LCC10	KF986549
				Dicyma pulvinat	KF986550
E	Female	4	VS	*Aspergillus versicolor*	KF986551
				Aureobasidium pullulans	KF986552
				Diaporthe phaseolorum	KF986553
				Fusarium proliferatum	KF986554
F	Female	6	VS	*Trichosporon guehoae*	KF990133
				Penicillium marneffe	KF990134
				Penicillium commune	KF990135
				Botryotinia fuckeliana	KF990136
				Gliocladium roseum	KF990137
				Bjerkandera adusta	KJ152158
G	Female	7	VS	*Pestalotiopsis vismiae*	KF990138
				Thanatephorus cucumeris	KF990139
				Fusarium merismoides	KF990140
				Debaryomyces hansenii	KF990141
				Candida catenulata	KF990142
				Pseudocercosporella fraxini	KF990143

Table 2 Fungal strains identified in vaginal secretion, foreskin inclusion, and semen of giant pandas *(Continued)*

Name	Gender	Strain No. in sample	Sample type	Fungal taxon	GenBank accession number
				Xylariaceae sp.LCC28	KF990144
B	Female	2	VS	*Penicillium marneffei*	KF990145
				Phanerochaete sordid	KF990146
I	Female	14	VS	*Isaria farinose*	KF990147
				Penicillium digitatum	KF990148
				Penicillium brevicompactum	KF990149
				Aspergillus sclerotiorum	KF990150
				Alternaria alternata	KF990151
				Aspergillus ruber	KF990152
				Diaporthe phaseolorum	KF990153
				Ascomycota sp.LCC38	KF990154
				Epicoccum nigrum	KF990155
				Basidiomycota sp.LCC40	KF990156
				Plectosphaerella cucumerin	KF990157
				Trichosporon japonicum	KF990158
				Trichosporon brassicae	KF990159
				Trichosporon cutaneum	KF990160
C	Female	2	VS	*Aspergillus versicolor*	KJ531956
				Bjerkandera adusta	KJ531957
K	Male	1	FI	*Alternaria alternata*	KC896385
L	Male	1	FI	*Candida catenulata*	KJ152159
O	Male	1	FI	*Sordariomycetes* sp.LCC03–1	KJ531958
T	Male	4	FI	*Aspergillus fumigatus*	KJ531960
				Cladosporium cladosporioides	KJ531961
				Trichosporon asteroides	KJ531962
				Meyerozyma guilliermondii	KJ531963
M	Male	1	FI	*Meyerozyma guilliermondii*	KJ152160
S	Male	4	FI	*Aspergillus versicolor*	KJ152161

Table 2 Fungal strains identified in vaginal secretion, foreskin inclusion, and semen of giant pandas *(Continued)*

Name	Gender	Strain No. in sample	Sample type	Fungal taxon	GenBank accession number
				Schizophyllum commune	KJ152162
				Rhizoctonia solani	KJ152163
				Trichosporon japonicum	KJ152164
N	Male	3	FI	*Plectosphaerella cucumerina*	KJ152165
				Beauveria bassiana	KJ152166
				Sordariomycetes sp.LCC07-3	KJ152167
Q	Male	7	FI	*Cladosporium tenuissimum*	KJ152168
				Ceriporia lacerate	KJ152169
				Colletotrichum gloeosporioides	KJ152170
				Tritirachium sp.LCC08-4	KJ152171
				Trichosporon jirovecii	KJ152172
				Nigrospora sp.LCC08-6	KJ152173
				Aspergillus versicolor	KJ152174
R	Male	2	FI	*Arthrinium phaeospermum*	KJ152175
				Periconia byssoides	KJ152176
U	Male	0	FI	–	–
O	Male	2	SE	*Trametes versicolor*	KJ531965
				Leptosphaeria sp.LCC1-2	KJ531966
P	Male	2	SE	*Thanatephorus cucumeris*	KJ531967
				Chaetomium globosum	KJ531968
	Male	1	SE	*Trametes versicolor*	KJ531969

Note: in the sample type, "VS" represents vaginal secretion, "FI" represent foreskin inclusion, and "SE" represents semen

Analysis of strain composition

Analysis of strains at the species level

Several species, such as *Alternaria alternate, Aspergillus versicolor,* and *Candida catenulate,* were present in more than one sample. After removing identical strains in the samples, 60 fungal species were identified in the giant panda's genital tract. Several species, including *A. alternate, A. versicolor, C. catenulate, Chaetomium globosum, Cladosporium cladosporioides, Plectosphaerella cucumerina, Thanatephorus cucumeris,* and *Trichosporon japonicum,* were isolated from both male and female giant pandas.

The 47 strains in the vaginal samples were identified as 42 species; the 24 strains in the foreskin samples were identified as 22 species; and the 5 strains in the semen samples were identified as 4 species (Table 2).

Analysis of strains at the genus level

The 76 strains belong to 42 genera. The predominant genera were *Aspergillus* (10.53%, 8/76), *Trichosporon* (9.21%, 7/76), and *Penicillium* (6.58%, 5/76). *Cladosporium, Diaporthe,* and *Sordariomycetes* accounted for 3.95% (3/76), while *Alternaria, Arthrinium, Bjerkandera, Chaetomium, Fusarium, Meyerozyma, Plectosphaerella, Thanatephorus,* and *Trametes* accounted for 2.63% (2/76). The other genera were represented by one strain each (1/76) (Table 3).

Comparison between the proportion of samples with mycetes and with yeasts

A total of 47 different strains were found in the vaginal samples, including 39 mycetes (51.32%, 39/76) and 8 yeasts (10.53%, 8/76). A total of 24 different strains were found in the foreskin samples, including 18 mycetes (23.68%, 18/76) and 6 yeasts (7.89%, 6/76). A total of 5 mycetes (6.58%, 5/76) were isolated in semen samples. In brief, among the 76 strains, the number of mycetes (62) was significantly higher than the number of yeasts (14) in all three sample types ($p = 0.0002$) (Fig. 2, Table 2).

Differences in strain number distribution among the three sample types

The number of strains and the range of variation were compared among the three sample types. A large range of strain numbers, from 1 to 14, was found in the vaginal samples. However, only 1 sample was found to have 14 strains; the remaining samples had 2~7 strains. A total of 24 strains were isolated from the foreskin samples, ranging from 0 to 7 per animal. Only 1 sample was found to have 7 strains, and 1 sample had no fungus. The others had 1~4 strains. In the 3 semen samples, only 5 strains (with 1, 2, and 2 strains) were isolated. Our results indicate that the number of fungi in the genital tract was significantly higher in the female pandas than in the male pandas ($p = 0.042$). (Table 2).

Regarding the number of strains from the three sample types, we found that the vaginal secretion had the highest number of fungal strains with an average of 5.67 isolates per animal. The average strains from foreskin inclusion and semen were 3.71 and 1.57, respectively. Additionally, several species, including *Fusarium* spp. and *Penicillium* spp., were present in multiple female

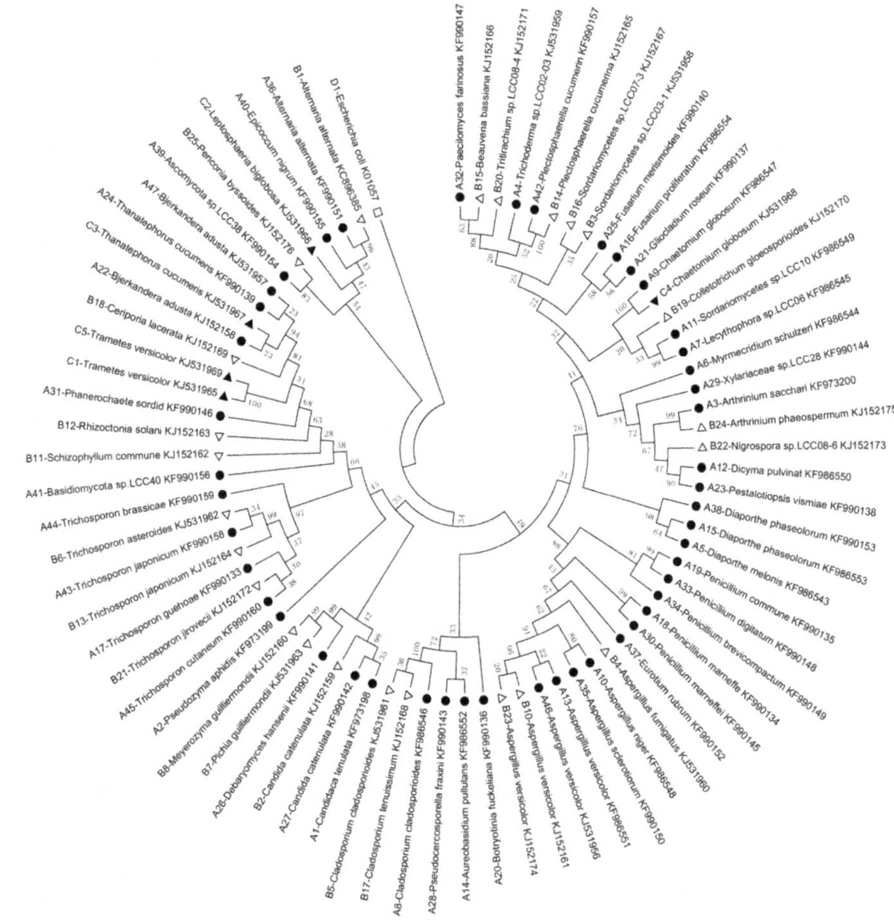

Fig. 1 Neighbor-joining phylogenic tree of 76 strains isolated from each sample. Solid circles (●) indicate strains isolated from vaginas; hollow triangles (Δ) indicate strains isolated from foreskins; solid triangles (▲) indicate strains isolated from semen; hollow squares (□) indicate reference sequences from GenBank

samples; *Meyerozyma guilliermondii* and *Trametes versicolor* were present in multiple male pandas.

Analysis of variation of fungal constitution between pregnant and nonpregnant female pandas

Of the 10 female pandas, 4 had already undergone successful pregnancy and 6 had never undergone successful breeding. There were distinct differences in the strains and species between these two groups. There were 1, 2, 2, and 5 strains in the vaginas of the pregnant pandas and 3, 3, 4, 6, 7, and 14 strains in the non-pregnant pandas. The average number of strains in the nonpregnant group (average: 6.2 strains) was higher than in the pregnant group (average: 2.5 strains), but the difference was not statistically significant ($p = 0.054$) (Tables 1, 2). Whether the high number of fungi in the vagina is related to non-pregnancy remains unclear.

The composition of fungal species between the pregnant and nonpregnant pandas was analyzed. There were 42 species in female pandas, and only a few species (4/42) were common between the two groups, including *A. versicolor, Bjerkandera adusta, C. catenulate*, and *Penicillium marneffei*. All other species(38/42)differed between these two groups.

Analysis of fungal constitution between younger and older pandas

To determine whether fungal constitution is related to age, the female giant pandas were divided into an older (age > 10 years, 4 pandas) and younger group (age < 10 years, 6 pandas). The average strain count was 4.0 per animal for the younger group and 5.75 per animal for the older group. There were 1, 3, 5, and 14 strains in the older group, and 2, 2, 3, 4, 6, and 7 strains in the younger group. However, there were no significant differences between the older and younger groups according to the ANOVA test

Table 3 Genus distribution of all strains

Genus level	strain No.	percentage of all strains (%)	Vaginal No.	Foreskin No.	Semen No.
Aspergillus	8	10.53	5	3	0
Trichosporon	7	9.21	4	3	0
Penicillium	5	6.58	5	0	0
Candida	3	3.95	2	1	0
Cladosporium	3	3.95	1	2	0
Diaporthe	3	3.95	3	0	0
Sordariomycetes	3	3.95	1	2	0
Alternaria	2	2.63	1	1	0
Arthrinium	2	2.63	1	1	0
Bjerkandera	2	2.63	2	0	0
Chaetomium	2	2.63	1	0	1
Fusarium	2	2.63	2	0	0
Meyerozyma	2	2.63	0	2	0
Plectosphaerella	2	2.63	1	1	0
Thanatephorus	2	2.63	1	0	1
Trametes	2	2.63	0	0	2
Ascomycota	1	1.32	1	0	0
Aureobasidium	1	1.32	1	0	0
Basidiomycota	1	1.32	1	0	0
Beauveria	1	1.32	0	1	0
Gliocladium	1	1.32	1	0	0
Botryotinia	1	1.32	1	0	0
Ceriporia	1	1.32	0	1	0
Colletotrichum	1	1.32	0	1	0
Debaryomyces	1	1.32	1	0	0
Dicyma	1	1.32	1	0	0
Epicoccum	1	1.32	1	0	0
Isaria	1	1.32	1	0	0
Lecythophora	1	1.32	1	0	0
Leptosphaeria	1	1.32	0	0	1
Myrmecridium	1	1.32	1	0	0
Nigrospora	1	1.32	0	1	0
Periconia	1	1.32	0	1	0
Pestalotiopsis	1	1.32	1	0	0
Phanerochaete	1	1.32	1	0	0
Pseudocercosporella	1	1.32	1	0	0
Pseudozyma	1	1.32	1	0	0
Rhizoctonia	1	1.32	0	1	0
Schizophyllum	1	1.32	0	1	0
Tritirachium	1	1.32	0	1	0
Xylariaceae	1	1.32	1	0	0
Trichoderma	1	1.32	1	0	0

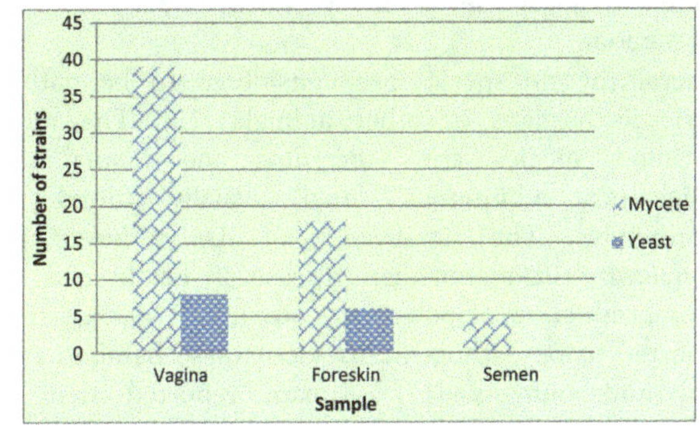

Fig. 2 Prevalence of mycetes and yeasts isolated from different types of samples

(p = *0.505*). Considering the composition of fungi between the older and younger female pandas, only 5 common genera were found between the two groups, including *Aspergillus, Candida, Penicillium, Diaporthe,* and *Trichosporon.* The other 26 genera differed (Tables 1, 2).

The 10 male pandas also were divided into an older (age > 10 years, 5 pandas) and younger group (age < 10 years, 5 pandas). There were 1, 1, 1, 2, and 3 strains from the foreskin of the older group and 0, 3, 4, 4 and 7 strains from the foreskin of the younger group. The younger pandas (average 3.6 fungal strains) had more fungal strains than the older pandas (average 1.6 fungal strains). Due to the small sample size, this difference was not statistically significant (p = *0.151*). However, the composition of fungal species differed between the older and younger male pandas, with the exception of the strain *Meyerozyma guilliermondii,* which was present in both an 8-year-old (T) and a 10-year-old (M) (Tables 1, 2).

Discussion

The fungal diversity of the giant panda genitals and semen

Previous studies performed isolation and identification of bacteria from the vaginas, foreskins, and semen of giant pandas [11, 14]. This study investigated the fungal flora in these samples. A total of 76 culturable fungal strains were identified. Our data indicates that the fungi are common in captive giant pandas (in 100% of the examined vaginal and semen samples, and in 90% of the examined foreskin samples). Our results show that there were significantly more mycete species (64/76) than yeasts (12/76) in the vaginas, foreskins, and semen of giant pandas. The mycetes were 5-fold higher than yeasts in the vaginas and 2.67-fold higher in the foreskins. However, no yeast was found in semen, which is similar to a previous report showing no yeast in the semen of 11 healthy male stallions [10].

Normal fungal species in the reproductive tract of the giant panda

Several mycete species are considered to be pathogenic in humans or other animals [15]. The most common species are *Aspergillus* and *Penicillium*, which are ubiquitous fungi, usually found as saprophytes. The significance of *Aspergillums* and *Penicillium* in mammalian disease is heightened by their production of potent mycotoxins. *P. marneffei* is reported to be pathogenic to Vietnamese bamboo rats [16] and humans [17]. Annam reported that *P. marneffei* caused genital ulcers in an HIV-infected patient [18]. However, no studies have shown *P. marneffei* to cause disease in giant pandas. In this study, *P. marneffei* was isolated from both breeding and non-breeding female pandas.

In this study, *A. fumigatus* was isolated from the foreskin inclusion of a healthy male panda, and *A. niger* was isolated from the vaginal secretion of a healthy female panda that had been successfully bred. *Aspergillus* spp. has also been reported to be associated with reproductive disorders. *Aspergillus* was responsible for mycotic abortion in cattle [3]. *A. fumigatus* was the most frequent isolate (62%) in bovine mycotic abortion [19], and *A. niger* is the most common isolate in 120 bovine animals that have had clinical histories of reproductive disorders [20]. In this study, however, *A. fumigatus* was isolated from the foreskin inclusion of a healthy male panda and *A. niger* from the vaginal secretion of a healthy female panda that had been successfully bred. It is unlikely that these *Aspergillus* spp. cause miscarriage or other reproductive disorders in giant pandas.

Cladosporium cladosporioides, which causes reproductive disorders in cows [20] and phaeohyphomycosis in humans [21] and giant pandas [12], was also isolated from the vagina and foreskin samples.

The microbial flora of giant pandas are significantly different from those of other animals due to their unique diet and habitat [22]. The identification of these fungal species from the healthy pandas suggests that they may be part of the normal fungal flora of the reproductive tract and that they may serve as a barrier against infectious agents [14]. These species may otherwise cause diseases when they reach and grow in locations different from the reproductive tract [23].

The yeast species in the reproductive tract of giant pandas

In this study, we found fewer yeast species, and none were cultured from semen, suggesting that yeasts may be less culturable. Our results showed that 20% of the isolated fungi consisted of yeast, including one species of *Candida* and six species of *Trichosporon*. *Candida spp.* often cause mucocutaneous syndromes and invasive candidiasis in certain settings [24], suggesting that they may be genital tract (mucosas system) pathogens. *Trichosporon spp.* are considered the second most common agent of yeast-disseminated infections [25]. In this study, *Trichosporon* was found in multiple pandas. Three species, including *T. japonicum*, *T. brassicae*, and *T. cutaneum*, were identified in one panda that had years of infertility. Whether *Trichosporon* can harm the vaginas and foreskins of giant pandas, or whether they are part of the normal fungal flora of the reproductive tract, warrants further study.

Fungi isolated from an older female panda

Older women are reported to be more susceptible to mycotic vaginitis [26]. Interestingly, 14 strains were isolated from the 18-year-old giant panda named "I", which had remained nonpregnant for the 5 preceding years. This is significantly higher than the average strains isolated from the female pandas (5.67 per animal). Although inconclusive due to the small sample size, it would be valuable to determine whether the number of fungi correlates with the age of giant pandas, which typically live approximately 20 years in the wild and approximately 30 years in captivity.

The difference of fungi between pregnant and non-pregnant groups

No significant difference was found in species number between pregnant and non-pregnant groups. This may be due to the small sample size. A larger sample size, although difficult to obtain with giant pandas, would greatly help better understand the possible difference.

Study of the dominance index of species in humans [27] suggests that the dominance index change may lead to reproductive barriers. Further study of the role of dominance index and different fungi species, along with larger sample sizes, may help uncover the role of fungi in panda breeding and health.

Conclusion

This study identified a total of 76 fungal strains, representing 42 genera and 60 species, from the gentital tracts (vagina, foreskin) and semen of healthy giant pandas. These fungal strains likely represent the normal fungal flora in their reproductive systems. These findings provide previsouly unavialble information on the fungal community, which will facilitate our understanding of the roles of fungi in the overall health and reproduction of giant pandas.

Acknowledgements
The authors thank Mr. Chengdong Wang, Yuliang Liu, and Mrs. Shanshan Lin for sampling.

Funding
This study was supported by the Applied Basic Research Project in Sichuan Province (2013JY0175), and international cooperation funds for giant pandas (AD1415).

Authors' contributions
XM carried out the collection of the vaginal sample of the giant pandas, isolated fungi, conceived the study, and drafted the manuscript. CL and YG participated in the sequence alignment, carried out the molecular genetic studies, and participated in the data analysis. JH conceived the study, participated in its design and coordination, and helped draft the manuscript. All authors read and approved the final manuscript.

Consent for publication
Not applicable.

Competing interests
The authors declare that they have no competing interests.

Author details
[1]College of Veterinary Medicine, Nanjing Agricultural University, Nanjing 210095, China. [2]College of Veterinary Medicine, Sichuan Agricultural University, Chengdu 611130, China. [3]College of Life Sciences, Sichuan Agricultural University, Ya'an 625014, China.

References

1. Peng J, Jiang Z, Hu J. Status and conservation of giant panda (Ailuropoda Melanoleuca): a review. Folia Zool. 2001;50(2):81–8.
2. Ran J, Du B, Yue B. Conservation of the endangered giant panda Ailuropoda Melanoleuca in China: successes and challenges. Oryx. 2009; 43(02):176–8.
3. Knudtson WU, Kirkbride CA. Fungi associated with bovine abortion in the northern plains states (USA). J Vet Diagn Invest. 1992;4(2):181–5.
4. Cafarchia C, Figueredo LA, Otranto D. Fungal diseases of horses. Vet Microbiol. 2013;167(1–2):215–34.
5. Lockhart SR, Pham CD, Gade L, Iqbal N, Scheel CM, Cleveland AA, Whitney AM, Noble-Wang J, Chiller TM, Park BJ, et al. Preliminary laboratory report of fungal infections associated with contaminated methylprednisolone injections. J Clin Microbiol. 2013;51(8):2654–61.
6. Castellani A. Urethromycoses of the male, and vulvovaginomycoses. J trop Med. 1929;32:357–8.
7. Guze LB, Haley LD. Fungus infections of the urinary tract. Yale J Biol Med. 1958;30(4):292–305.
8. Moraes IA, Stussi JS, Lilenbaum W, Pissinatti A, Luz FP, Ferreira AMR. Isolation and identification of fungi from vaginal flora in three species of captive Leontopithecus. Am J Primatol. 2004;64(3):337–43.
9. Shokri H, Khosravi A, Sharifzadeh A, Tootian Z. Isolation and identification of yeast flora from genital tract in healthy female camels (Camelus Dromedarius). Vet Microbiol. 2010;144(1–2):183–6.
10. Rota A, Calicchio E, Nardoni S, Fratini F, Ebani VV, Sgorbini M, Panzani D, Camillo F, Mancianti F. Presence and distribution of fungi and bacteria in the reproductive tract of healthy stallions. Theriogenology. 2011;76(3):464–70.
11. LEI L, YU MX, ZENG W, Song FL, Qiang W. Survey vaginal microorganism Flora of the Giant panda. Chin J Vet Sci Technol. 2001;31:10–1.
12. Ma XP, Gu Y, Liu XM, Li D, Ling S, Hou J, Wang C, Cao S, Huang X, Wen X. Phaeohyphomycotic dermatitis in a giant panda (Ailuropoda Melanoleuca) caused by Cladosporium cladosporioides. Med Mycol Case Rep. 2013;2:119–21.
13. Edita CFCSAS: Flora Fungorum Sinicorum. In: Flora Fungorum Sinicorum. Edited by Edita CFCSAS, vol. 1–42. Beijing: Science Press; 1987–2013.
14. Yang X, Yang J, Wang H, Li C, He Y, Jin S, Zhang H, Li D, Wang P, Xu Y, Xu C, Fan C, Xu L, Huang S, Qu C, Li G. Normal vaginal bacterial flora of giant pandas (ailuropoda melanoleuca) and the antimicrobial susceptibility patterns of the isolates. J Zoo Wildl Med. 2016;47(1):374–8.
15. Pitt J. The current role of Aspergillus and Penicillium in human and animal health. Med Mycol. 1994;32(S1):17–32.
16. Segretain G. Description d'une nouvelle espece de penicillium: Penicillium marneffei n. sp. Bull Soc Mycol France. 1959;75:412–6.
17. Segretain G. Penicillium marneffei n. Sp., agent of a mycosis of the reticuloendothelial system. Mycopathologia. 1959;11:327–53.
18. Annam V, Inamadar AC, Palit A, Koppad M, Peerapur B, Yelikar B. Genital ulcer caused by *Penicillium marneffei* in an HIV-infected patient. Sex Transm Infect. 2007;83(3):249–50.
19. Knudtson WU, Kirkbride CA. Fungi associated with bovine abortion in the northern plains states (USA). J Vet Diagn Investig. 1992;4(2):181–5.
20. Sirohi N, Khar S: Mycotic infection in some reproductive disorders of bovine. Indian J Dairy Sci 2000, 53(2):108–111.
21. Vieira M, Milheiro A, Pacheco F. Phaeohyphomycosis due to *Cladosporium cladosporioides*. Med Mycol. 2001;39(1):135–7.
22. Zhang Z, He G, Wang X, Zhong S, Zhang A, Guanghan L. The study on the giant panda's intestinal flora. Acta Theriologica Sinica. 1995;15(3):170–5.
23. Zambrano-Nava S, Boscán-Ocando J, Nava J. Normal bacterial flora from vaginas of Criollo Limonero cows. Trop Anim Health Prod. 2011;43(2):291–4.
24. Ostrosky-Zeichner L, Rex JH, Bennett J, Kullberg B-J. Deeply invasive candidiasis. Infect Dis Clin N Am. 2002;16(4):821–35.
25. Chagas-Neto TC, Chaves GM, Colombo AL. Update on the genus Trichosporon. Mycopathologia. 2008;166(3):121–32.
26. Changqing L, Jianying W, Shaoquan S, Cheng H, Feng W. Clinical analysis of fungal vaginitis in middle -aged women. Chin J Nosocomiol. 2011;21(15):3185–7.
27. Guo R, Zheng N, Lu H, Yin H, Yao J, Chen Y. Increased diversity of fungal flora in the vagina of patients with recurrent vaginal candidiasis and allergic rhinitis. Microb Ecol. 2012;64(4):918–27.

10

Normal computed tomographic features and reference values for the coelomic cavity in pet parrots

Irene A. Veladiano[1], Tommaso Banzato[1], Luca Bellini[1], Alessandro Montani[2], Salvatore Catania[3] and Alessandro Zotti[1*]

Abstract

Background: The increasing popularity gained by pet birds over recent decades has highlighted the role of avian medicine and surgery in the global veterinary scenario; such a need for speciality avian medical practice reflects the rising expectation for high-standard diagnostic imaging procedures. The aim of this study is to provide an atlas of matched anatomical cross-sections and contrast-enhanced CT images of the coelomic cavity in three highly diffused psittacine species.

Results: Contrast-enhanced computed tomographic studies of the coelomic cavity were performed in 5 blue-and-gold macaws, 4 African grey parrots and 6 monk parakeets by means of a 4-multidetector-row CT scanner. Both pre- and post-contrast scans were acquired. Anatomical reference cross-sections were obtained from 5 blue-and-gold macaw, 7 African grey parrot, and 9 monk parakeet cadavers. The specimens were stored in a −20 °C freezer until completely frozen and then sliced at 5-mm intervals by means of a band saw. All the slices were photographed on both sides. Individual anatomical structures were identified by means of the available literature. Pre- and post-contrast attenuation reference values for the main coelomic organs are reported in Hounsfield units (HU).

Conclusions: The results provide an atlas of matched anatomical cross-sections and contrast-enhanced CT images of the coelomic cavity in three highly diffused psittacine species.

Keywords: Monk parakeet, African grey parrot, Blue-and-gold macaw, Coelomic cavity, Computed tomography

Abbreviations: CT, Computed tomographic

Background

The increasing popularity gained by pet birds over recent decades has highlighted the role of avian medicine and surgery in the global veterinary scenario. The success of birds as pets is likely due both to the strong emotional connection linking such animals to their owners and to the high economical value of some species [1]. Among birds, psittacines have become one of the most diffused avian pet species; their appealing appearance, their deep interaction with the owner and the long lifespan expectation typical of some species represent the main reasons for their spread.

* Correspondence: alessandro.zotti@unipd.it
[1]Department of Animal Medicine, Production and Health, University of Padua, Viale dell'Università 16, Legnaro (PD) 35020, Italy
Full list of author information is available at the end of the article

The increasing need for speciality avian medical procedures during recent decade reflects the rising expectation among owners for high-standard medical treatment for their pets.

Most parrots are so-called "stoic" animals; to avoid predation these animals evolved to mask signs of illness [2]. Accordingly, clinical signs are difficult to notice during routine examination, the role of ancillary diagnostic techniques becomes vital in the diagnosis of several different diseases.

Diagnostic imaging plays a key role in exotic pet medicine and several references aimed at standardizing normal features through different imaging techniques in exotic and wild mammals [3–8], reptiles [9–15], and birds [16–21] are currently available.

Some references describing the CT (computed tomographic) features of the coelomic cavity of avian species are currently available [16–21]. However, to the best of the authors' knowledge, no specific references regarding the coelomic cavity in psittacines have yet been published. Moreover, little information is available regarding the use of contrast medium to enhance the visibility of individual coelomic organs in avian patients [22].

The aim of this study is to provide an atlas of matched anatomical cross-sections and contrast-enhanced CT images of the coelomic cavity in three highly diffused psittacine species (monk parakeet, African grey parrot, and blue-and-gold macaw). In addition, pre- and post-contrast attenuation reference values for the main coelomic organs are reported in Hounsfield units (HU).

Methods

Animals

Three different species of parrots were selected for the present study: blue-and-gold macaw (*Ara ararauna*), African grey parrot (*Pittacus erithacus*) and monk parakeet (*Myiopsitta monachus*). Five blue-and-gold macaws (Two males and Three females, mean weight 1000gr ± 14gr, mean length 86 cm ± 3.5 cm), Four African grey parrots (Three males and One females, mean weight 371gr ± 5gr, mean length 35 cm ± 1.5 cm) and Six monk parakeets (Three males and Three females, mean weight 130gr ± 2.5gr, mean length 28.5 cm ± 1 cm) presented to the University Veterinary Teaching Hospital of the University of Padua (Padua, Italy) were included in the study*. All the animals enrolled for the study were affected by head or limb pathologies (Seven head traumas and Eight leg fractures). Upon owner consent, whole body CT scans were performed.

Anatomical procedures

The cadavers of Five adult-blue-and-gold macaws (Three males and Two females, mean weight 1003gr ± 13.5gr, mean length 85 cm ± 2 cm), Seven adult African grey parrots (Three males and Four females, mean weight 345gr ± 4.5, mean length 32 ± 2 cm), and Nine monk parakeets (Six males and Three females, mean weight 126gr ± 3gr, mean length 29 ± 0.5 cm) were used in this study. Within 24–36 h of death the cadavers were fixed in prone position on a plastic support and stored in a freezer (−20 °C) for 48 h. Consecutive 5-mm transverse slices were obtained by means of an electric band saw, from the inlet of the coelomic cavity to the cloaca. The slices were then numbered, cleaned with water and photographed on both sides. All the above animals died soon after hospitalization or were euthanized because of advanced medical conditions and their bodies were donated to the Veterinary Teaching Hospital of the University of Padua (Padua, Italy) or to the Clinic for Exotic Animals (Rome, Italy) by the owners.

Imaging procedures

Computed tomography examinations were performed by means of a 4-multidetector-row CT scanner (Asteion S4, Toshiba Medical System, Amsterdam, NL). All live animals were anaesthetized with sevoflurane and oxygen administered via a facial mask, then intubated with an appropriate endotracheal tube; anaesthesia was maintained with sevoflurane carried by a mixture of medical air and oxygen. Computed tomographic studies were performed following a cranio-caudal direction with the animal in a prone position. Pre- and post-contrast sequences were acquired. Contrast medium (Optiray® 350 mg/ml, Covidien Spa, Italy) was injected in the right jugular vein with a 28-gauge needle at a dose of 660 mg/kg. The CT parameters were: helical acquisition mode, exposure time of 0.725 s, voltage of 120 kV, amperage of 150 mA, slice thickness of 1 mm.

The images were reconstructed with a soft tissue kernel and displayed in bone (window length 1000, window width 4000), pulmonary (window length −500, window width 1400) and abdomen (window length 40, window width 350) windows.

Attenuation was measured in Hounsfield units (HU) in the lungs, air sacs, liver, spleen, ventriculus, intestine and kidney in pre- and post-contrast scans using a commercially available DICOM processing software (Osirix, pixmeo SARL, Switzerland). Measurements were repeated three times using a region of interest of the same dimensions both in the pre and post-contrast images, and then averaged.

Statistical analysis

Normality was graphically assessed by means of the Q-Q plot. Normally distributed data were reported as mean ± standard deviation whereas non-normally distributed variables were reported as median with the limits for the overall range. Differences among species were calculated through analysis of variance (ANOVA) in normally distributed data whereas differences were calculated utilizing the Kruskal-Wallis H Test in the non-normally distributed data.

Results

All the CT scans were performed on live animals and therefore a direct comparison with the anatomical images was not possible; nevertheless, visual inspections reveal a high correlation of both as shown in Figs. 1, 2, 3, 4, 5 and 6. Only post-contrast images are displayed. Individual anatomic structures were identified and labelled on the basis of the anatomical references [23–25], both in the anatomical cross-sections and in the corresponding CT images. All the main organs of the respiratory,

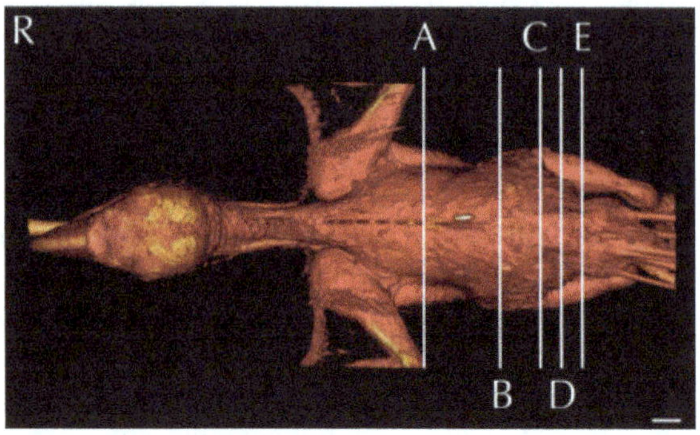

Fig. 1 Three-dimensional reconstruction of the body of a blue-and-gold macaw. Lines A-E indicate the level of the matched cross-sections and CT images displayed in Figs. 2, 3, 4, 5, 6 and 7

digestive, urinary (including the ureters) and reproductive systems were visible both in the anatomical sections and in the corresponding CT images.

The approximate level of the reported matching cross-sections and CT images are shown in Fig. 1. The displayed matched cross-sectional images and CT scans shown in Figs. 2, 3, 4, 5, 6 and 7 are approximately at the same level in all the considered species, and the same structures are present in almost all the corresponding slices of different species.

All the considered HU values were non-normally distributed; hence the differences among species were calculated by means of the Kruskal-Wallis H test. As no statistically significant differences among species were evident for any organ, only descriptive statistics of the pooled data have been reported. Medians with the limits for the overall range of HU values, for the selected coelomic organs are reported in Table 1.

Discussion

The coelomic cavity in the avian species is a single cavity with no further partitioning. Most of the coelomic cavity is filled by a very complex respiratory system that is composed of nine air sacs, six of which are in the coelomic cavity, plus two relatively small and non-expandable lungs.

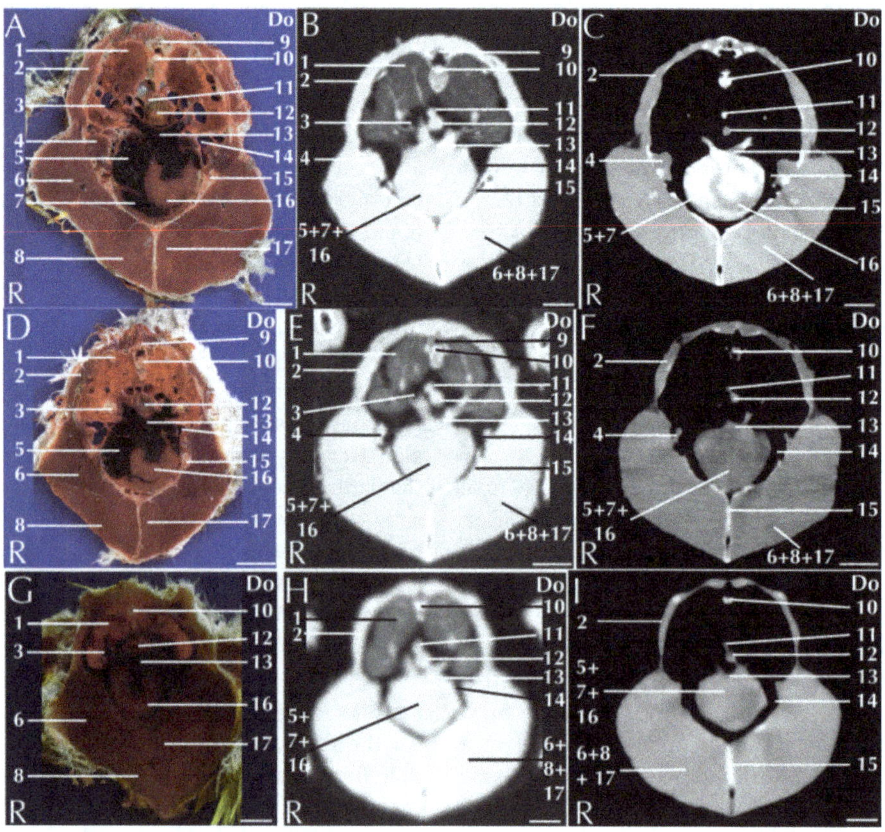

Fig. 2 Matched cross-sections and CT images at the level of the heart corresponding to line A in Fig. 1. Matched cross-sections and CT images of blue-and-gold macaw (**a-c**), African grey parrot (**d-f**) and monk parakeet (**g-i**). The CT images have been reconstructed with a soft tissue kernel and displayed in pulmonary (**b-e-h**) and abdomen (**c-f-i**) window. Do is dorsal and R are right. Bar = 1 cm. 1. Lung; 2. Scapulohumeralis muscle; 3. Intrapulmonary primary bronchus; 4. Scapulohumeral caudal muscle; 5. Right atrium; 6. Pectoral muscle (thoracobrachialis portion); 7. Right ventricle; 8. Pectoral muscle (sternobrachialis portion); 9. Vertebra; 10. Spinal cord; 11. Aorta; 12. Oesophagus; 13. Pulmonary trunk; 14. Cranial thoracic air sac; 15. Carina sterni; 16. Cardiac muscle, left ventricle; 17. Supracoracoid muscle

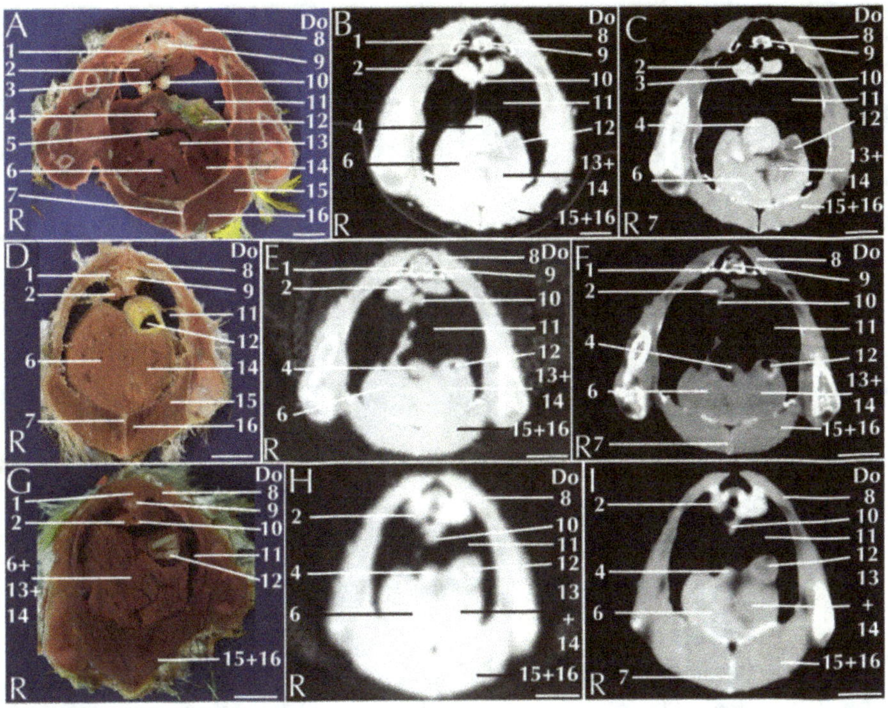

Fig. 3 Matched cross-sections and CT images at the level of the liver corresponding to line B in Fig. 1. Matched cross-sections and CT images of blue-and-gold macaw (**a-c**), African grey parrot (**d-f**) and monk parakeet (**g-i**). The CT images have been reconstructed with a soft tissue kernel and displayed in pulmonary (**b-e-h**) and abdomen (**c-f-i**) window. Do is dorsal and R are right. Bar = 1 cm. 1. Vertebra; 2. Kidney (cranial lobe); 3. Common iliac vein; 4. Spleen; 5. Caudal vena cava; 6. Liver, right lobe; 7. Carina Sterni; 8. Longissimus dorsi muscle; 9. Spinal cord; 10. Gonads; 11. Air sac; 12. Proventriculus; 13. Liver, medial part of the left lobe; 14. Liver, lateral part of the left lobe; 15. Pectoral muscle; 16. Supracoracoid muscle

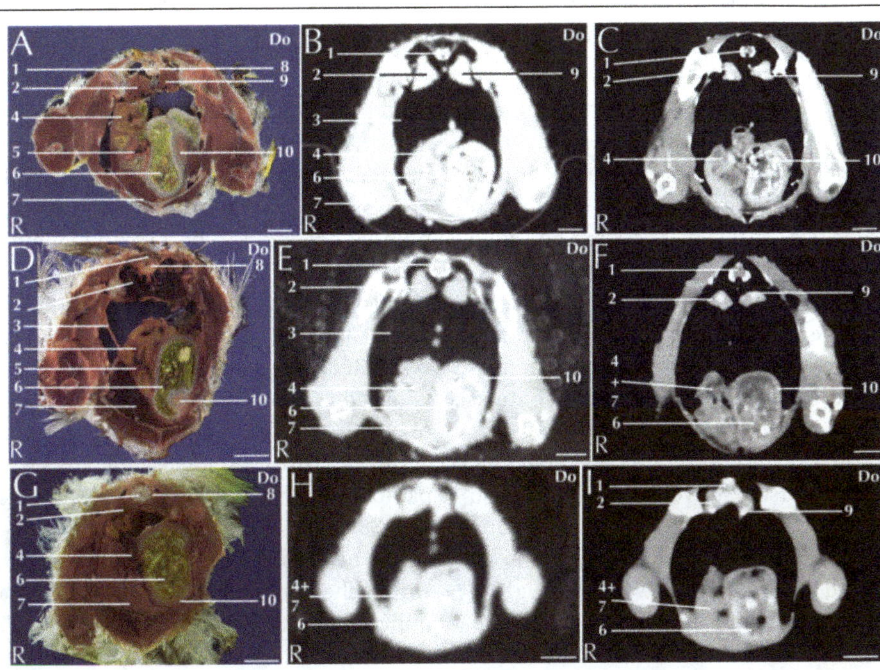

Fig. 4 Matched cross-sections and CT images at the level of the ventriculus corresponding to line C in Fig. 1. Matched cross-sections and CT images of blue-and-gold macaw (**a-c**), African grey parrot (**d-f**) and monk parakeet (**g-i**). The CT images have been reconstructed with a soft tissue kernel and displayed in pulmonary (**b-e-h**) and abdomen (**c-f-i**) window. Do is dorsal and R are right. Bar = 1 cm. 1. Spinal cord; 2. Medial lobe of the right kidney; 3. Air sac wall; 4. Small intestine; 5. Pancreas. 6. Ingesta; 7. Liver; 8. Vertebra; 9. Left ureter; 10. Ventriculus, muscular wall

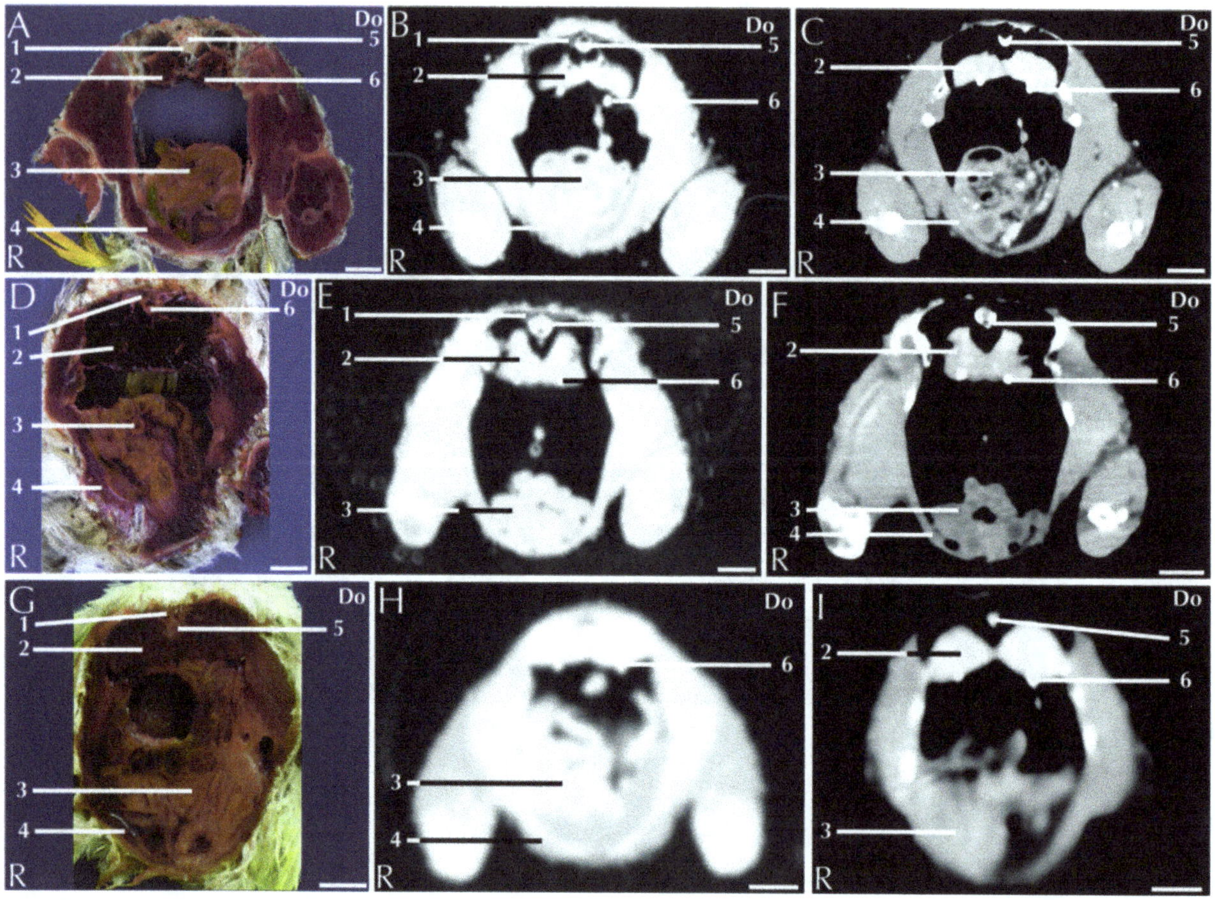

Fig. 5 Matched cross-sections and CT images at the level of the kidneys corresponding to line D in Fig. 1. Matched cross-sections and CT images of blue-and-gold macaw (**a-c**), African grey parrot (**d-f**) and monk parakeet (**g-i**). The CT images have been reconstructed with a soft tissue kernel and displayed in pulmonary (**b-e-h**) and abdomen (**c-f-i**) window. Do is dorsal and R are right. Bar = 1 cm. 1. Vertebra; 2. Medial lobe of the right kidney; 3. Intestine; 4. Pectoral muscle (thoracic portion); 5. Spinal cord; 6. Left ureter

The air sacs are air-filled structures covered by a thin pavimentous or cubical epithelium. This epithelium was clearly visible in CT scans of the blue-and-gold macaw and in the African grey parrot, but was not visible in monk parakeet (likely due to the small size of the animal) (Figs. 3b, e, h, 4b, e, h). The very limited vascularization of these structures brings differences that are undetectable between pre- and post-contrast scans [26].

The lungs are located cranio-dorsally in the coelomic cavity and are attached dorsally to vertebrae and ribs so that impressions of the ribs can be seen in isolated lung specimens [26]. These features were clearly visible in all the CT scans displayed in a pulmonary window (Fig. 2b, e, h). The trachea, the mainstem bronchi and the pulmonary arteries and veins could be clearly identified in all the examined species (Fig. 2b, e, h). No differences in the attenuation of the lung parenchyma after contrast medium injection could be noticed (Table 1). A high prevalence of respiratory diseases, both of bacterial and mycotic origin, is reported in pet parrots [26]. Although neoplastic pathologies are less frequent, a case of pulmonary adenocarcinoma in a blue-and-gold macaw has been reported [27]. It is also possible to find metastatic neoplasia in the lung parenchyma [28]. The use of CT in the diagnosis of respiratory diseases has been widely investigated in snakes [29] but, to the best of the authors' knowledge, no references reporting the CT appearance of respiratory diseases in avian patients are currently available. However, thickened air sacs are a common pathological finding associated with respiratory disease [26–30].

The heart is located along the central axis of the body within the coelomic cavity in an indentation of the sternum, cranial to the liver (Fig. 2c, f, i). The four distinct chambers were visible in the CT images, displayed in an abdominal window in the blue-and-gold macaw (Fig. 2c). The aorta and pulmonary arteries were identified in all the examined species (Fig. 2c, f, i). It was possible to follow the aorta for its entire length. In birds, the aorta

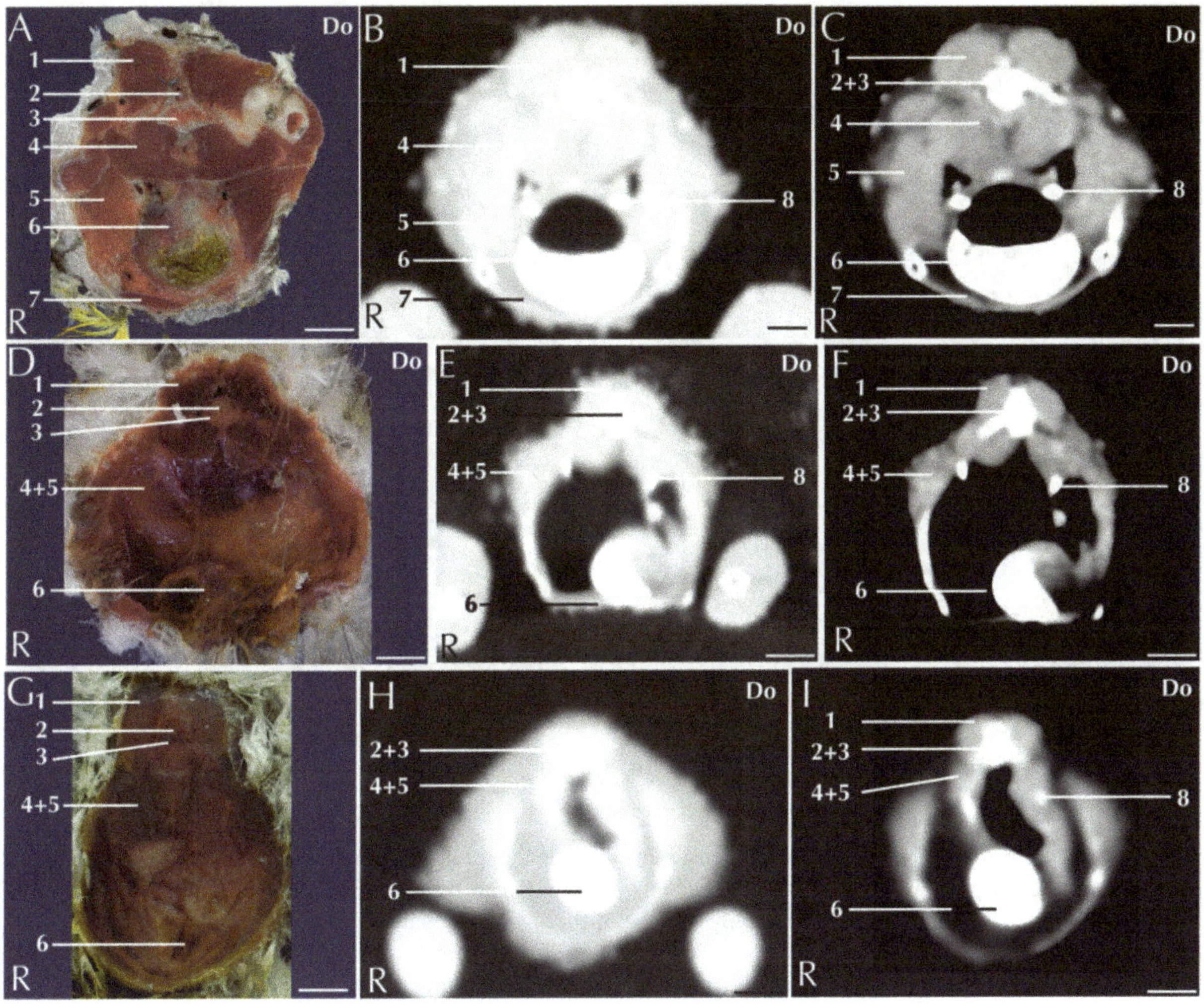

Fig. 6 Matched cross-sections and CT images at the level of the cloaca corresponding to line E in Fig. 1. Matched cross-sections and CT images of blue-and-gold macaw (**a-c**), African grey parrot (**d-f**) and monk paraket (**g-i**). The CT images have been reconstructed with a soft tissue kernel and displayed in pulmonary (**b-e-h**) and abdomen (**c-f-i**) window. Do is dorsal and R are right. Bar = 1 cm. 1. Musculus levator caudae; 2. Spinal cord; 3. Vertebra; 4. Musculus levator cloacae; 5. Musculus transversus cloacae; 6. Cloaca; 7. Pectoral muscle (abdominal portion); 8. Left ureter

traces a curvy path turning to the right immediately after its ascending portion [31] (Fig. 2c, f, i).

The avian liver is a bi-lobed structure that lies on the sternum, wrapping cranially around the heart and dorsally around the lateral margin of the proventriculus. The right lobe is generally bigger than the left in parrots [32] (Fig. 3c, f, i). Most parrot species, including all the study species, lack gallbladder [32]. In the contrast-enhanced CT images displayed in an abdominal window, the main lobar veins were well visible within a homogeneous parenchyma (Figs. 3c, f, i, 4c, f, i). Pre- and post-contrast densities of the liver are reported in Table 1. The liver is a common target for metabolic lipidosis and for bacterial and viral disorders that affect the entire parenchyma or cause disseminated focal necrosis [30].

The avian stomach is composed of the proventriculus, a glandular portion located after the junction with the oesophagus and the ventriculus, a muscular portion located caudally in the digestive system [33]. The junction between the proventriculus and the ventriculus is called the isthmus. The proventriculus and the ventriculus are clearly visible in the left portion of the coelomic cavity (Figs. 3c, f, i, 4c, f, i). The ventriculus has a thick muscular layer that was clearly visible in all the examined species (Fig. 4c, f, i). In all the study subjects the ventriculus was filled with *ingesta* that appeared as a mixture of air and dense material with an ill-defined shape (Fig. 4c, f, i). It was possible to distinguish the grit as a highly attenuating element. Alteration of the stomach, specifically of the proventriculus, can be caused by infective pathologies. In particular, proventricular dilatation disease [34] and *Machrorabdus ornitogaster* infection could be considered as the most common infection related to alteration of the proventriculus shape. The isthmus is a

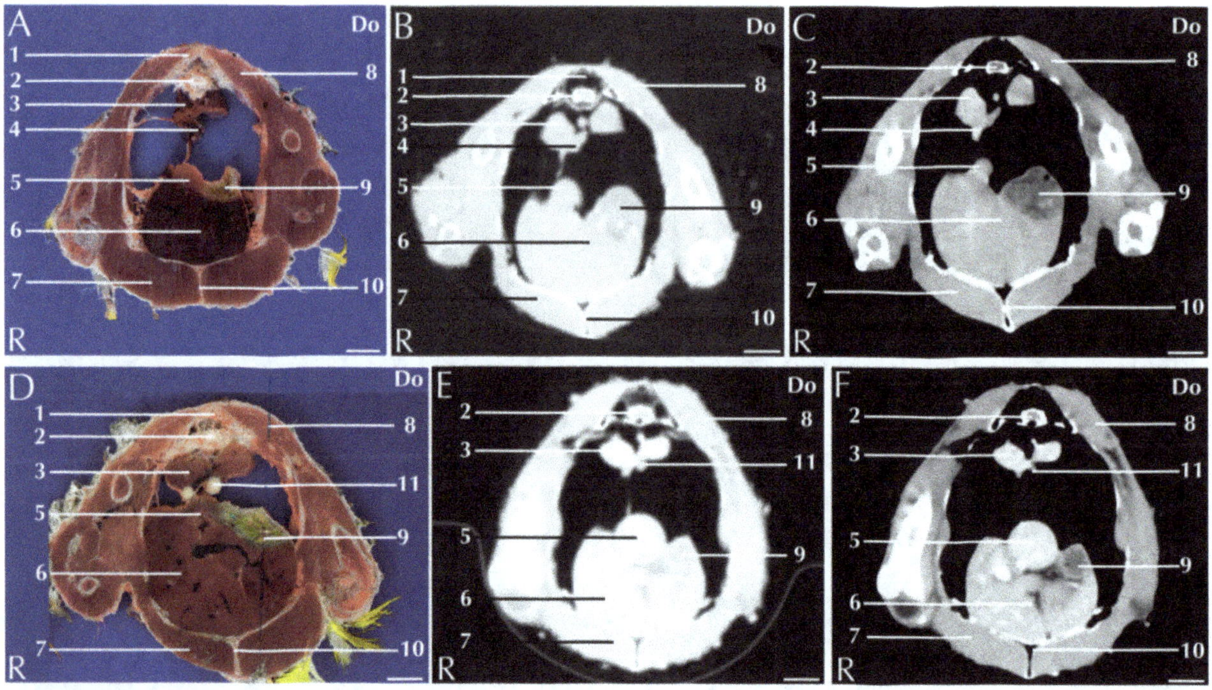

Fig. 7 Matched cross-sections and CT images at the level of the gonads corresponding to line E in Fig. 1. Matched cross-sections and CT images of female blue-and-gold macaw (**a-c**), and male blue-and-gold macaw (**d-f**). The CT images have been reconstructed with a soft tissue kernel and displayed in pulmonary (**b-e**) and abdomen (**c-f**) window. Do is dorsal and R are right. Bar = 1 cm. 1. Vertebra; 2. Spinal cord; 3. Kidney; 4. Ovary; 5. Spleen; 6. Liver; 7. Pectoral muscle; 8. Longissimus dorsi muscle; 9. Proventriculus; 10. Coracoid bone; 11. Testicles

common localization of *Machrorabdus ornitogaster* infection and gastric carcinoma [30].

Individual intestinal loops were visible only in the blue-and-gold macaw (Fig. 5c). Intestinal loop attenuation was difficult to evaluate both because of the presence of a mixture of *ingesta* and air and due to the limited dimensions of the intestinal wall. Nevertheless, the intestines appeared more attenuating in post-contrast scans (Table 1). Intestinal impaction, volvulus and intussusception have been described in avian patients [33]; although mycobacterial lesion (granulomas) can be relatively often recovered in the gut [35] there were no pathologies in our specimens.

Table 1 Attenuation values measured in the CT scans of some selected coelomic organs, calculated in pre- and post-contrast CT scans. Pooled data from the considered species are reported

	Pre-contrast HU values	Post-contrast HU values
LIVER[a]	57.20 (33.14–104.66)	122.99 (86.85–172.83)
VENTRICULUS[a]	64.78 (36.19–91)	116.43 (92.37–143.13)
KIDNEY[a]	34.92 (12.39–74.86)	178.44 (151.52–378.97)
SPLEEN[a]	54.55 (23.11–81.3)	141.70 (123.90–181.95)
INTESTINE[a]	28.73 (10.8–59.53)	77.16 (32.92–102.09)
LUNG[a]	−589.47 (−677.26 - -478.48)	−579.97 (−690.50 - -385.73)
AIR SACS[a]	−957.84 (−969 - -929.32)	−982.06 (−1021 - -947.63)
TESTICLE[a]	22.20 (16.93–25.31)	47.60 (38.85–63.95)
OVARY[a]	15.94 (11.86–20.73)	80.97 (65.2–91.51)

[a]Data are reported as medians (with the limits of the overall range)

The pancreas was located between the descending and ascending duodenal loops and was clearly visible in the anatomical section of blue-and-gold macaw and African grey parrot (Fig. 4a, d), but was not clearly distinguishable in the CT of any of the considered species.

The spleen was visible as a round structure lying to the left of the ventriculus (Fig. 3b, e, h, c, f, i). Pre- and post-contrast attenuation values of the spleen are reported in Table 1. Several infectious pathologies lead to increased overall dimensions of the spleen [30], but no reference have been made available to date.

Paired kidneys are located lateral to the spine and ventral to the pelvis. Although not clearly distinguishable in transversal CT images, multiplanar reconstructions (not shown in present paper) enabled to individually identify the three distinct lobes of the kidneys (Fig. 5c, f, i). A corticomedullary distinction was not evident. The ureters were visible, after contrast medium injection, in all the examined species and could be followed from the caudal pole of the kidney to the inlet in the cloaca (Fig. 6b, c, e, f, i). Pre- and post-contrast HU values are reported in Table 1. Renal pathologies are very common in avian patients; changes in shape and size of the renal parenchyma are associated with infections (acute or chronic), or chronic degenerative pathologies [30]. A case of renal tubule neoplasia has been reported in a channel-billed Toucan [36].

The gonads are located ventral to the cranial lobe of the kidney (Fig. 7c, f). When visible, the testicles appeared as moderately enhancing rounded paired structures whereas the ovaries appeared as single small, slightly elongated structures. In all the considered species, only the left ovary is functional. The gonads were clearly distinguishable only in sexually mature animals of the largest species (4 African grey parrots and 5 blue-and-gold macaw) (Fig. 7c, f). Although the gonads were clearly visible, the sex of the animal could not be determined in the smallest species (monk parakeet) because both the ovaries and the testicles had the same CT appearance. The oviduct was not visible in the anatomical images or CT scans. Pre- and post-contrast HU values are reported in Table 1. The reproductive organs of birds undergo cyclic atrophy and enlargement during the year in sexually mature animals [37]. Indeed, the male animals (2 african grey parrots, 1 monk parakeet) scanned during the reproductive season had remarkably larger testicles than the animals (2 blue-and-gold macaws, 1 African grey parrot, 2 monk parakeets) scanned during the non-reproductive period. Testicular and ovarian neoplasia are reported in avian patients [38, 39].

Although limited, the use of ultrasonography has been described in birds. The limited dimensions of the coupling sites and the presence of feathers act as limiting factors in the development of this imaging technique in avian patients. Some pathologic conditions, such as fluid accumulation, organ enlargement or displacement of the air sacs, enlarge the coupling site and therefore improve image quality. Ultrasonography is reported to be a useful diagnostic tool in the differentiation between cardiomegaly and hydropericardium in the investigation of masses involving the female reproductive tract and in the assessment of liver parenchymal changes. Gender determination through ultrasonography is possible only in mature animals during the breeding season; during the rest of the year and in immature animals the visibility of the gonads is hindered by the interposition of air sacs [40].

The lack of superimpositions and the fine anatomical resolution make CT the diagnostic imaging technique of choice when a pathology involving a coelomic organ is suspected. However, the clinician should also bear in mind both the potential risks associated with the general anaesthesia and the possible diagnostic information retrieved from a CT scan.

Conclusions

The matched anatomical cross-sections and CT images presented in this study are a useful reference for the interpretation of CT examination of the blue-and-gold macaw, African grey parrot and monk parakeet.

All the images and descriptions presented in this paper relate only to the above-mentioned species. This atlas can be used as reference for other psittaccine species only if the clinician is aware of the anatomical and physiological differences occurring between the species under investigation and the species considered in this paper.

The complex anatomy of the coelomic cavity and the lack of intracoelomatic fat make the interpretation of plain radiographs often challenging in avian patients; on the other hand, the fine anatomical detail and the scope to evaluate coelomic organ vascularization make CT the gold standard diagnostic imaging modality if a pathology involving the coelomic cavity is suspected.

Authors' contributions

IAV: conceived the study, performed CT scans, drafted the manuscript; TB: participated in the design of the study, performed the CT scans and drafted the manuscript; LB: performed the anesthesia during the CT scans and drafted the manuscript; AM, SC: matched the anatomical images with the radiographs and the CT scans, performed the anatomical recognition of the structures indicated in the figures; AZ: conceived the study, supervised the selection of patients, drafted the manuscript. All authors read and approved the final manuscript.

Competing interests

The authors declare that they have no competing interests.

Author details

[1]Department of Animal Medicine, Production and Health, University of Padua, Viale dell'Università 16, Legnaro (PD) 35020, Italy. [2]Clinic for Exotic Animals, CVS, Rome 00137, Italy. [3]Avian Medicine Laboratory, Istituto Zooprofilattico Sperimentale delle Venezie, Legnaro 35020, Italy.

References

1. Groskin R. Prologue. In: Ritchie BW, Harrison GJ, Harrison LR, editors. Avian medicine: principle and application. 1st ed. Lake Worth: Wingers publishing inc; 1994. p. 17–25.
2. Raftery A. The initial presentation: triage and critical care. In: Harcourt-Brown N, Chitty J, editors. BSAVA Manual of Psittacine Birds. 2nd ed. Gloucester: British small animal veterinary association; 2005. p. 35–49.
3. Alonso-Farré JM, Gonzalo-Orden M, Barreiro-Vázquez JD, Ajenjio JM, Barreiro-Lois A, Llarena-Reino M, Degollada E. Cross-sectional anatomy, computed tomography and magnetic resonance imaging of the thoracic region of common dolphin (Delphinus delphis) and striped dolphin (Stenella coeruleoalba). Anat Histol Embryol. 2014;43(3):221–9.
4. Endo H, Sasaki H, Hayashi Y, Petrov EA, Amano M, Suzuki N, Miyazaki N. CT examination of the head of the Baikal seal (*Phoca sibirica*). J Anat. 1999; 194(1):119–26.
5. Zotti A, Banzato T, Cozzi B. Cross-sectional anatomy of the rabbit neck and trunk: Comparison of computed tomography and cadaver anatomy. Res Vet Sci. 2009;87(2):171–6.
6. de Rycke LM, Boone MN, Van Caelenberg AI, Dierick M, Van Hoorebeke L, van Bree H, Gielen IM. Micro-computed tomography of the head and dentition in cadavers of clinically normal rabbits. Am J Vet Res. 2012;73(2):227–32.
7. Banzato T, Bellini L, Contiero B, Martin A, Balikçi S, Zotti A. Abdominal anatomic features and reference values determined by use of

ultrasonography in healthy common rats (*Rattus norvegicus*). Am J Vet Res. 2014;75(1):67–76.
8. Banzato T, Bellini L, Contiero B, Selleri P, Zotti A. Abdominal ultrasound features and reference values in 21 healthy rabbits. Vet Rec. 2015;176(4):176–01.
9. Schumacher J, Toal RL. Advanced radiography and ultrasonography in reptiles. Semin Avian Exot Pet. 2001;10(4):162–8.
10. Arencibia A, Rivero MA, De Miguel I, Contreras S, Cabrero A, Oro S. Computed tomographic anatomy of the head of the loggerhead sea turtle (*Caretta caretta*). Res Vet Sci. 2006;81(2):65–169.
11. Putterill JF, Soley JT. Morphology of the Gular Valve of the Nile Crocodile, Crocodylus niloticus. J Morphol. 2006;267(8):924–39.
12. Banzato T, Russo E, Toma A, Palmisano G, Zotti A. Evaluation of radiographic, computed tomographic, and cadaveric anatomy of the head of boa constrictors. Am J Vet Res. 2011;72(12):1592–9.
13. Banzato T, Russo E, Finotti L, Zotti A. Development of a technique for contrast radiographic examination of the gastrointestinal tract in ball pythons *(Python regius)*. Am J Vet Res. 2012;73(7):996–1001.
14. Banzato T, Selleri P, Veladiano IA, Martin A, Zanetti E, Zotti A. Comparative evaluation of the cadaveric, radiographic and computed tomographic anatomy of the heads of green iguana (*Iguana iguana*), common tegu (*Tupinambis merianae*) and bearded dragon (*Pogona vitticeps*). BMC Vet Res. 2012;8:53.
15. Banzato T, Selleri P, Veladiano IA, Zotti A. Comparative evaluation of the cadaveric and computed tomographic features of the coelomic cavity in the green iguana (*Iguana iguana*), black and white tegu (*Tupinambis merianae*) and bearded dragon (*Pogona vitticeps*). Anat Histol Embriol. 2013; 42(6):453–60.
16. Orosz SE, Toal R. Tomographic anatomy of the golden eagle (*Aquila chrysaetos*). J Zoo Wildl Med. 1992;23(1):39–46.
17. Krautwald-Junghanns ME, Kostka V, Dorsch B. Comparative studies on the diagnostic value of conventional radiography and computed tomography in evaluating the heads of psittacine and raptorial birds. Avian Med Surg. 1998;12(3):149–57.
18. Krautwald-Junghanns ME, Valerius K, Duncker H, Sohn HG. CT-assisted versus silicone rubber cast morphometry of the lower respiratory tract in healthy amazons (*Genus amazona*) and grey parrots (*Genus psittacus*). Res Vet Sci. 1998;65(1):17–22.
19. Pepperberg IM, Howell KS, Banta PA, Patterson DK, Meisser M. Measurement of grey parrot (*Psittacus erithacus*) trachea via magnetic resonance imaging, dissection, and electron beam computed tomography. J Morphol. 1998; 238(1):81–91.
20. Gumpenberger M, Kolm G. Ultrasonographic and computed tomographic examinations of the avian eye: physiologic appearance, pathologic findings, and comparative biometric measurement. Vet Radiol Ultrasound. 2006;47(5):492–502.
21. Gumpenberger M. Avian. In: Tobias S, Saunders JH, editors. Veterinary computed tomography. 1st ed. Wiley-Blackwell: Chichester, West Sussex, England; 2011. p. 571–32.
22. Krautwald-Junghanns ME, Schroff S, Bartels T. Radiographic investigations. In: Krautwald- Junghanns ME, Pees M, Reese S, Tully T, editors. Diagnostic Imaging of Exotic Pets: Birds, Small Mammals, Reptiles. Hannover: Schluetersche Verlagsgesellschaft mbH & Co KG; 2011. p. 2–35.
23. McLelland J. A colour atlas of avian anatomy. Aylesbury: Wolfe Publishing; 1990. p. 1–127.
24. Baumel JJ, King AS, Breazile JE, Evans HE, Vanden Berge JC, editors. Handbook of avian anatomy: Nomina Anatomica Avium. 2nd ed. Cambridge: Nuttall Ornithological Club; 1993. p. 1–591.
25. Canova M, Clavenzani P, Bombardi C, Mazzoni M, Bedoni C, Grandis A. Anatomy of the shoulder and arm musculature of the common buzzard (Buteo buteo Linnaeus, 1758) and the European honey buzzard (Pernis apivorus Linnaeus, 1758). Zoomorphol. 2015;134:291–308.
26. Thully Jr TN, Harrison GJ. Pneumology. In: Ritchie BW, Harrison GJ, Harrison LR, editors. Avian medicine: principle and application. 1st ed. Lake Worth: Wingers publishing inc; 1994. p. 556–81.
27. Fredholm DV, Carpenter JW, Schumecher LL, Moon RS. Pulmonary adenocarcinoma with osseous metastasis and secondary paresis in a blue-and-gold macaw (*Ara ararauna*). J Zoo Wildl Med. 2012;43(4):909–1013.
28. Lamb S, Reavill D, Wojcieszyn J, Sitinas N. Osteosarcoma of the tibiotarsus with possible pulmonary metastasis in a ring-necked dove (Streptopelia risoria). J Avian Med Surg. 2014;28(1):50–6.
29. Pees M, Kiefer I, Oechtering G, Krautwald-Junghanns ME. Computed tomography for the diagnosis and treatment monitoring of bacterial pneumonia in Indian pythons (*Python molurus*). Vet Rec. 2008;163(5):152–6.
30. Dorrestein GM, de Wit M. Clinical pathology and necropsy. In: Harcourt-Brown N, Chitty J, editors. BSAVA Manual of Psittacine Birds. 2nd ed. Gloucester: British small animal veterinary association; 2005. p. 60–86.
31. Lumeij JT, Branson WR. Cardiology. In: Ritchie BW, Harrison GJ, Harrison LR, editors. Avian medicine: principle and application. 1st ed. Lake Worth: Wingers publishing inc; 1994. p. 695–722.
32. Lumeij JT. Hepatology. In: Ritchie BW, Harrison GJ, Harrison LR, editors. Avian medicine: principle and application. 1st ed. Lake Worth: Wingers publishing inc; 1994. p. 522–37.
33. Lumeij JT. Gastroenterology. In: Ritchie BW, Harrison GJ, Harrison LR, editors. Avian medicine: principle and application. 1st ed. Lake Worth: Wingers publishing inc; 1994. p. 482–521.
34. Staeheli P, Rinder M, Kaspers B. Avian bornavirus associated with fatal disease in psittacine birds. J Virol. 2010;84(13):6269–75.
35. Panigrahy B, Clark FD, Hall CF. Mycobacteriosis in psittacine birds. Avian Dis. 1983;27(4):1166–8.
36. Mainez M, Cardona T, Such R, Juan-Sallés C, Garner MM. Bilateral Renal Tubular Neoplasm in a Channel-billed Toucan (Ramphastos vitellinus). J Avian Med Surg. 2015;29(1):46–50.
37. Taylor M. Endoscopic examination and biopsy techniques. In: Ritchie BW, Harrison GJ, Harrison LR, editors. Avian medicine: principle and application. 1st ed. Lake Worth: Wingers publishing inc; 1994. p. 343.
38. Campbell TW. Citology. In: Ritchie BW, Harrison GJ, Harrison LR, editors. Avian medicine: principles and application. 1st ed. Lake Worth: Wingers publishing inc; 1994. p. 199–222.
39. Uetsuka K, Suzuki T, Doi K, Nunoya T. Malignant sertoli cell tumor in a goose (Anser cygnoides domesticus). Avian Dis. 2012;56(4):781–5.
40. Krautwald-Junghanns ME, Pees M. Ultrasonographic examination. In: Krautwald- Junghanns ME, Pees M, Reese S, Tully T, editors. Diagnostic Imaging of Exotic Pets: Birds, Small Mammals, Reptiles. Hannover: Schluetersche Verlagsgesellschaft mbH & Co KG; 2011. p. 36–136.

Redundant contribution of a Transient Receptor Potential cation channel Member 1 exon 11 single nucleotide polymorphism to equine congenital stationary night blindness

Michelle L. Scott[1], Emily E. John[1], Rebecca R. Bellone[2], John C. H. Ching[1], Matthew E. Loewen[1], Lynne S. Sandmeyer[3], Bruce H. Grahn[3] and George W. Forsyth[1*]

Abstract

Background: Congenital stationary night-blindness (CSNB) is a recessive autosomal defect in low-light vision in Appaloosa and other horse breeds. This condition has been mapped by linkage analysis to a gene coding for the Transient Receptor Potential cation channel Member 1 (*TRPM1*). TRPM1 is normally expressed in the ON-bipolar cells of the inner nuclear layer of the retina. Down-regulation of TRPM1 expression in CSNB results from a transposon-like insertion in intron 1 of the *TRPM1* gene. Stop transcription signals in this transposon significantly reduce TRPM1 primary transcript levels in CSNB horses. This study describes additional contributions by a second mutation of the TRPM1 gene, the ECA1 108,249,293 C > T SNP, to down-regulation of transcription of the TRPM1 gene in night-blind horses. This *TRPM1* SNP introduces a consensus binding site for neuro-oncological ventral antigen 1 (Nova-1) protein in the primary transcript. Nova-1 binding disrupts normal splicing signals, producing unstable, non-functional mRNA transcripts.

Results: Retinal bipolar cells express both TRPM1 and Nova-1 proteins. In vitro addition of Nova-1 protein retards electrophoretic migration of TRPM1 RNA containing the ECA1 108,249,293 C > T SNP. Up-regulating Nova-1 expression in primary cultures of choroidal melanocytes carrying the intron 11 SNP caused an average log 2-fold reduction of ~6 (64-fold) of TRPM1 mRNA expression.

Conclusions: These finding suggest that the equine TRPM1 SNP can act independently to reduce survival of TRPM1 mRNA escaping the intron 1 transcriptional stop signals in CSNB horses. Coexistence and co-inheritance of two independent TRPM1 mutations across 1000 equine generations suggests a selective advantage for the apparently deleterious CSNB trait.

Keywords: Appaloosa, Congenital stationary night blindness, Transient Receptor Potential cation channel Member 1

* Correspondence: george.forsyth@usask.ca
[1]Veterinary Biomedical Sciences, Western College of Veterinary Medicine, University of Saskatchewan, Saskatoon, SK S7N 5B4, Canada
Full list of author information is available at the end of the article

Background

Reduced expression of the transient receptor potential cation channel, subfamily M, member 1 (*TRPM1*) in retinal ON bipolar cells causes congenital stationary night-blindness (CSNB) in Appaloosa, Knabstrupper and other horse breeds. We have reported an 1800-fold reduction of *TRPM1* mRNA expression in CSNB retinal tissue [1]. ON bipolar cells lacking the *TRPM1* cation channel are unable to depolarize in response to mGlu R6 receptor interaction with its coupled Gαo protein, interrupting signal transmission to the optic nerve [2, 3]. This failure of depolarization eliminates the b wave in the electroretinogram, providing a distinctive clinical signature for impaired night-vision in affected horses. Inherited defects in *TRPM1* channel expression or function produce this CSNB phenotype.

TRPM1 protein is also expressed in equine skin melanocytes where it participates in melanin production [4]. However, expression of *TRPM1* mRNA is only reduced ~300 fold in non-pigmented skin from CSNB horses. The coat pattern spotting of heterozygotes and the "snow cap" phenotype of homozygous CSNB horses typified in the Appaloosa breed appears to have some connection to the reduced *TRPM1* expression in CSNB skin [1]. The distinctive spotted coat pattern characteristic of heterozygotes with a single functional TRPM1 gene accounts for the selective breeding for reduced *TRPM1* expression. But the homozygous *TRPM1*-negative Snowcap stallion guaranteed to produce spotted offspring on a solid Bay mare is night-blind [5]. Interest in the molecular basis for tissue-specific effects of the equine *TRPM1* gene is enhanced by their different modes of inheritance and the divergent tissue phenotypes attending heterozygous and homozygous *TRPM1* mutations.

Sequencing the coding and flanking regions of the *TRPM1* gene did not identify a credible cause for reduced levels of transcript in CSNB horses [6, 7]. However, analysis of the CSNB retinal transcriptome revealed the transposon-like insertion of a retroviral LTR in intron 1 of the *TRPM1* gene [8]. This insertion introduces multiple polyadenylation signals likely to prematurely truncate the primary CSNB TRPM1 transcript. This finding accounts for decreased TRPM1 expression, but fails to explain tissue-specific differences (retina vs skin) in the extent of reduced TRPM1 expression in homozygous CSNB horses or in tissue specificity for the dominance pattern of the retinal and skin phenotypes of the TRPM1 mutations. Partial dominance of the Leopard coat pattern spotting phenotype, but recessive inheritance of night blindness could be connected to tissue-specific differences in TRPM1 mRNA expression or tissue processing.

Previous to discovery of the retroviral LTR insertion in intron 1 of the *TRPM1* gene we had identified an intronic mutation associated with CSNB and coat pattern phenotypes. This ECA1 108,249,293 C > T SNP located in intron 11 of the TRPM1 transcript [6] introduces a binding site for the tissue-specific neuro-oncological ventral antigen 1 (Nova-1). Nova-1 protein is a splice enhancer which can reduce the survival of transcripts carrying its recognition motifs within their RNA sequence [9]. Nova-1 is expressed at highest levels in neural tissue such as retina [10] where TRPM1 expression is particularly affected in the CSNB condition. However, there is much less Nova-1 expression in skin; providing a basis for tissue-specific differences in survival of the TRPM1 transcript carrying the intron 11 SNP.

This manuscript reports in vitro and in situ Nova-1 protein interactions with, and effects on the survival of mutant mRNA carrying the *TRPM1* intron 11 C > T SNP.

Methods

Primary choroidal melanocyte cultures

Retinal and skin tissue samples were obtained from horses humanely euthanized for other purposes at the Veterinary Medical Center of the University of Saskatchewan following the Canadian Council on Animal Care Guidelines for Experimental Animal Use and approved by the University of Saskatchewan Animal Care Committee. Samples for choroidal cell culture, for immunohistochemistry, and retinal and skin samples for RNA isolation were collected from an unaffected (homozygous WT) Appaloosa horse. Tissue was also collected from a CSNB-affected (homozygous for the *TRPM1* intron 11 SNP) horse for RNA isolation and choroidal cell culture. Collected choroidal cells were placed in cell culture media (DMEM media containing 10 % fetal bovine serum, 2 mM L-glutamine, 0.1 mM 3-isobutyl-1-methylxanthine, 16.2 nM phorbol 12-myristate 13-acetate, and 50 μg/mL and 50 units/mL of Penicilllin-Streptomycin) in six-well plates. Cells were incubated in 5 % CO_2 at 37 °C. Upon reaching 90–100 % confluency (7–10 days) cells were trypsinized and passaged into 75 cm^2 flasks. Cells from passage number 5 (p5) were used in all comparisons between the two genotypes of choroidal melanocytes.

Transfection constructs

Nova 1 expression in cultured choroidal melanocytes was increased by transfecting cells with human Nova-1 in Origene's pCMV6-XL5 expression vector. Microphthalmia-associated transcription factor, subtype M (MITF-M) expression was up-regulated by transfecting with an expression plasmid containing human MITF-M cDNA under control of a cytomegaloviral (CMV) promoter (a gift of Dr. Shigeki Shibahara of Tohoku University School of Medicine, Sendai, Japan) [11].

Transfections

P5 choroidal melanocytes from a normal and a night blind Appaloosa horse were plated at a density of 6×10^6 cells per flask and incubated 24 h. Media was exchanged 2 h before transfecting with 30 μg of plasmid DNA (Nova-1 pCMV6-XL5 cDNA or MITF-M pRc/CMV). Plasmid DNA solutions in 2.25 mL 2x BES buffer were mixed with 225 ul saturated $CaPO_4$, incubated exactly 20 min at 20 °C and added dropwise to recipient cells [12] to produce three biological replicates for each transfection condition. Transfected cells were incubated overnight prior to RNA isolation, cDNA synthesis and q-PCR.

q-PCR

RNA was isolated from tissues and cultured cells using the Trizol protocol and treated with the Turbo DNase according to manufacturer's recommended procedure (Invitrogen). RNA quantity and quality were tested for A260/280 absorbance and for size (Agilent 2100 bioanalyser). First strand cDNA synthesis was carried out with ThermoScript reverse transcriptase (Invitrogen) according to the manufacturer's protocol. Intron-spanning primer pairs specific for TRPM1, Nova-1, MITF-M and β-actin were designed and tested for efficiency and for production of respective unique products (Table 1). qPCR was carried out on an Agilent Mx3005P instrument using SYBR Green for product detection. Relative quantification (RQ) was calculated using $2^{-\Delta\Delta CT}$ method [13] on 6 replicated RT reactions for each condition. qRT-PCR data were analyzed according Schmittgen and Livak [14].

Immunohistochemistry

Immunohistochemical staining was conducted at Prairie Diagnostic Services, Saskatoon, SK on an automated staining platform (Code-On Histomatic Stainer, Fisher Scientific, Edmonton, AB, Canada). Heat-induced epitope retrieval was performed (sodium citrate buffer, pH 6.1) and primary goat polyclonal antibody (goat anti-Nova-1, Santa Cruz Biotechnology Inc, Dallas, TX) was used at dilutions of 1:10 and 1:20. Primary antibody-dependent binding of rabbit anti-goat immunoglobulins was detected with an avidin-biotin immunoperoxidase complex reagent (Vector Labs; Burlingame, CA), with 3,3′-diaminobenzidine tetrahydrochloride (Electron Microscopy Science, Ft. Washington, PA) as chromogen.

Gel shift assay

Custom RNA oligomers corresponding to 60 bases spanning the *TRPM1* intron 11 SNP, or to the positive control RNA used in Nova-1 binding protocol (Table 2) were purchased from GE Healthcare Dharmacon. 10 ng of each RNA oligomer was denatured at 80 °C for 5 min, cooled to room temperature, then incubated for 30 min @ 20° with 500 ng of wheat germ recombinant human Nova-1 protein (Abcam, Toronto, ON Canada) in buffer containing 0.5 M LiCl, 1 mM $MgCl_2$, 20 mM Tris–HCl pH 7.6, and 20 ng of yeast tRNA per reaction. Samples were electrophoresed in TBE running buffer on non-denaturing Tris-glycine-buffered 8 % polyacrylamide gels at 75 V for 1.5 h. Four replicate gels were stained in SYBR gold for 35 min, then imaged for 8 s exposures. Pixel intensity of fluorescent bands was quantitated with Image Pro Plus 7.0 software by Media Cybernetics. GraphPad Prism software was used for unpaired *T*-test analyses of output data.

Results

Differences in expression of TRPM1 mRNA reported previously between retinal tissues from CSNB and control horses [1] were confirmed in tissues sourced for this study. TRPM1 mRNA expression (normalized to β-actin) in

Table 1 PCR primers used to amplify human (H s) and equine (E c) cDNA templates

Primer	5′ – 3′ sequence	Product bp	Efficiency
E c Nova-1 F16	CAA ACT ACC ACC AAG TCC TC		
E c Nova-1 R224	CTC ACA GTG ACA ACC CTC TC	209	110 %
E c Nova-1 F1024	GGG ACA TTT GCA TTA GGT AG		
E c Nova-1 R1454	ATG GGG TAA AGG AGG GGT TA	431	
H s Nova-1 F310	ACA TTG CCA TCT TCC CCA AC		
H s Nova 1 R371	TGG AGG TGG TCA TGG GAT CA	62	
E c MITF-M F 408	CTT GAT GGA TCC TGC CTT G		
E c MITF-M R573	GGG AAA AAT ACA CGC TGT GA	166	110 %
E c βactin F55	GCC GTC TTC CCC TCC AT		
E c βactin R135	GCC C AC GTA TGA GTC CTT CTG	81	121 %
E c TRPM1 F2254	GAC GAC ATC TCC CAG GAT CT		
E c TRPM1 R2326	TGC TCG TCG TGC TTA TAG GA	73	113 %

Table 2 RNA oligomer sequences tested in gel shift assay for interaction with Nova-1 protein. Highlighted –UCAU- motifs are predicted to interact with the Nova-1 protein

60 bp TRPM1 CSNB Intron 11 SNP (position 41 A) RNA oligo; **5'-GGAAGAUCGAGCUGCUGAACUGGGUAUGUGGAAAGCCCUCAUCCCAUUGCUUGGGAUCAU-3'**
60 bp TRPM1 WT Intron 11 RNA (position 41 G) RNA oligo; **5'- GGAAGAUCGAGCUGCUGAACUGGGUAUGUGGAAAGCCCUCGUCCCAUUGCUUGGGAUCAU-3'**
Positive control RNA oligo (9) designed for optimal Nova-1 binding; 53 bp **5'-CCUUAUCAUGCUGACUCACGUCAUUUCAUCUCAUCAAGGGAGUCAGUGGGAUA-3'**

retinal tissue from the ERG-confirmed night-blind (CSNB) horse used in this study was 0.26 ± .022 % of the expression level measured in retina of a control horse (Fig. 1).

Expression of mRNA coding for the choroidal melanocyte marker protein (and TRPM1 transcription factor) MITF-M [15, 16], was similar in WT and CSNB retinal tissue and also between WT and CSNB cultured melanocytes.

Buckanovich et al. reported that Nova-1 expression is confined to tissues of neural origin [9]. In this study Nova 1 cDNA template was identified in retinal RNA by agarose gel electrophoresis (Fig. 2. lane 1) but was not detectable after 30 pcr cycles with intron-spanning primers with equal amounts of cDNA template prepared from equine skin RNA (lane 2). PCR amplification from the same cDNA template with a primer pair spanning the stop codon revealed DNA contamination of the cDNA template made from RNA treated with DNase. This difference in Nova 1 mRNA expression between retina and skin shown in Fig. 2 has been confirmed by qrtPCR (E.J. data not shown).

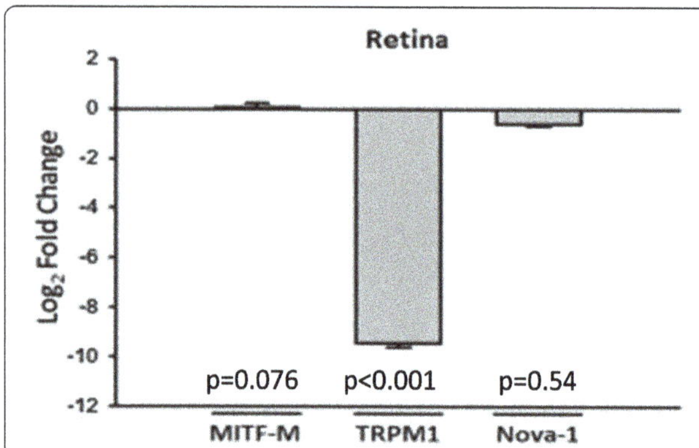

Fig. 1 mRNA expression in night-blind equine retina. Relative expression of mRNA coding for the three proteins of interest from retina of a night blind (CSNB) horse, compared to expression in a control horse with normal night vision. Triplicate qrt-pcr reactions were carried out on single RNA samples

Nova-1 expression must co-localize with TRPM1 in the retinal ON-bipolar cell in order for the Nova-1 binding site created by the TRPM1 intron 11 SNP to affect processing/stability of TRPM1 transcripts. Immunohistochemistry with goat anti-equine Nova-1 antibody shows the presence of Nova-1 antigen in a subpopulation of bipolar cells in the inner nuclear layer of equine retina (Fig. 3).

Nova-1 is reported to prefer binding to RNA containing 2 or 3 repeats of the -UCAU- recognition sequence motif [10]. Nova-1 binding may also be facilitated by secondary RNA structure where 5′-UCAU-3′ motifs occur in the predicted loop of stem-loop structures. M-fold software predicts that the ECA1 108,249,293 C > T SNP will lie close to the tip of a loop of a predicted secondary "hairpin" structure in the primary TRPM1 transcript (Fig. 4). The -UCAU- motif produced by the SNP is in an exposed location (position 39 in the 60-mer)

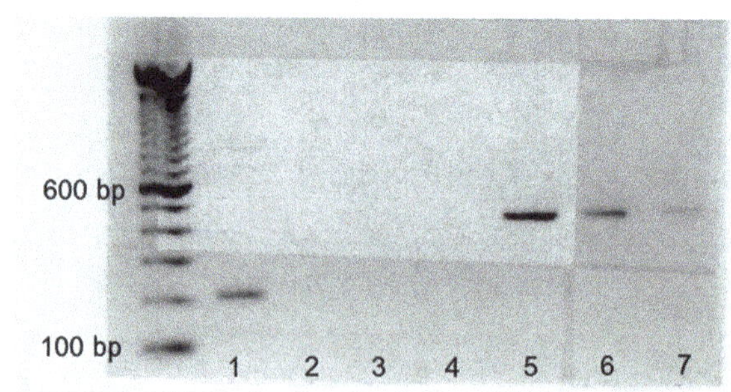

Fig. 2 Tissue-specific Nova-1 expression. RNA from retina (lanes 1 & 5), pigmented (lanes 2 & 6) and unpigmented skin (lanes 3 & 7) from a normal horse was reverse-transcribed using equal amounts of cDNA template in 30 cycles of PCR. PCR products were separated on agarose gel electrophoresis and identified by fluorescence with ethidium bromide. Lanes 1–3 were amplified with intron-spanning primers E c Nova-1 F16 – R224, product length = 209 bp. Lanes 5–7 were amplified with E c Nova-1 F1024 – R1454 primers spanning the stop codon, ;product length = 431 bp

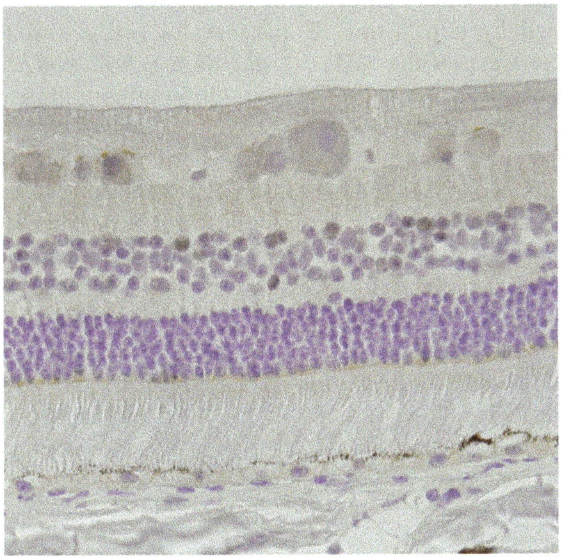

Fig. 3 Nova-1 expression in equine retina. Immunohistochemical identification of Nova-1 in equine retinal pigment epithelial cells and in bipolar cells in the inner nuclear layer. Orientation of retinal cross-section from lower to upper region is as follows: Choroid, retinal pigment epithelia, rod and cone photoreceptors, outer nuclear layer, inner nuclear layer (containing the ON-bipolar cells), ganglionic cell layer, inner limiting membrane

which is likely to be stabilized by extensive complementary base pairing in the stem region of the oligomer.

5'-GGAAGAUCGAGCUGCUGAACUGGGUAUGUGGAAAGCCCUCAUCCCAUUGCUUGGGAUCAU-3'

UCGU

The other consensus Nova-1 site at position 57 in the 60-mer occurs in the presumably less accessible stem of the hairpin in the native WT transcript.

The gel-shift assay result shown in Fig. 5 was used to test the three synthetic RNA oligonucleotides described in Table 2 for possible in vitro interactions with Nova-1 protein. Small 53-60-mer synthetic RNA oligomers migrated more rapidly than the yeast tRNA (73–93 nucleotides) used to prevent non-specific RNA-protein binding to Nova-1, and were lost from the bottom of each lane prior to staining. The excess yeast tRNA appears as the intensely-stained band at the bottom of each lane.

Preincubation of Nova 1 protein with a 53 base "positive control" RNA oligomer containing three tandem repeats of UCAU recognition sequence (Fig. 5 lane 7) formed a complex which retarded migration of this oligomer in polyacrylamide media under the non-denaturing conditions used for electrophoresis. Even a single occurrence of the UCAU motif in the WT TRPM1 oligomer (lane 3) was apparently sufficient to allow Nova-1-dependent-RNA complex formation and retarded electrophoretic migration.

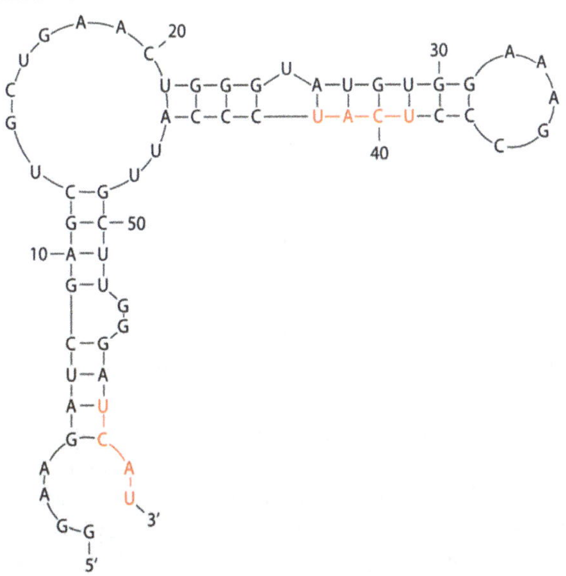

Fig. 4 M-fold minimal energy model of RNA secondary structure. Predicted two-dimensional secondary structure with base-pairing of a synthetic 60-mer transcript spanning the ECA1 108,249,293 C > T TRPM1 intron 11 SNP. Transcription of the SNP produces the adenine residue at position 41 in the RNA oligomer

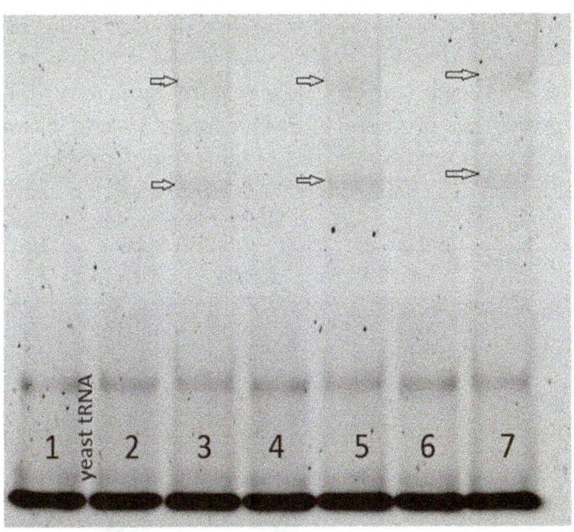

Fig. 5 The effect of the presence of Nova-1 protein on electrophoretic migration of synthetic RNA oligomers. RNA bands were visualized after electrophoresis by SYBR-gold fluorescence. Lane 1; Background yeast tRNA only. Lane 2; TRPM1 WT intron 11 60-mer RNA oligo. Lane 3; TRPM1 WT intron 11 60-mer RNA oligo plus Nova-1 protein. Lane 4; TRPM1 CSNB Intron 11 SNP 60mer RNA oligo. Lane 5; TRPM1 CSNB Intron 11 SNP 60mer RNA oligo plus Nova-1. Lane 6; positive control 60-mer oligo containing 3 UCAU motifs. Lane 7; positive control 60-mer oligo plus Nova-1. Location of RNA-Nova-1 complex with retarded mobility is indicated by open arrows

Quantitative pixel intensity measurements of the CYBR Gold fluorescence products in Fig. 5 showed a 154 ± 34 % increase in fluorescence intensity for the retarded positive control RNA bands containing 3 repeats of the Nova-1 binding motif (lane 7) in four replicates of this gel-shift assay compared to the native TRPM1 oligomer bands (lane 3) containing a single copy of the motif. Insertion of a second –UCAU- Nova-1 target motif corresponding to the transcript of the intron 11 SNP into the pyrimidine-rich area of the 60-mer increased the fluorescence intensity of the Nova-1- RNA complex in lane 5 to 157 ± 17 % of that of the native TRPM1 oligomer in the 4 gel-shift replicates. Limits to precise quantitation in this assay make the extent of Nova-1 binding to the 60-mer TRPM1 oligo containing the CSNB SNP indistinguishable from Nova-1 binding to the positive control 53-mer RNA of Buckanovich and Darnell [10] identified in Table 1.

Evidence for the presence of Nova-1 in retinal inner nuclear bipolar cells and for physical interactions of Nova-1 protein with TRPM1 mRNA suggests the possibility of in vivo effects of Nova-1 on TRPM1 mRNA containing the transcript of the intron 11 SNP. The cultured primary choroidal melanocytes obtained from the CSNB and from the normal horse were used to investigate this possibility. Melanocyte passage to P5 was necessary to obtain sufficient cell numbers for replicate transfections. However melanocyte mRNA expression diminished significantly ($p < 0.001$) with successive choroidal melanocyte passage for all three marker genes used in this study (Fig. 6).

An in situ cell culture model requires sufficient MITF-M protein to promote TRPM1 expression and Nova-1 protein to interact with the binding motif provided by the intron 11 SNP. Increased expression of marker mRNA in de-differentiated melanocyte cultures was obtained by transfecting P5 melanocytes singly with the vectors expressing MITF-M and Nova-1, and then with dual transfection to increase expression of both proteins. Single transfections with MITF-M increased TRPM1 expression ~4-fold in 3 biological replicate transfections of WT melanocytes and ~2-fold in CSNB melanocyte cultures (Table 3). Single transfections with Nova-1 had the opposite effect on TRPM1 mRNA expression, decreasing WT melanocyte TRPM1 expression 5-fold and decreasing CSNB melanocyte TRPM1 expression 55-fold. The combined dual transfection reduced WT melanocyte TRPM1 mRNA expression 14-fold (1/0.072) and CSNB melanocyte TRPM1 mRNA by ~150-fold (1/0.0068) (Table 3). These genotype differences in response to dual transfection were significant at the $p < 0.001$ level.

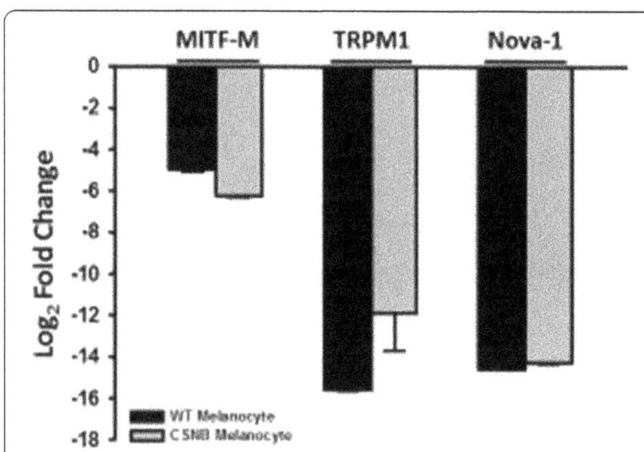

Fig. 6 Reduced expression of tissue-specific choroidal melanocyte marker genes with cell passage. ΔΔCT values compare mRNA expression levels measured by q-RT-PCR from six separate flasks of each genotype of melanocytes at the 5th passage to fresh retinal tissue relative to β-actin

Discussion

Nova-1 is a neuron-specific RNA splicing factor that favors alternative exon inclusion during transcript maturation. Mutations inserting Nova-1 recognition sites into transcripts expressed in neural tissue could significantly disrupt normal transcript processing/maturation. Co-expression of Nova-1 with TRPM1 in bipolar cells in the neural retina indicates potential trouble for the mutant TRPM1 transcripts containing the novel Nova-1 binding site. However, the degree of jeopardy attending generation of a new Nova-1 binding site could be influenced by accessibility of the new site to its protein ligand. M-fold structure predictions for synthetic oligomers constructed for this study suggest that the TRPM1 intron 11 SNP lies in an exposed loop area of the nascent transcript, and that the SNP-induced G > A change to the TRPM1 transcript helps stabilize this exposed target loop by adding an extra base pair to the proposed secondary structure. This conjectured importance of a new Nova-1 binding site on the side of a modelled exposed loop is supported by the outcome of the gel shift results reported above.

The existence of a native WT Nova-1 binding site distal to the intron 11 SNP is of interest because M-fold software predicts this Nova-1 binding site to be relatively inaccessible, located at the base of a "stem" in the secondary structure. The gel shift finding of enhanced binding of the mutant CSNB oligomer containing a second site supports in vivo validity of the M-fold model as the single Nova-1 site in the stem permits the binding of less oligomer than the combined two sites corresponding to the CSNB mutant transcript. As observed by Buckanovich and Darnell [9], it is also possible that the combination of two Nova-1 sites on the SNP-containing oligomer outweighs the importance of Nova-1 accessibility to any single site.

One could speculate that greater down-regulation of TRPM1 mRNA expression in CSNB retina (~1800-fold)

Table 3 Relative amount of TRPM1 mRNA detected in cultured choroidal melanocytes transfected with expression vectors coding for MITF-M and/or Nova-1 expression. $n = 6$ replicate rt q-pcr reactions

	Effect of transfection on relative TRPM1 mRNA level				
	Wild type melanocytes		LP/LP melanocytes		*P*
	ΔΔCT	Fold change	ΔΔCT	Fold change	
MITF-M	−2.1 ± 0.8	4.3	−0.8 ± 1.9	1.74	0.14
Nova-1	2.3 ± 0.8	0.20	5.8 ± 1.1	0.018	<0.001
MITF-M & Nova-1	3.8 ± 0.3	0.072	7.2 ± 0.9	0.0068	<0.001

compared to skin (~300-fold) might be partially attributed to localized Nova-1 expression in ON-bipolar cells in the retina. However, connections of tissue differences in Nova-1 expression to the dominance of coat pattern and the recessive inheritance of night blindness are not apparent.

Transcriptome analysis unequivocally demonstrates termination of TRPM1 transcripts at polyadenylation sites in the long terminal repeat (LTR) insertion in intron 1 [8]. This study documents the existence of a second mutation that can apparently decrease the production of TRPM1 mRNA in the CSNB horse. The co-existence of these two mutations in modern horse breeds, each of which may be able to independently reduce or eliminate the TRPM1 transcript in the ON-bipolar cell of the retina, is an untoward situation. Linkage between the intron 1 LTR insertion and the intron 11 SNP has been documented to exist in equine DNA samples dating to 16,000 years BP [17]. Other than a genomic proximity of ~60 kb, there is no obvious selection pressure to preserve this linkage for over 1000 equine generations. The recent finding that some modern Noriker horses carrying the LTR insert lack the intron 11 SNP demonstrates that a crossover between the two loci does occur, and that the predicted coat pattern phenotype expression exists without the intron 11 SNP [6]. We are not aware of any documented observations of progeny carrying the other crossover product; the intron 11 SNP without the LTR insert. Such horses should exist, but may lack the coat color phenotype to attract attention? So the coat pattern and night-blindness phenotypes of the isolated intron 11 SNP remain an issue for future resolution.

Conclusions

The C > T SNP in intron 11 of the TRPM1 transcript (ECA1 position 108,249,293) found in CSNB Appaloosa horses introduces a functional binding site for the tissue-specific neuro-oncological ventral antigen 1 (Nova-1). The electrophoretic migration of RNA oligomers containing the translation product of the SNP is retarded in the presence of Nova-1 protein. Up-regulating Nova-1 expression in cell lines containing the intron 11 SNP significantly reduces TRPM1 expression. Hence, night-blind Appaloosa horses have a second independent mutation which may contribute to reducing the amount of functional TRPM1 transcript in retinal ON-bipolar cells.

Abbreviations

CMV, cytomegalovirus; CSNB, congenital stationary night blindness; ECA1, horse chromosome one; LTR, long terminal repeat; Nova-1, neuro-oncological ventral antigen 1; SNP, single nucleotide polymorphism; TRPM1, Transient Receptor Potential cation channel Member 1

Funding

Research grants from a Class Action Vitamins Settlement to the University of Saskatchewan and by the Equine Health Research Fund of the Western College of Veterinary Medicine at the University of Saskatchewan provided financial support for the execution of this study. The study design was completely independent of these funding sources. Data analysis, interpretation and manuscript preparation were provided by GF as a part of the assigned duties of his appointment to the Department of Veterinary Biomedical Sciences at the University of Saskatchewan.

Authors' contributions

All authors have read and approved the final version of the manuscript. MS and EJ carried out the tissue culture and molecular studies. RB sequenced TRPM1 intron 11 and identified the Nova-1 site created by the SNP. JC and ML assisted with the data analysis. BG and LS verified the night-blind status of horses and obtained the skin and the ocular tissues used to start primary cell cultures. GF conceived the study, obtained research funding, was the PI and supervisor of MS and EJ.

Competing interests

The authors declare that they have no competing interests.

Consent to publish

Not applicable.

Author details

[1]Veterinary Biomedical Sciences, Western College of Veterinary Medicine, University of Saskatchewan, Saskatoon, SK S7N 5B4, Canada. [2]Department of Biology, University of Tampa, Tampa, FL 33606, USA. [3]Small Animal Clinical Sciences, Western College of Veterinary Medicine, University of Saskatchewan, Saskatoon, Canada.

References

1. Bellone RR, Brooks SA, Sandmeyer LS, Murphy BA, Forsyth GW, Archer S, Bailey E. Differential gene expression of TRPM1, the potential cause of congenital stationary night blindness and coat spotting patterns (LP) in the Appaloosa horse (Equus caballus). Genetics. 2008;179:1861–70.
2. Koike C, Numata T, Ueda H, Mori Y, Furukawa T. TRPM1: a vertebrate TRP channel responsible for retinal ON bipolar function. Cell Calcium. 2010;48:95–101.

3. Morgans CW, Brown RL, Duvoisin RM. TRPM1: The endpoint of the mGluR6 signal transduction cascade in retinal ON-bipolar cells. Bioessays. 2010;32: 609–14.
4. Oancea E, Vriens J, Brauchi S, Jun J, Splawski I, Clapham DE. TRPM1 forms ion channels associated with melanin content in melanocytes. Sci Signal. 2009;2:ra21.
5. Sandmeyer LS, Breaux CB, Archer S, Grahn BH. Clinical and electroretinographic characteristics of congenital stationary night blindness in the Appaloosa and the association with the leopard complex. Vet Ophthalmol. 2007;10:368–75.
6. Bellone RR, Forsyth GW, Leeb T, Archer S, Biagi T, Sigurdsson S, Maucelli E, Engensteiner M, Bailey E, Sandmeyer LS, Lindblad-Toh K, Wade C, Grahn BH. Fine-mapping and mutation analysis of TRPM1: a candidate gene for leopard complex (LP) spotting and congenital stationary night blindness in horses. Brief Funct Genomics. 2010;9:193–207.
7. Bellone RR, Archer S, Wade CM, Cuka-Lawson C, Haase B, Leeb T, Forsyth GW, Sandmeyer LS, Grahn BH. Association analysis of candidate SNPs in TRPM1 with leopard complex spotting (LP) and congenital stationary night blindness (CSNB) in horses. Anim Genet. 2010;41:207.
8. Bellone RR, Holl H, Setaluri V, Devi S, Maddodi N, Archer S, Sandmeyer L, Ludwig A, Foerster D, Pruvost M, Reissmann M, Bortfeldt R, Adelson DL, Lim SL, Nelson J, Haase B, Engensteiner M, Leeb T, Forsyth GW, Mienaltowski MJ, Mahadevan P, Hofreiter M, Paijmans JL, Gonzalez-Fortes G, Grahn BH, Brooks SA. Evidence for a retroviral insertion in TRPM1 as the cause of congenital stationary night blindness and leopard complex spotting in the horse. PLoS One. 2013;8(10):e78280.
9. Buckanovich RJ, Posner JB, Darnell RB. Nova, the paraneoplastic Ri antigen, is homologous to an RNA binding protein and is specifically expressed in the developing motor system. Neuron. 1993;11:657–72.
10. Buckanovich RJ, Darnell RB. The neuronal RNA binding protein Nova-1 recognizes specific RNA targets in vitro and in vivo. Mol Cell Biol. 1997;17:3194–201.
11. Yasumoto K, Yokoyama K, Shibata K, Tomita Y, Shibahara S. Microphthalmia-associated transcription factor as a regulator for melanocyte-specific transcription of the human tyrosinase gene. Mol Cell Biol. 1994;14:8058–70.
12. Graham FL, van der Eb AJ. A new technique for the assay of infectivity of human adenovirus 5 DNA. Virology. 1973;52(2):456–67.
13. Livak KJ, Schmittgen TD. Analysis of relative gene expression data using real-time quantitative PCR and the $2^{-\Delta\Delta CT}$ method. Methods. 2001;25:402–8.
14. Schmittgen TD, Livak K. Analyzing real-time PCR data by the comparative C(T) method. Nat Protoc. 2008;3:1101–8.
15. Watanabe K, Takeda K, Yasumoto K, Udono T, Saito H, Ikeda K, Takasaka T, Takahashi K, Kobayashi T, Tachibana M, Shibahara S. Identification of a distal enhancer for the melanocyte-specific promoter of the MITF gene. Pigment Cell Res. 2002;15:201–11.
16. Miller AJ, Du J, Rowan S, Hershey CL, Widlund HR, Fisher DE. Transcriptional regulation of the melanoma prognostic marker melastatin (TRPM1) by MITF in melanocytes and melanoma. Cancer Res. 2004;64:509–16.
17. Pruvost M, Bellone RR, Beneke N, Sandoval-Castellanos E, Cieslak M, Kuznetzova T, Morales-Muñiz A, O'Connor T, Reissmann M, Hofreiter M, Ludwig A. Genotypes of predomestic horses match phenotypes painted in Paleolithic works of cave art. Proc Natl Acad Sci. 2011;108:18626–30.

12

Frequency of canine nt230(del4) MDR1 mutation in prone pure breeds, their crosses and mongrels in Israel - insights from a worldwide comparative perspective

Yaron Dekel[1,2,4*], Yossy Machluf[5], Aviad Stoler[4], Arava Aderet[4], Daniel Baumel[4], Efrat Kellerman[4], Yoram Plotsky[4], Oshrat Noked Partouche[1,3], Gal Elhalal[6], Izhar Ben-Shlomo[2,7] and Dani Bercovich[3,4]

Abstract

Background: Sensitivity to macrocyclic lactones, which are commonly used in veterinary clinics, was first found in Rough Collies, and was attributed in 2001 to a 4 bp deletion in the MDR1 gene. The list of affected breeds currently includes 13 breeds. Researchers from different countries and continents examined the allelic frequencies of the nt230(del4) MDR1 mutation, emphasizing the clinical importance of this test not only to mutation-prone dogs, but also to their crosses and mongrels, since treatment of a deletion carrier with these compounds may lead to its death.
In this study, the allelic frequencies of nt230(del4) MDR1 mutation in affected breeds, their crosses, unrelated pure breeds and mongrels are reported for the state of Israel ($n = 1416$ dogs). The Israeli data were compared with reports from the US, Europe, UK, Australia and Japan.

Results: The allelic frequencies of nt230(del4) MDR1 mutation in Israel for Australian, Swiss and German Shepherds (31%, 17% and 2.4%, respectively) are similar to the corresponding frequencies worldwide, much higher for Border Collies (4.8%), twice lower for Rough Collies (28%, compared to 55% or more elsewhere), and ~1% for mongrels. The frequencies for crosses of Australian Shepherd and Border Collies in Israel are 4 and 1.6 times lower, respectively, compared to the frequencies for the respective pure breeds.

Conclusions: This work, that for the first time presents the frequency of nt230(del4) MDR1 mutation in Israel, along with a worldwide survey, has implications for clinicians, owners and breeders of sheepdogs and their crosses and supports the need for extra care in treatment and in future breeding. Of note, the relative proportion of affected breeds, in the overall tested dogs, might be higher than their actual proportion in Israel due to directed samples collection by veterinarians for clinical purposes, as these are mainly limited to certain affected breeds or dogs that resemble them.

Keywords: nt230(del) MDR1 mutation, Macrocyclic lactones, Sheepdogs, Drug sensitivity, Taqman assay

* Correspondence: Yarond@gri.org.il
[1]Shamir Research Institute, University of Haifa, P.O.Box 97, 1290000 Kazerin, Israel
[2]Zefat Academic College, Zefat, Israel
Full list of author information is available at the end of the article

Background

The multi drug resistance 1 (MDR1) gene, a member of the ATP-binding cassette (ABC) transporters superfamily, is a highly conserved ATP-dependent P-glycoprotein (P-gp) membrane transporter [1]. In eukaryotes, the extrusion transporters have a fundamental function as eliminators of several toxic compounds, mainly hydrophilic and amphiphatic ones [2–4]. ABCB1 (ABC subfamily B member 1, also referred to as MDR1 and PGY1) transporters are expressed in several organs and their role in the gut epithelia and the blood-tissue barriers (blood-brain barrier, blood-testis barrier and placenta) of mammals has been studied extensively [5]. While MDR1 activity in the small intestine can limit the bioavailability of various drugs, its inactivity in the luminal membranes of the endothelial cells of the brain can lead to toxic accumulation of xenobiotics in the central nervous system (CNS) and to severe adverse effects, including death [6, 7].

Since the early 1980s, sheepdogs were reported to have sensitivity to ivermectin, a relatively new macrocyclic lactone parasiticide drug [8, 9]. Elevated concentrations of ivermectin were found in the CNS of affected dogs [10]. In 2001, ivermectin sensitivity in Rough Collies was associated with a 4-base pair (bp) deletion mutation in the fourth exon of the canine ABCB1 gene [11]. The deletion, usually annotated *ABCB1:c.227_230delATAG* or ABCB1–1Δ (MDR1) mutation (hereafter nt230(del4) MDR1 mutation), causes a frameshift that leads to a premature stop codon and a truncated transporter of 91 amino acids as opposed to 1281 amino acids, i.e. only 7.1% of the full-length mature P-gp protein [12]. Later studies showed that nt230(del4) MDR1 mutation heterozygous dogs can be regarded as having an intermediate macrocyclic lactone sensitive phenotype. This is a relevant clinical notion in cases of high-dose protocols [6, 13]. Pertinent macrocyclic lactones include ivermectin, doramectin, moxidectin and milbemycin oxime. Other drugs commonly used in the veterinary clinic, such as P-glycoprotein substrates of the non-macrocyclic lactones type, were also reported as toxic to nt230(del4) MDR1 mutation homozygote dogs (–/–). These include vincristine, digoxin, mexiletine, quinidine, fexofenadine, vinblastine, and loperamide, cyclosporine A, verapamil, paclitexal, doxorubicin, dexamethasone and others [14–19]. Moreover, treating nt230(del4) MDR1 mutation heterozygote dogs (+/–) with reduced doses of P-glycoprotein substrates such as vincristine, vinblastine and doxorubicin (but not a full dosage treatment of a non-P-glycoprotein substrate) may cause delayed drug excretion, and consequently drug toxicosis and myelosuppression [20]. Recently, a collie affected (homozygote) by the Nt230(del4) MDR1 mutation mutation experienced exaggerated CNS depression when treated with apomorphine [21], an opioid which has not been described as a P-glycoprotein substrate. Yet, other opioids, including loperamide and butorphanol, are known substrates for canine P-glycoprotein [22]. A cell line for assessing drugs as canine P-gp substrates was recently developed [23]. Noteworthy, based on its anti-parasitic and anti-inflammatory activities, ivermectin has recently received US Food and Drug Administration (FDA) and EU approval for the treatment of adult human patients for a growing number of indications [24].

The nt230(del4) MDR1 mutation has to date been detected in diverse dog breeds, including Rough Collies and other related sheepdogs, such as Australian Shepherds, miniature Australian Shepherds, Border Collies, Shetland Sheepdogs, Old English Sheepdogs, English Shepherd, German Shepherd, White Swiss Shepherd, McNab as well as Wäller and two sight-hounds, Longhaired Whippet and Silken Windhound. From a genealogy perspective, all of the above breeds share a common ancestor that lived in Great Britain before the breeds were classified and registered in 1873 [15, 25]. This notion is consistent with genomic data that cluster these breeds in common clusters or sometimes even fail to differentiate between close varieties that may have undergone recent selection based on size, such as in the case of Rough Collies and Shetland Sheepdogs [26, 27].

A fast and simple detection method using allele-specific loop-mediated isothermal amplification (AS-LAMP) [28] as well as PCR-based diagnostic tests [29, 30] and the TaqMan allelic discrimination assay [15] were designed as a result of the high clinical importance of nt230(del4) MDR1 mutation detection. Efforts to map allele frequencies in affected pure breed dogs, some of their crosses, and unrelated purebred dogs have been made in different parts of the world [19, 25, 31–40]. These studies supply clinicians with regional information on the mutation distribution in their countries and highlight the need for a genetic test prior to any treatment involving common parasiticides in affected breeds and their crosses.

In Israel, spirocercosis is a widespread disease and dogs are routinely treated with macrocyclic lactones parasiticide. On average, more than 20 dogs are diagnosed annually, with the highest infection rates in the center of the country [41, 42]. The aim of this study was to determine the frequency of the mutant allele in Israel in the affected breeds, their crosses and undefined dogs, and to compare the data with recent worldwide studies. To the best of our knowledge, this is the first report on nt230(del4) MDR1 mutation frequency in Israel and it may provide a comparative perspective. It should be noted that the evaluation of nt230(del4) MDR1 mutation genetic disposition in diverse canine breeds was performed in order to inform medical and clinical professionals, rather than to illuminate the relationship of different genotypes with the clinical signs in each breed. The latter is not within the scope of this study.

Methods

Animals

Biological samples from 1416 dogs (blood, blood on paper and hair roots) were voluntarily and non-selectively obtained from veterinarians, breeders and owners from all regions of the country, and analyzed for the nt230(del4) MDR1 mutation as part of the diagnostic research service at our institute. A total of 481 samples from 7 purebred breeds known to bear the nt230(del4) MDR1 mutation allele (including 5 crosses of two of these breeds) and 280 crosses of these same breeds (dogs for which one parent was known to be a purebred dog, often either Australian Shepherd or Border Collie), 61 unrelated purebred dogs and 594 unclassified crosses (mongrels, dogs for which either both parents were known to be non-purebred dogs or the parentage was unclassified) were obtained. Breed status was reported by the veterinarian or owner, and was not confirmed by other inspection.

DNA extraction

DNA from blood and blood on paper samples was extracted with the Chelex method using Bio-Rad, 'InstaGeneTM Matrix'. Briefly, 5 μL of whole blood (or 0.25 cm^2 paper with blood) were incubated at room temperature for 15–30 min and then centrifuged at 12,000 rpm for 3 min. The supernatant was carefully withdrawn and 200 μL of InstaGene matrix were added to the pellet and incubated at 56 °C for 15–30 min, vortexed and incubated in a 100 °C heat block for 8 min. After incubation, spin down was performed at 12,000 rpm for 3 min. The resulting supernatant contained the DNA. DNA from hair roots was extracted with the nexttec 'Special Protocol DNA Isolation Hair by nexttec™ 1-Step'. Briefly, three to five hair roots were dissolved with Proteinase K and DTT. Samples were then incubated in a shaker (at 56 °C, 200 rpm for 2 h). Then, 100 μL of the lysates were incubated for 3 min at room temperature and later centrifuged and eluted at 700×g for 1 min. All procedures were performed according to these kits' extraction manuals and according to the facility guidelines.

Genotyping by Taqman assay

nt230(del4) MDR1 mutation was screened using the Fluidigm BioMark apparatus (Fluidigm Corporation US) with an Assay-specific TaqMan fluorescence probe mix. The probe sequences, which were designed following NC_006596.3, are as follows: VIC Probe Sequence was ATGACAGATAGCTTTGCAA (wt), FAM Probe Sequence AACATGACAGCTTTGCAAA (mutant); the forward and reverse primers are CCATCATCCATG GAGCTGC and CACAAATAATACTTACTTTCATTA ATTATAACTGG, respectively, amplicon size 133 bp. Assay along with PCR master mix were run in duplicate by loading 5 μl into each well of the primed 96.96 Fluidigm Chip. The chip was then placed in the integrated fluidic circuit controller and loaded before analysis with the BioMark reader. The following thermal cycling protocol was used: 50°C (2 min), 70°C (30 min), 25°C (10 min), 50°C (2 min), and 95°C (4 min). This was followed by 40 cycles of 95°C (10 s) and 61°C (30 s). The initial cycle [50°C (2 min), 70°C (30 min), 25°C (10 min)]. Data were analyzed and cycle threshold (CT) values were determined using BioMark real-time PCR analysis software (Fluidigm Corp.), and automated mutation calling was carried out using an algorithm based on the change in CT (DCT) values between the wild-type and the mutant.

Validation by PCR and Sanger sequencing

Each nt230(del4) MDR1 mutated allele was validated by PCR and Sanger sequencing. The nt230(del4) MDR1 mutation region was amplified using a touchdown reaction (4 cycles: 94°C (30 s), 58°C (30 s), 72°C (30 s); 30 cycles: 94°C (30 s), 56°C (30 s), 72°C (30 s)) with the following forward and reverse primers: TTTTTAGTTT CGCTATTCAAATTGGC and CAAACTTATTACCAA TATTAACTGTAGCTC, respectively. Sequencing reactions for both DNA strands were performed with BigDye Terminator Cycle Sequencing Ready Reaction Kit (Applied Biosystems, Foster City, CA) and analyzed with an automatic sequencer (Applied Biosystems).

Data analysis

Breeds were classified into two main groups according to nt230(del4) MDR1 mutated allele breed genealogy: Related (as detailed in the introduction) and non-related (all others). Within each group, breeds were subsequently separated into pure breeds and mix breeds. Worldwide mapping of the allelic frequency of nt230(del4) MDR1 mutation only includes breeds for which at least 50 dogs were genotyped.

Results and discussion

nt230(del4) MDR1 mutation allelic frequencies in Israel

Raw data is provided in Additional file 1 (for each sample ID, the breed and MDR1 genotype status are indicated). Table 1 summarizes the allelic frequencies of the canine nt230(del4) MDR1 mutation in Israel in all mentioned subgroups. The nt230(del4) MDR1 mutation frequency varied markedly by breed. Among the relatively abundant breeds (sample size greater than 10 dogs, not including 37.5% for Old English Sheepdog where the sample size was only 4 dogs), it was highest for Australian Shepherds

Table 1 Observed frequencies of nt230(del4) MDR1 mutation in related (affected known breeds, pure and crossed ones), and non-related (un-affected known breeds and mongrels) breeds in Israel

nt230(del4) MDR1 mutation allele breed genealogy	Breed			Frequency of nt230(del4) MDR1 mutation allele status [%]			
	Name	Status	Sample size	Homozygote (−/−)	Heterozygote (+/−)	Normal (+/+)	Frequency of nt230(del4) MDR1 mutation allele
Related	Australian Shepherd	Pure	145	9.0%	44.8%	46.2%	31.4%
	Australian Shepherd	Crosses	32	0.0%	15.6%	84.4%	7.8%
	Border Collie	Pure	261	2.3%	5.0%	92.7%	4.8%
	Border Collie	Crosses	183	0.0%	6.0%	94.0%	3.0%
	Border Collie X Australian Shepherd	Pure	5	0.0%	20.0%	80.0%	10.0%
	Rough Collie	Pure	20	5.0%	45.0%	50.0%	27.5%
	Rough Collie	Crosses	49	2.0%	4.1%	93.9%	4.1%
	German Shepherd	Pure	21	0.0%	4.8%	95.2%	2.4%
	German Shepherd	Crosses	11	0.0%	0.0%	90.9%	0.0%
	White Swiss Shepherd	Pure	12	8.3%	16.7%	75.0%	16.7%
	White Swiss Shepherd	Crosses	4	0.0%	0.0%	75.0%	0.0%
	Shetland Sheepdog	Pure	13	0.0%	53.8%	46.2%	26.9%
	Shetland Sheepdog	Crosses	1	0.0%	0.0%	100.0%	0.0%
	Old English Sheepdog	Pure	4	0.0%	75.0%	25.0%	37.5%
	Old English Sheepdog	Crosses	0	0%	0.0%	0.0%	0%
Non-Related	Others	Pure	61	0.0%	0.0%	100.0%	0.0%
	Others (mongrels)	Crosses	594	0.0%	1.9%	98.1%	0.9%

'+' stands for WT allele; '-' stands for nt230(del4) MDR1 mutation allele

(31.4%, where 9.0% of 145 dogs were homozygotes for the mutation), Rough Collies (27.5%, $n = 20$ and 5.0%, respectively), and Shetland Sheepdog (26.9%, $n = 13$ and 0%, respectively), followed by White Swiss Shepherd (16.7%, $n = 12$ and 8.3%, respectively), Border Collie (4.8%, $n = 269$ and 2.3%, respectively), and German Shepherd (2.4%, $n = 21$ and 0%, respectively). As expected, an intermediate frequency (10.0%) was observed in crosses of pure Australian Shepherds and pure Border Collies ($n = 5$). The respective allelic frequencies among crosses of these breeds were much lower compared to their purebred counterpart, as expected: 4 and 1.6 times lower in Australian Shepherd (7.8%, $n = 32$) and Border Collie (3.0%, $n = 183$), respectively. The nt230(del4) MDR1 mutation allele was not detected in any of the unrelated purebred dogs ($n = 61$), as expected [43]. Almost 2% ($n = 594$) of the mongrels are affected (heterozygotes for the mutation, allelic frequency of almost 0.9%), a finding that justifies a more cautious approach in the clinic in case of unspecified dogs. This value is at the lower end of the previously reported 2–7% [32, 37].

A worldwide view – Comparative perspective

Figure 1 presents a comparative view of the Israeli and the worldwide nt230(del4) MDR1 mutation allelic frequencies. In most cases, the frequencies in Israel seem to be similar to those in other countries, whereas in other cases the range of frequencies is wide [also see 6]. These values might also be biased by the sample size, which varied greatly in different studies, and/or by the collection method. The frequencies observed for Australian Shepherd dogs living in Israel, US, Europe and Japan are similar, ranging from 25% to 33%, while higher frequencies were observed in the UK and Australia (~45%). Allelic frequencies for Border Collie are below 1% across the world, except 2.3% in the UK, compared to a much higher frequency in Israel (4.8%). This might be an indication for over inbreeding of carrier dogs in Israel. In contradistinction, the worldwide frequencies for Rough Collies are very high (55% or higher) compared to an almost 2-fold lower rate in Israel (28%, however the sample size was small). This study provides evidence for the existence of the mutation in the popular German Shepherd, for the first time outside the US, with frequencies ranging from ~2.5% to ~4%. Similarly the nt230(del4) MDR1 mutation allele is reported in White Swiss Shepherd outside Europe, for the first time, with a similar frequency in Israel (~15%). These two latter pure breeds, the German Shepherd and the White Swiss Shepherd, arise from the same lineage, as older breed standards of the German Shepherd allowed all color varieties, including white [38]. The differences in allelic frequencies between these breeds

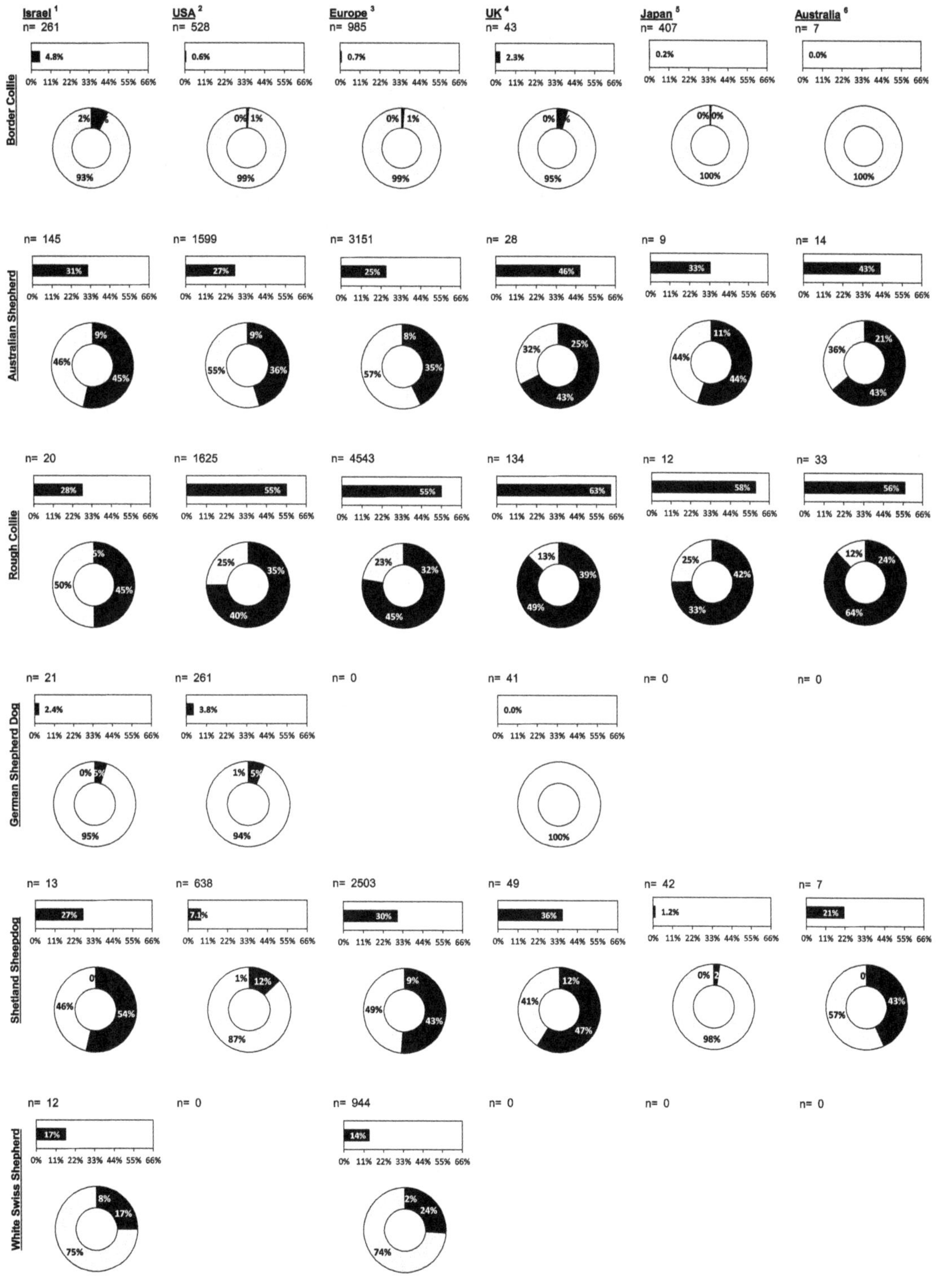

1 This study
2 References: [Neff et al., 2004; Mealey et al., 2002; Mealey and Meurs, 2008]
3 References: [Baars et al., 2008; Firdova et al., 2016; Geyer et al., 2005a; Geyer et al., 2007; Gramer et al., 2011; Hugnet et al., 2004]
4 References: [Parker, 2012; Tappin et al., 2012]
5 References: [Kawabata et al., 2005; Mizukami et al., 2012]
6 References: [Mealey et al., 2005]

Fig. 1 (See legend on next page.)

(See figure on previous page.)
Fig. 1 Allelic frequencies of nt230(del4) MDR1 mutation in six related breeds (from top to bottom: Border Collie, Australian Shepherd, Collie, German Shepherd Dog, Shetland Sheepdog and White Swiss Shepherd) in Israel, USA, Europe, UK, Japan and Australia (footnotes 1 to 6 respectively with the relevant literature in the bottom of the panel). Dogs number is given on top of each panel as n. Bar graph indicate allele frequency of each breed, pie graph indicate allelic frequencies of nt230(del4) MDR1 mutation as follows: pale gray for normal (+/+), gray for heterozygote (+/−) and black for homozygote (−/−)

might indicate over inbreeding in the case of the White Swiss Shepherd or for a founder effect in the breeds founding stock, back in the 1960s and 1970s [38]. The allelic frequency observed for Shetland Sheepdogs in Israel is very similar to that in Europe (27% and 30%, respectively), close to that in Australia (21%) and the UK (36%), while the frequencies in the US (7.1%) and Japan (1.2%) are much lower.

It is pertinent to state that the relative proportion of affected (predominantly pure) breeds, in the overall tested dogs in this study, might be higher than their actual proportion in Israel. The bias is related to samples collection by professional veterinarians for clinical purposes, as these are mainly limited to certain affected breeds, or dogs that resemble these breeds, from specific areas of the country where spirocercosis is more widespread [41]. Nevertheless, the allelic frequency of nt230(del4) MDR1 mutation within each affected breed is probably not significantly (if at all) affected by this bias, while it can be affected in the non-related breeds.

Conclusions

Here, we report for the first time on the allelic frequencies of the nt230(del4) MDR1 mutation in affected breeds, as well as in their crosses and even in mongrels, in Israel. The Israeli data was compared to a worldwide literature survey which summarizes the corresponding allele status in the USA, Europe, UK, Australia and Japan. The main findings are:

- nt230(del4) MDR1 mutation allele frequencies in Israel resemble, per breed, the status in the world. Exceptions to this finding are the Israeli Border Collies and Rough Collies which have the highest (4.8%) and lowest (28%) frequency rates in the world.
- The first report on the existence of the nt230(del4) MDR1 mutated allele outside the USA and Europe on German Shepherd Dogs and White Swiss Shepherds, respectively.
- High prevalence rate of the nt230(del4) MDR1 mutated allele in mixes of prone breeds.
- The nt230(del4) MDR1 mutation frequency in dogs which were described as unrelated mongrels is 1%.

Noteworthy, due to inherent bias in the sample collection by veterinarians for clinical purposes, the relative proportion of affected breeds, in the overall tested dogs, might be higher than their actual proportion in Israel. Nevertheless, the allelic frequency of nt230(del4) MDR1 mutation within each affected breed is probably not significantly affected by this bias, while it can be affected in the non-related breeds.

The allelic frequencies of the nt230(del4) MDR1 mutation in affected breeds seems to vary slightly across the world. This notion is in agreement with the strict registry breeding procedures in breeding clubs that do not permit "new genes" to enter the breeding stock. The breeding aims at meeting the breed standard, which is a combination of phenotypic and characteristic traits with less emphasis on genetic predisposition for ailments.

This work, that for the first time presents the nt230(del4) MDR1 mutation frequency status in Israel, along with a worldwide survey, has implications for clinicians, owners and breeders of sheepdogs and their crosses and supports the need for extra care in treatment and in future breeding.

Abbreviations

ABC: ATP-Binding Cassette transporters superfamily;; *ABCB1*: ABC subfamily B member 1; *AS-LAMP*: Allele-Specific Loop-Mediated isothermal amplification; *CNS*: Central Nervous System; *FDA*: Food and Drug Administration; *MDR1*: Multi Drug Resistance 1; *P-gp*: P-glycoprotein

Acknowledgements

The authors thank Mrs. Esther Furman for linguistic editing and editorial assistance.

Funding

This research received no specific grant from any funding agency in the public, commercial, or not-for-profit sectors.

Authors' contributions

We hereby declare that all authors made substantial contributions to conception and design / acquisition of data / analysis and interpretation of data; were involved in drafting the article / revising it critically for important intellectual content; gave final approval of the version to be published. Therefore, each of the authors takes public responsibility for the content, and agrees to be accountable for all aspects of the work in ensuring that questions related to the accuracy or integrity of any part of the work are appropriately investigated and resolved. More specifically, these authors led the following tasks: Conceptualization: YD DB(2). Formal analysis and interpretation of data: YM YD. Investigation: AS DB(1) AA EK ONP YD DB(2) YP. Project administration: YD DB(2) YP. Resources: GE YD YP. Supervision: YD DB(2) IBS YP. Validation: YD YM. Visualization: YM. Writing – original draft: YD YM. Writing – review and editing: YD YM DB(2) ISB YP EK AS AA DB(1) ONP GE. All authors read and approved the final manuscript.

Consent for publication

Not applicable.

Competing interests

The author declares that he/she has no competing interests.

Author details

[1]Shamir Research Institute, University of Haifa, P.O.Box 97, 1290000 Kazerin, Israel. [2]Zefat Academic College, Zefat, Israel. [3]Tel Hai College, 12210 Tel-Hai, Israel. [4]GGA – Galil Genetic Analysis Ltd, P.O.Box 3664, 12900 Kazerin, Israel. [5]Specialist in the Fields of Genetics, Epidemiology and Molecular Biology, Rehovot, Israel. [6]Vetmarket Ltd. Industrial Park Hevel Modiin, P.O.Box 960, 6085001 Shoham, Israel. [7]Faculty of Medicine in the Galilee, Bar-Ilan University & Baruch Padeh Medical Center, Poria, Israel.

References

1. Saier MH Jr, Paulsen IT, Sliwinski MK, Pao SS, Skurray RA, Nikaido H. Evolutionary origins of multidrug and drug-specific efflux pumps in bacteria. FASEB J. 1998;12(3):265–74.
2. Annilo T, Chen ZQ, Shulenin S, Costantino J, Thomas L, Lou H, Stefanov S, Dean M. Evolution of the vertebrate ABC gene family: analysis of gene birth and death. Genomics. 2006;88(1):1–11.
3. Dean M, Annilo T. Evolution of the ATP-binding cassette (ABC) transporter superfamily in vertebrates. Annu Rev Genomics Hum Genet. 2005;6:123–42.
4. Fromm MF. P-glycoprotein: a defense mechanism limiting oral bioavailability and CNS accumulation of drugs. Int J Clin Pharmacol Ther. 2000;38(2):69–74.
5. Fromm MF. Importance of P-glycoprotein at blood-tissue barriers. Trends Pharmacol Sci. 2004;25(8):423–9.
6. Geyer J, Janko C. Treatment of MDR1 mutant dogs with macrocyclic lactones. Curr Pharm Biotechnol. 2012;13(6):969–86.
7. Thuerauf N, Fromm MF. The role of the transporter P-glycoprotein for disposition and effects of centrally acting drugs and for the pathogenesis of CNS diseases. Eur Arch Psychiatry Clin Neurosci. 2006;256(5):281–6.
8. Preston JM. Adverse reactions to unapproved applications. The Veterinary record. 1983;112(12):286.
9. Seward RL. Reactions in dogs given ivermectin. J Am Vet Med Assoc. 1983; 183(5):493.
10. Pulliam JD, Seward RL, Henry RT, Steinberg SA. Investigating ivermectin toxicity in collies. Veterinary Medicine. 1985;80(7):33–40.
11. Mealey KL, Bentjen SA, Gay JM, Cantor GH. Ivermectin sensitivity in collies is associated with a deletion mutation of the mdr1 gene. Pharmacogenetics. 2001;11(8):727–33.
12. Roulet A, Puel O, Gesta S, Lepage JF, Drag M, Soll M, Alvinerie M, Pineau T. MDR1-deficient genotype in collie dogs hypersensitive to the P-glycoprotein substrate ivermectin. Eur J Pharmacol. 2003;460(2–3):85–91.
13. Bissonnette S, Paradis M, Daneau I, Silversides DW. The ABCB1-1Delta mutation is not responsible for subchronic neurotoxicity seen in dogs of non-collie breeds following macrocyclic lactone treatment for generalized demodicosis. Vet Dermatol. 2009;20(1):60–6.
14. Kitamura Y, Koto H, Matsuura S, Kawabata T, Tsuchiya H, Kusuhara H, Tsujimoto H, Sugiyama Y. Modest effect of impaired P-glycoprotein on the plasma concentrations of fexofenadine, quinidine, and loperamide following oral administration in collies. Drug metabolism and disposition: the biological fate of chemicals. 2008;36(5):807–10.
15. Klintzsch S, Meerkamp K, Doring B, Geyer J. Detection of the nt230[del4] MDR1 mutation in dogs by a fluorogenic 5′ nuclease TaqMan allelic discrimination method. Veterinary journal (London, England : 1997). 2010; 185(3):272–7.
16. Krugman L, Bryan JN, Mealey KL, Chen A. Vincristine-induced central neurotoxicity in a collie homozygous for the ABCB1Delta mutation. J Small Anim Pract. 2012;53(3):185–7.
17. Henik RA, Kellum HB, Bentjen SA, Mealey KL. Digoxin and mexiletine sensitivity in a collie with the MDR1 mutation. Journal of veterinary internal medicine / American College of Veterinary Internal Medicine. 2006;20(2):415–7.
18. Sartor LL, Bentjen SA, Trepanier L, Mealey KL. Loperamide toxicity in a collie with the MDR1 mutation associated with ivermectin sensitivity. Journal of veterinary internal medicine / American College of Veterinary Internal Medicine. 2004;18(1):117–8.
19. Geyer J, Doring B, Godoy JR, Leidolf R, Moritz A, Petzinger E. Frequency of the nt230 (del4) MDR1 mutation in collies and related dog breeds in Germany. J Vet Pharmacol Ther. 2005;28(6):545–51.
20. Mealey KL, Northrup NC, Bentjen SA. Increased toxicity of P-glycoprotein-substrate chemotherapeutic agents in a dog with the MDR1 deletion mutation associated with ivermectin sensitivity. J Am Vet Med Assoc. 2003; 223(10):1453. -1455, 1434
21. Campbell O, de Lorimier LP, Mealey KL. Adverse reaction to apomorphine in a collie homozygous for the ABCB1-1 (MDR1) mutation. J Small Anim Pract. 2017;58(2):119.
22. Mealey KL, Fidel J. P-glycoprotein mediated drug interactions in animals and humans with cancer. Journal of veterinary internal medicine / American College of Veterinary Internal Medicine. 2015;29(1):1–6.
23. Mealey KL, Dassanayake S, Burke NS. Establishment of a cell line for assessing drugs as canine P-glycoprotein substrates: proof of principle. J Vet Pharmacol Ther. 2017;40(5):545–51.
24. Kircik LH, Del Rosso JQ, Layton AM, Schauber J. Over 25 years of clinical experience with Ivermectin: an overview of safety for an increasing number of indications. Journal of drugs in dermatology. 2016;15(3):325–32.
25. Neff MW, Robertson KR, Wong AK, Safra N, Broman KW, Slatkin M, Mealey KL, Pedersen NC. Breed distribution and history of canine mdr1-1Delta, a pharmacogenetic mutation that marks the emergence of breeds from the collie lineage. Proc Natl Acad Sci U S A. 2004;101(32):11725–30.
26. Parker HG, Kim LV, Sutter NB, Carlson S, Lorentzen TD, Malek TB, Johnson GS, DeFrance HB, Ostrander EA, Kruglyak L. Genetic structure of the purebred domestic dog. Science (New York, NY). 2004;304(5674):1160–4.
27. Parker HG. Genomic analyses of modern dog breeds. Mamm Genome. 2012;23(1–2):19–27.
28. Stiedl CP, Weber K. Fast and simple detection methods for the 4-base pair deletion of canine MDR1/ ABCB1 gene by PCR and isothermal amplification. J Vet Diagn Investig. 2017;29(2):176–80.
29. Geyer J, Doring B, Godoy JR, Moritz A, Petzinger E. Development of a PCR-based diagnostic test detecting a nt230(del4) MDR1 mutation in dogs: verification in a moxidectin-sensitive Australian shepherd. J Vet Pharmacol Ther. 2005;28(1):95–9.
30. Baars C, Leeb T, von Klopmann T, Tipold A, Potschka H. Allele-specific polymerase chain reaction diagnostic test for the functional MDR1 polymorphism in dogs. Veterinary journal (London, England : 1997). 2008; 177(3):394–7.
31. Firdova Z, Turnova E, Bielikova M, Turna J, Dudas A. The prevalence of ABCB1:c.227_230delATAG mutation in affected dog breeds from European countries. Res Vet Sci. 2016;106:89–92.
32. Gramer I, Leidolf R, Doring B, Klintzsch S, Kramer EM, Yalcin E, Petzinger E, Geyer J. Breed distribution of the nt230(del4) MDR1 mutation in dogs. Veterinary journal (London, England : 1997). 2011;189(1):67–71.
33. Hugnet C, Bentjen SA, Mealey KL. Frequency of the mutant MDR1 allele associated with multidrug sensitivity in a sample of collies from France. J Vet Pharmacol Ther. 2004;27(4):227–9.
34. Mealey KL, Bentjen SA, Waiting DK. Frequency of the mutant MDR1 allele associated with ivermectin sensitivity in a sample population of collies from the northwestern United States. Am J Vet Res. 2002;63(4):479–81.
35. Mizukami K, Chang HS, Yabuki A, Kawamichi T, Hossain MA, Rahman MM, Uddin MM, Yamato O. Rapid genotyping assays for the 4-base pair deletion of canine MDR1/ABCB1 gene and low frequency of the mutant allele in border collie dogs. J Vet Diagn Investig. 2012;24(1):127–34.
36. Tappin SW, Goodfellow MR, Peters IR, Day MJ, Hall EJ, Mealey KL. Frequency of the mutant MDR1 allele in dogs in the UK. The Veterinary record. 2012; 171(3):72.

37. Mealey KL, Meurs KM. Breed distribution of the ABCB1-1Delta (multidrug sensitivity) polymorphism among dogs undergoing ABCB1 genotyping. J Am Vet Med Assoc. 2008;233(6):921–4.
38. Geyer J, Klintzsch S, Meerkamp K, Wohlke A, Distl O, Moritz A, Petzinger E. Detection of the nt230(del4) MDR1 mutation in white Swiss shepherd dogs: case reports of doramectin toxicosis, breed predisposition, and microsatellite analysis. J Vet Pharmacol Ther. 2007;30(5):482–5.
39. Kawabata A, Momoi Y, Inoue-Murayama M, Iwasaki T. Canine mdr1 gene mutation in Japan. The Journal of veterinary medical science / the Japanese Society of Veterinary Science. 2005;67(11):1103–7.
40. Mealey KL, Munyard KA, Bentjen SA. Frequency of the mutant MDR1 allele associated with multidrug sensitivity in a sample of herding breed dogs living in Australia. Vet Parasitol. 2005;131(3–4):193–6.
41. Aroch I, Markovics A, Mazaki-Tovi M, Kuzi S, Harrus S, Yas E, Baneth G, Bar-El M, Bdolah-Abram T, Segev G, et al. Spirocercosis in dogs in Israel: a retrospective case-control study (2004-2009). Vet Parasitol. 2015;211(3–4): 234–40.
42. Gottlieb Y, Lavy E, Kaufman M, Markovics A, Ghanim M, Aroch I. A novel bacterial symbiont in the nematode Spirocerca lupi. BMC Microbiol. 2012;12:133.
43. Merola VM, Eubig PA. Toxicology of avermectins and milbemycins (macrocylic lactones) and the role of P-glycoprotein in dogs and cats. Vet Clin North Am Small Anim Pract. 2012;42(2):313–33. vii

13

Escherichia coli-derived recombinant human bone morphogenetic protein-2 combined with bone marrow-derived mesenchymal stromal cells improves bone regeneration in canine segmental ulnar defects

Takamasa Itoi[1*], Yasuji Harada[1], Hiroyuki Irie[2], Michiko Sakamoto[2], Katsutoshi Tamura[3], Takuya Yogo[1], Satoshi Soeta[4], Hajime Amasaki[4], Yasushi Hara[1] and Masahiro Tagawa[1]

Abstract

Background: Large bone defects in canines usually require assistance to achieve healing. Implantation of osteoinductive factors can promote bone healing, while transplantation of osteoprogenitor cells can enhance bone regeneration. We hypothesized that implantation of an osteoinductive factor, recombinant human bone morphogenetic protein-2 (rhBMP-2), combined with osteoprogenitor cells, bone marrow-derived mesenchymal stromal cells (BMSCs), would synergistically promote bone healing. In this study, we examined the combined effects of *Escherichia coli*-derived rhBMP-2 and BMSCs on bone healing after implantation into canine ulnar defects.

Results: Critical-sized osteoperiosteal segmental defects (2.5 cm) were created in the ulnae of healthy female beagle dogs, and implanted with combinations of *E. coli*-derived rhBMP-2 (560 or 140 μg) and autologous BMSCs (10^7, 10^5, or 0 cells). In the present study,18 forelimbs of nine healthy purpose-bred female beagles were used. All six treatment groups contained three forelimbs, and the animals were euthanized after 12 weeks. The control groups (560 and 140 μg/0 cells) were cited from our previous study to reduce the number of experimental animals. Radiographically, the regenerated bone width was significantly increased in the 560 or 140 μg with 10^7 and 10^5 cells groups compared with the 0 cells groups. By quantitative CT, the bone mineral density was higher in the 560 μg with 10^7 and 10^5 cells groups, while non-uniformity of the bone mineral density was improved in the 560 μg with 10^7 and 10^5 cells groups and 140 μg/10^7 cells group. Mechanically, the maximum loads at failure were significantly higher in the 560 μg with 10^7 and 10^5 cells groups. Histologically, the regenerated bone was well-developed and contained osteocyte-like cells marrow cavities, and vessels. However, the osteoclasts and osteoblasts were hardly observed. The osteocyte-like cell numbers were significantly higher in the 560 μg with 10^7 and 10^5 cells and 140 μg with 10^7 and 10^5 cells groups.

Conclusions: Implantation of *E. coli*-derived rhBMP-2 and BMSCs led to significantly enhanced bone formation, with improved bone mineral density and reduced non-uniformity of the regenerated bone. Combined implantation of rhBMP-2 and BMSCs may be useful for promotion of bone healing in critical-sized defects in canines.

Keywords: Recombinant human bone morphogenetic protein-2, Bone marrow-derived mesenchymal stromal cells, Bone regeneration, Canine, Ulnar defect

* Correspondence: takamasa.itoi@hotmail.co.jp
[1]Division of Veterinary Surgery, Nippon Veterinary and Life Science University, 1-7-1 Kyonan-cho, Musashino, Tokyo 180-8602, Japan
Full list of author information is available at the end of the article

Background

Many studies have suggested that osteoinductive factors, such as bone morphogenetic proteins (BMPs), can greatly increase bone regeneration [1–7]. Currently, recombinant human bone morphogenetic protein-2 (rhBMP-2) is used in veterinary medicine for treatment of canines with non-unions [8, 9], arthrodesis [10, 11], and mandibular defects [12, 13].

In a previous study, we evaluated the healing efficacy of *Escherichia coli*-derived rhBMP-2 in a canine model [14]. The animals administered higher doses of rhBMP-2 (560 μg/site or more) showed larger callus formation and integration with the host bone, while those administered lower doses (140 μg/site or less) showed smaller callus formation and incomplete integration the host bone. However, the higher doses of rhBMP-2 also led to transient decreases in bone mineral density during the early stage of treatment. Because rhBMP-2 promotes bone regeneration by activating progenitor cell recruitment, proliferation, and differentiation [15–19], we hypothesized that implantation of rhBMP-2 combined with osteoprogenitor cells would improve bone regeneration.

Bone marrow-derived mesenchymal stromal cells (BMSCs) comprise a heterogeneous population of multipotent cells, including mesenchymal stem cells, which have frequently been investigated as a cell source for regenerative medicine applications [20–23]. Mesenchymal stem cells were first isolated from bone marrow in 1991 by Caplan [24], and have the potential to differentiate into multilineage cells, including osteoblasts. Several studies have examined the regeneration of bone defects following transplantation of BMSCs combined with artificial bone ceramics [25, 26]. Thus, we hypothesized that the combination of *E. coli*-derived rhBMP-2 and BMSCs would synergistically affect bone regeneration. The purpose of this study was to determine the effects of implantation of rhBMP-2 combined with BMSCs on the regeneration of segmental canine ulnar defects. The newly formed bone structures and mechanical strengths were evaluated by X-rays, computed tomography (CT), mechanical testing, and histology.

Methods

Experimental design

Because this study was performed using identical conditions to our previous study [14] and we wanted to reduce the number of experimental animals, the data for the two control groups not implanted with cells are cited from our previous study.

In the study, 18 forelimbs of nine healthy purpose-bred female beagle dogs (age: 1 year; body weight: 9.4–11.0 kg) were used. The animals were maintained under uniform conditions in our institutional animal laboratory. The surgical techniques were described previously [14]. Briefly, at 15 min after administration of droperidol (0.25 mg/kg, intramuscular; Sankyo Co., Tokyo, Japan), anesthesia was induced with propofol (7 mg/kg, intravenous; Fuji Pharma Co. Ltd., Toyama, Japan) and maintained with inhalation of isoflurane (1.5–2.0 %; Mylan Inc., Osaka, Japan) and oxygen. Before surgery, 2 % lidocaine hydrochloride (1 mL/4.5 kg; AstraZeneca, Osaka, Japan) and 0.5 % bupivacaine hydrochloride (1 mL/4.5 kg; AstraZeneca) were injected around the brachial plexus to induce local anesthesia. Critical-sized osteoperiosteal segmental defects of 2.5 cm were created on the ulnae of the canines distal to the interosseous ligament using an oscillating saw. The defects were approximately three times larger than the diameter of the ulnar shaft at its mid-point, reported as a critical size that does not heal spontaneously [27].

After defect creation, 700 mg of β-tricalcium phosphate granules containing *E. coli*-derived rhBMP-2 and autologous BMSCs was implanted into the defect. The experimental forelimbs were divided into six groups of three forelimbs treated with 560 or 140 μg of rhBMP-2 and 10^7, 10^5, or 0 BMSCs, designated 560 μg/10^7 cells, 560 μg/10^5 cells, 560 μg/0 cells, 140 μg/10^7 cells, 140 μg/10^5 cells, and 140 μg/0 cells. The perioperative analgesic management included preoperative and postoperative administration of buprenorphine (20 μg/kg, intramuscular; Otsuka Pharmaceutical Co. Ltd., Tokyo, Japan). Buprenorphine was administered twice a day for 3 days postoperatively. For 7 days postoperatively, 25 mg/kg ampicillin was administered orally twice daily. The forelimbs underwent radiographic examinations preoperatively and postoperatively, and then weekly thereafter using a lateral view, and the width of the regenerated bone was measured. CT scanning was performed with 1.0-mm slice thickness in the axial plane at time 0 (post-operation) and at 4, 8, and 12 weeks postoperatively with the canines under general anesthesia. At 12 weeks postoperatively, the animals were euthanized with an overdose of injected pentobarbital sodium (Somnopentyl; Kyoritsu Seiyaku Co., Tokyo, Japan). The tissues, including the regenerated bones, were harvested for mechanical and histological examinations. As noted above, the data for the two control groups not treated with cells are cited from our previous study [14], and thus mechanical testing was not performed on these two groups.

Preparation of the implants

The *E. coli*-derived rhBMP-2 used in this study was supplied by Osteopharma Inc. (Osaka, Japan). Although *E. coli*-derived rhBMP-2 is not glycosylated, unlike Chinese hamster ovary cell-derived rhBMP-2, a previous in vitro study suggested that the biological activities of rhBMP-2 derived from these two different cellular origins are similar [28]. The biodegradable artificial bone β-tricalcium phosphate granules used were produced by HOYA Technosurgical Corporation (Tokyo, Japan). The granules had diameters of 2–4 mm, and were composed of interconnecting porous structures (pore size: 50–300 μm; porosity: 75 %). Freeze-dried *E. coli*-derived rhBMP-2 powder (140 or 560 μg) was reconstituted in 0.32 mL of sterile distilled water before use. Approximately 15 min before implantation, 0.32 mL of rhBMP-2 solution was dripped onto 700 mg of β-tricalcium phosphate granules and allowed to infiltrate.

Autologous BMSCs were isolated from the bone marrow of each animal at 10 days before transplantation. Under general anesthesia, bone marrow was aspirated from the proximal humerus using standard bone marrow biopsy techniques. A sterile 13-gauge Jamshidi needle was used to aspirate 5 mL of bone marrow into a syringe containing 5 mL of heparinized (1,000 U/mL) saline solution. The techniques reported by Kadiyala et al. [29] were used for bone marrow harvesting and BMSC isolation. To obtain BMSC-enriched nucleated cells, density separation was performed using Lymphoprep (Axis-Shield, Oslo, Norway). Briefly, bone marrow cells in phosphate-buffered saline (10 mL) were carefully layered onto 5 mL of Lymphoprep, and separated by centrifugation at 800 × *g* for 30 min at room temperature. The nucleated cells were collected from the solution/Lymphoprep interface, washed in phosphate-buffered saline, and plated in T-75 cell culture flasks with 10 mL of Dulbecco's modified Eagle's medium supplemented with 10 % fetal bovine serum and 1 % antibiotic/antimycotic solution (control medium). The cells were incubated at 37 °C in a humidified 5 % CO_2 environment, and the medium was changed twice weekly. When the primary cultures reached 70–80 % confluency, the attached cells were passaged by exposure to 0.25 % trypsin/1 mM EDTA for 3 min. The detached cells were replated at 8.0×10^3 cells/cm^2. Either 10^7 or 10^5 BMSCs were suspended in 0.32 mL of saline and seeded onto the rhBMP-2-treated β-tricalcium phosphate granules immediately before implantation. Saline alone (0.32 mL) was seeded onto the rhBMP-2-treated β-tricalcium phosphate granules in the groups receiving 0 cells.

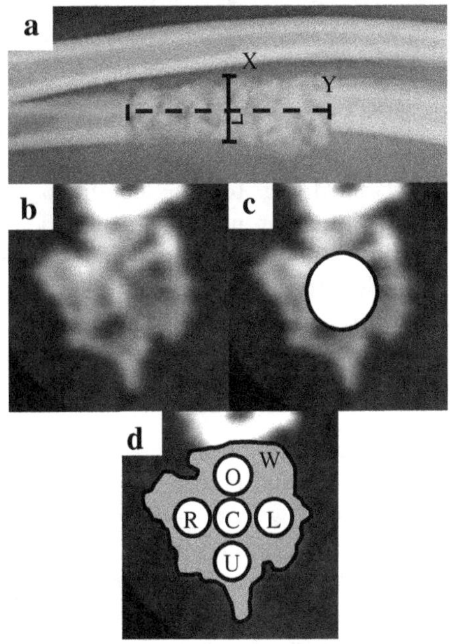

Fig. 1 Measurement methods for the experiments. **a** Lateral-view X-ray of the experimental region. The width of the regenerated bone was determined by calculating the length of the perpendicular line "X" at the midpoint of the longitudinal line "Y" in the defect. **b** Transverse-plane CT image of the central portion of the regenerated bone. **c** The bone mineral density was calculated by measuring the CT-determined Hounsfield units in the 5.5-mm diameter ROI at the center of the regenerated bone and the calibration phantom. **d** The non-uniformity of the bone mineral density was calculated by measuring the CT-determined Hounsfield units in the whole area W and in five points within the specified 1.5-mm diameter ROI

Width of the regenerated bone

The width of the regenerated bone was measured on a lateral view radiograph. An aluminum plate (25 mm × 74 mm) was exposed alongside the forelimbs to standardize the magnification and contrast for all X-ray images. A line perpendicular to the midpoint of the long axis of the regenerated bone was measured, and the distance between the outer edges of the intersections of the line was defined as the regenerated bone width (Fig. 1a).

Bone mineral density of the regenerated bone

The bone mineral density of the regenerated bone was measured using a quantitative CT method [30, 31] on a transverse plane reconstruction in the middle region of the defect. Quantitative CT is a volumetric method for estimating the mass of hydroxyapatite per cubic centimeter of bone tissue. The slice thickness was maintained at 1 mm, and the forelimbs were scanned along with a calibration phantom (B-MAS200; Kyoto Kagaku Co. Ltd., Kyoto, Japan). A multiplanar reconstruction mode was used for the analysis (Fig. 1b). Twenty-five slices of 1-mm thickness were reconstructed in each defect with correct alignment, and the thirteenth slice was defined as the center slice for assessment. The window width and window level were set at 1500 and 300 Hounsfield units, respectively. The mean Hounsfield units in a specified 5.5-mm diameter region of interest (ROI) were determined at the center of the regenerated bone and for the calibration phantom, after which the mean value of the bone mineral density was calculated (Fig. 1c).

Non-uniformity of the bone mineral density

The non-uniformity of the bone mineral density was calculated in the same CT image used to measure the bone mineral density. The mean bone mineral density for the whole area (W) and the mean bone mineral density inside a specified 1.5-mm diameter ROI based on five points were measured (Fig. 1d). The non-uniformity index was calculated as the root-mean-square deviation of the five measurement points, with W used as the "true" average. A completely uniform field resulted in a non-uniformity index of 0, and higher values indicated increased non-uniformity.

Mechanical testing

As noted above, the data for the two control groups not treated with cells are cited from our previous study [14], and thus mechanical testing was not performed on these two groups. After euthanasia of the animals at 12 weeks, the tissues including the regenerated bones were harvested with extra margins as necessary for mechanical testing. A three-point bending test was performed using a universal testing machine (858Mini Bionix II; MTS Systems Corporation, Tokyo, Japan). The crosshead speed was 2.5 mm/min, the distance between the fulcrum points was 60 mm, and the load was applied from the cranial side. The tests were destructive to allow determination of the maximum load at breaking point.

Histology

Immediately after the mechanical testing, the samples were fixed in 4 % paraformaldehyde for 2 days and then decalcified with EDTA. The decalcified samples were embedded in paraffin and sectioned in the sagittal plane at 3-μm thickness. The sections were stained with hematoxylin and eosin to show the structure of the regenerated bone. The density of osteocyte-like cells was calculated by counting the cell number and determining the area of newly formed trabecular bone within each field of view.

Statistical analysis

A two-way repeated measures ANOVA was used to investigate the effects of the different transplanted BMSC numbers with 560 μg or 140 μg of rhBMP-2 on the width of the regenerated bone, bone mineral density of the regenerated bone and non-uniformity of the bone mineral density. When a main effect was found, Tukey's honest significant difference test was used to compare the mean values between the groups at each time point.

A one-way repeated measures ANOVA was used to investigate the effects of the different transplanted BMSC numbers with 560 μg or 140 μg of rhBMP-2 on the mechanical testing and density of osteocyte-like cells. When a significant difference was found, Tukey's honest significant difference test was used to compare the mean values between the groups.

Values of $P < 0.05$ were considered statistically significant. All statistical analyses were performed using IBM SPSS Statistics, Version 16.0 (IBM Corp., Tokyo, Japan). All data are presented as mean ± SD.

Results

The surgery was performed smoothly with no postoperative pain in all groups. No complications developed in any of the groups during the study period.

X-ray analysis

Radiographs highlighting the postoperative changes in the six groups are shown in Fig. 2. At 4 weeks after surgery, the callus expansion peaked in all groups treated with 560 μg of rhBMP-2 and in the 140 μg/10^7 cells group, and the border between the regenerated bone and the host bone was nearly unidentifiable, especially in the distal region. In contrast, the 140 μg/10^5 cells group and one sample in the 140 μg/0 cells group showed relatively small callus formation. No external callus formation was observed in the other two samples in the 140 μg/0 cells group. A gap was visible between the graft and the host bone in the groups treated with 140 μg rhBMP-2 and 10^5 or 0 cells. The granularity of the implanted materials disappeared in all samples in all groups.

At 8 weeks after surgery, the remodeling process had progressed in all three groups treated with 560 μg rhBMP-2 and in the 140 μg/10^7 cells group, and the outline of the regenerated bone had adapted to fit the shape of the host bone, particularly on the distal side. In contrast, no changes were visible in the outline of the regenerated bone in the 140 μg groups with 10^5 and 0 cells. The distal side of the regenerated bone was completely integrated with the host bone in all three groups treated with 560 μg rhBMP-2 and in the 140 μg/10^7 cells group. On the proximal side, the regenerated bone was integrated for one sample in the 560 μg/10^7 cells group and two samples in the 560 μg/10^5 cells group. A radiolucent gap was observed at the proximal side for all samples in the 560 μg/0 cells group, but the cells were bridged to the host bone. Two samples in the 140 μg/10^5 cells group showed integration at the distal end, but all samples in the 140 μg/0 cells group showed a radiolucent gap on each side.

At 12 weeks after surgery, the distal part of the regenerated bone was completely integrated with the host bone in all samples in the three groups treated with 560 μg rhBMP-2 and in the 140 μg rhBMP-2 with 10^7 and 10^5 cells groups. The proximal part of the regenerated bone was also integrated with the host bone in all samples in the 560 μg with 10^7 and 10^5 cells groups, as

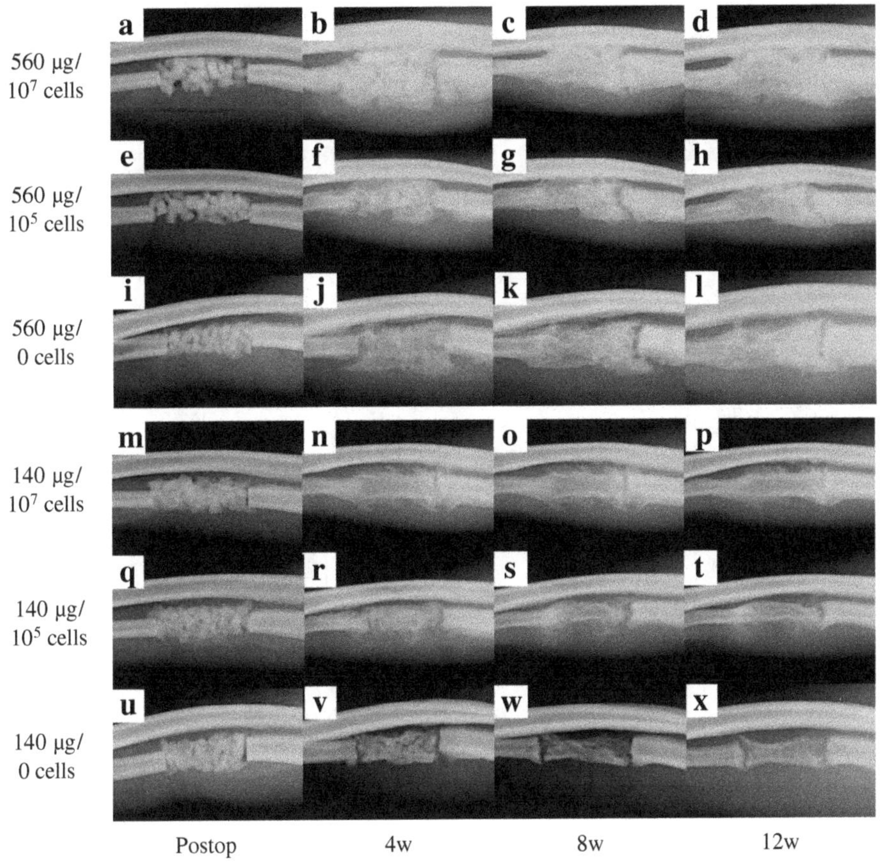

Fig. 2 Radiographs of the postoperative changes. **a**–**x** Postoperative images taken at 4, 8 and 12 weeks after surgery are shown for all six experimental groups: 560 µg rhBMP-2 with 10^7 (**a**–**d**), 10^5 (**e**–**h**), and 0 (**i**–**l**) cells, and 140 µg rhBMP-2 with 10^7 (**m**–**p**), 10^5 (**q**–**t**), and 0 (**u**–**x**) cells. The groups transplanted with BMSCs form more regenerated bone than the groups without cells at the same dose of rhBMP-2

well as in the 140 µg/10^7 cells group. Although a small gap was present at the proximal side of the lesion, it was covered by a callus in all samples in the 560 µg/0 cells group. The width of the regenerated bone was larger than or equal to that of the proximal ulna in all samples in the three groups treated with 560 µg and in the 140 µg with 10^7 and 10^5 cells groups. In two samples in the 140 µg/0 cells group, the regenerated bone was not integrated with the host bone and a distinct gap remained on each side. The width of the regenerated bone was nearly equal to or less than that of the proximal ulna.

Changes in the width of the regenerated bone over time

The sequential changes in the width of the regenerated bone over time after surgery measured on a lateral radiograph are shown in Fig. 3a. In the 560 µg/10^7 cells group, the width of the regenerated bone increased rapidly, peaked at 4 weeks, and then decreased slowly until 12 weeks. In the 560 µg/10^5 cells group, the width of the regenerated bone increased during the first 4 weeks, reached a peak, and then remained at the same level until 12 weeks. In the 560 µg/0 cells group, the regenerated bone width increased rapidly for 2 weeks, peaked at 4 weeks, and decreased slowly thereafter until 12 weeks. The widths of the regenerated bone in the 560 µg/10^7 cells group were significantly larger than those in the 560 µg/0 cells group at 1 to 12 weeks after transplantation. Furthermore, the width of the regenerated bone in the 560 µg/10^5 cells group was significantly larger than that in the 560 µg/0 cells group at 1 week after transplantation.

In the 140 µg/10^7 cells group, the regenerated bone width increased rapidly, peaked at 5 weeks, and then slowly decreased until 12 weeks. In the 140 µg/10^5 cells group, the regenerated bone width increased slowly, reached a peak at 3 weeks, and slowly decreased thereafter until 12 weeks. In the 140 µg/0 cells group, the regenerated bone width increased slightly, peaked at 2 weeks, and then decreased slowly until 12 weeks. The regenerated bone widths in the 140 µg/10^7 cells group were significantly larger than those in the 140 µg /0 cells group at 2 to 12 weeks after transplantation. Significant differences were found between the regenerated bone

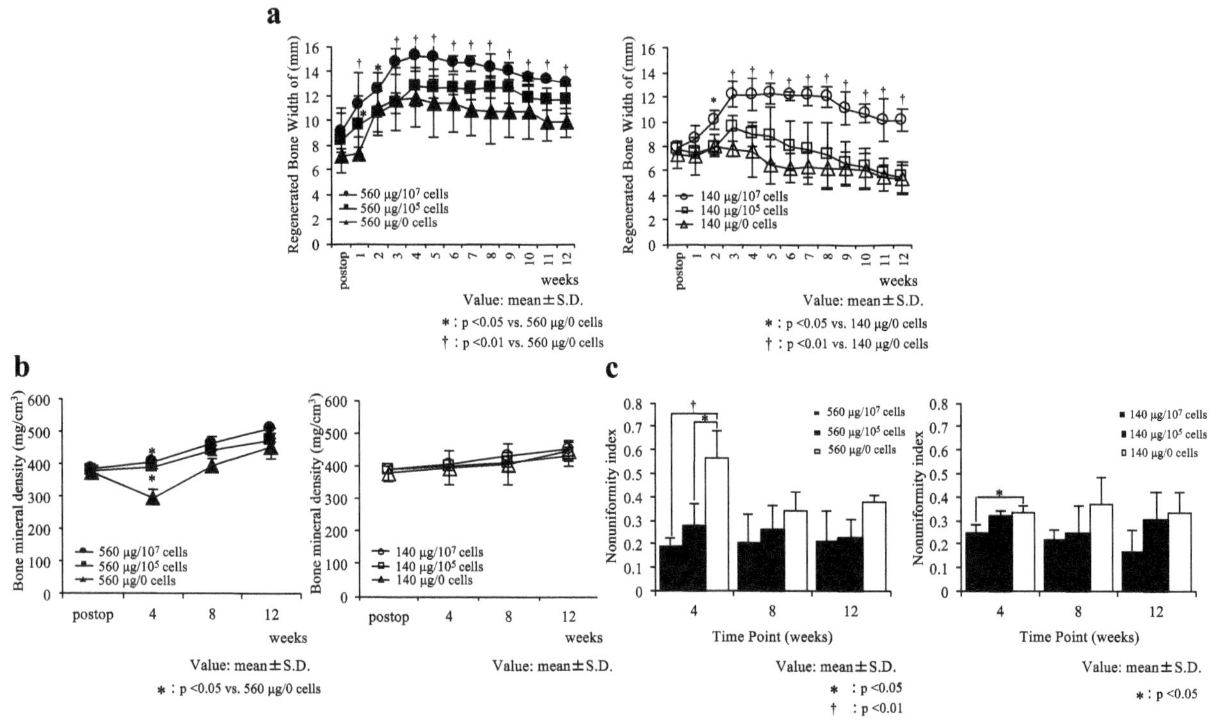

Fig. 3 X-ray examination. (Radiohraphic and CT examination). **a** Sequential changes in the width of the regenerated bone over time. The changes in the width of the regenerated bone (mean ± SD) over time are shown. The width of the regenerated bone is significantly larger in the groups treated with BMSCs than that in the groups treated with rhBMP-2 alone. *$P < 0.05$ vs 560 μg/0 cells or vs. 140 μg/0 cells. †$P < 0.01$ vs. 560 μg/0 cells or vs. 140 μg/0 cells. **b** Changes in the bone mineral density over time. The changes in the regenerated bone mineral density (mean ± SD) over time are shown. The inclusion of 10^7 and 10^5 BMSCs is able to prevent the transient decrease in the bone mineral density observed at 4 weeks after surgery for the high dose of rhBMP-2 without cells. The regenerated bone mineral densities in the 560 μg with 10^7 and 10^5 cells groups are significantly larger than that in the 560 μg/0 cells group at 4 weeks. No significant differences in the bone mineral density are found among the groups treated with 140 μg of rhBMP-2. *$P < 0.05$ vs. 560 μg/0 cells. **c** Non-uniformity index values of the bone mineral density in the regenerated bone. The changes in the non-uniformity index of the regenerated bone mineral density (mean ± SD) over time are shown. The non-uniformity index in the groups transplanted with both BMSCs and rhBMP-2 are significantly lower than those in the groups treated with rhBMP-2 alone at 4 weeks. The new bone in the 560 μg with 10^7 and 10^5 cells groups and in the 140 μg with 10^7 and 10^5 cells groups is more uniform than that in their respective control groups with 0 cells. *$P < 0.05$; †$P < 0.01$

widths in the 140 μg/10^7 cells and 560 μg/10^7 cells groups, but not between the 140 μg/10^7 cells and 560 μg/10^5 cells groups.

Changes in the bone mineral density of the regenerated bone over time

The changes in the bone mineral density over time after surgery, as measured by a quantitative CT method, are shown in Fig. 3b. The bone mineral densities of the implanted materials assessed postoperatively were nearly equal between- group. The bone mineral density in the 560 μg with 10^7 and 10^5 cells groups was slightly increased at 4 weeks and continued to increase until 12 weeks. The bone mineral density in the 560 μg/0 cells group showed a transient decrease at 4 weeks, but then increased until 12 weeks. The bone mineral density in the 560 μg/0 cells group was significantly lower than those in the 560 μg with 10^7 and 10^5 cells groups at 4 weeks. The bone mineral density in all three groups treated with 140 μg rhBMP-2 showed similar tendencies with no significant differences between the groups.

Non-uniformity of the bone mineral density

The non-uniformity index values for the bone mineral density of the regenerated bone after surgery in the different groups, as measured by the quantitative CT method, are shown in Fig. 3c. The non-uniformity index was significantly lower in the 560 μg with 10^7 and 10^5 cells groups than in the 560 μg/0 cells group at 4 weeks. Similarly, the non-uniformity index in the 140 μg/10^7 cells group was significantly lower than that in the 140 μg/0 cells group at 4 weeks.

Mechanical testing

The results of the mechanical testing are shown in Fig. 4. The maximum loads at failure in the 560 μg with 10^7

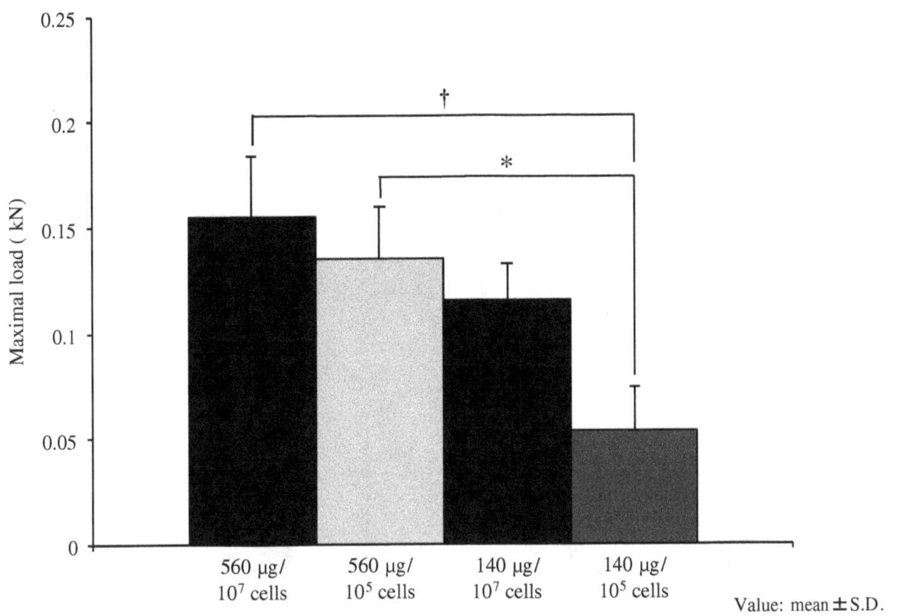

Fig. 4 Mechanical testing. This experiment was carried out in the 560 μg with 10^7 and 10^5 cells groups and the 140 μg with 10^7 and 10^5 cells groups, because the 560 μg/0 cells group and 560 μg/0 cells group are cited from our previous study The maximum loads at failure of the regenerated bone using a three-point bending test (mean ± SD) are shown. The regenerated bone in the 560 μg with 10^7 and 10^5 cells groups is mechanically stronger than that in the 140 μg/10^5 cells group. $^*P < 0.05$; $^\dagger P < 0.01$

and 10^5 cells groups were significantly higher than that in the 140 μg/10^5 cells group.

Histology

Representative images for the histology of the regenerated bone (magnification; ×400) are shown in Fig. 5a. The newly formed trabecular bone was well developed and contained osteocyte-like cells, marrow cavities, and vessels. The structure and thickness of the trabecular bone were similar among the different groups. In all samples, many flattened of spindle cells were observed, while osteoblasts that were activated and cuboidal were hardly observed. Osteoclasts that were multinuclear with large sizes were also hardly observed.

The numbers of osteocyte-like cells per trabecular bone area in the different groups are shown in Fig. 5b. The 560 μg with 10^7 and 10^5 cells groups had significantly more osteocyte-like cells than the 560 μg/0 cells group. Similarly, the numbers of osteocyte-like cells were significantly larger in the 140 μg with 10^7 and 10^5 cells groups than in the 140 μg/0 cells group.

Discussion

The results of the present study show that implantation of rhBMP-2 combined with BMSCs led to significantly larger amounts of bone formation than implantation of rhBMP-2 alone. The mechanism of action for the effects of BMPs involves regulation of gene expression by the transfer of bone-inducing signals, and induction of new bone formation by activating the proliferation and differentiation of mesenchymal stem cells into osteoblasts [15]. The results of the present study suggest that BMSCs were activated by rhBMP-2 following implantation BMSCs with rhBMP-2, thus promoting bone formation.

Meanwhile, although rhBMP-2 was reported to show an effect on bone formation induction in a dose-dependency manner [32], the promotion of bone resorption with its high-dose use is of concern. This phenomenon is thought to arise because BMP signaling is involved not only in osteoblast differentiation, but also in regulating osteoclast formation. Despite the fact that osteoclasts are formed by hematopoietic progenitors of the monocytic lineage, proper BMP-dependent maturation of osteoblasts is required for osteoclast differentiation to occur [33]. Seeherman et al. [34] reported rhBMP-2-induced transient bone resorption prior to bone formation after implantation of rhBMP-2 with an absorbable sponge in the metaphyseal region of femurs. Bone resorption around the defect was observed radiologically by 2 weeks after surgery, and histologically at 1 week after surgery. In the present study, the 560 μg/0 cells group showed a transient decrease in the bone mineral density at 4 weeks after surgery. This finding suggests that the high dose of rhBMP-2 increased bone resorption during the early phase of bone regeneration. However, the 560 μg rhBMP-2 with 10^7 and 10^5 cells groups did not show any transient decreases in the bone mineral density. In addition, the non-uniformity

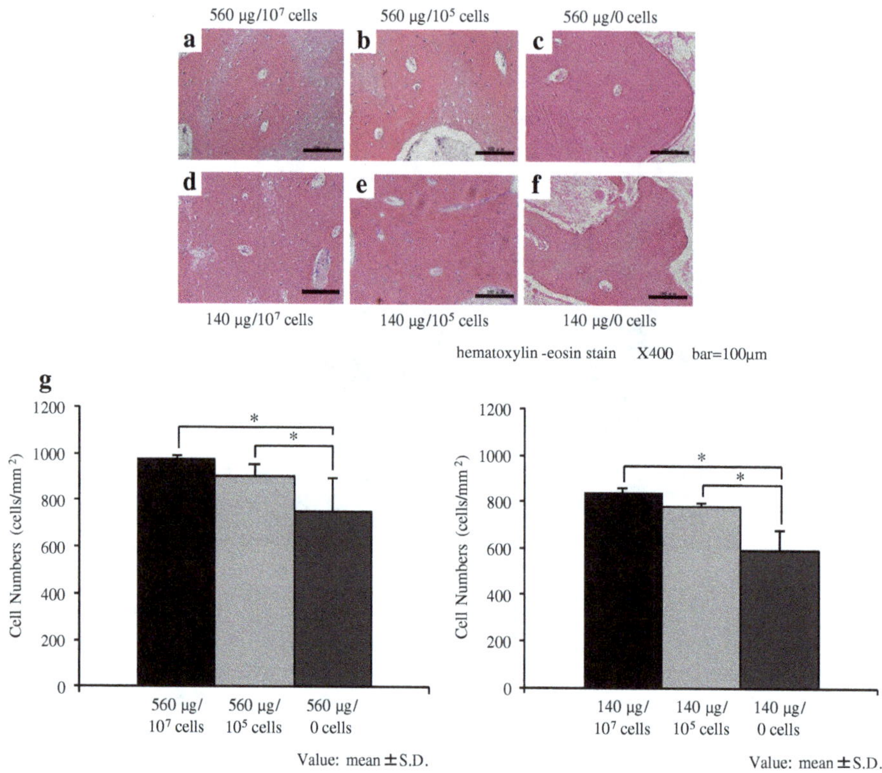

Fig. 5 Histology of the regenerated bone. **a**–**f** Representative histological sections of the regenerated bone at 12 weeks after surgery stained with hematoxylin and eosin (×400, scalebar = 100 μm). The groups treated with 560 μg rhBMP-2 with 10^7 (**a**), 10^5 (**b**), and 0 (**c**) cells, and 140 μg rhBMP-2 with 10^7 (**d**), 10^5 (**e**), and 0 (**f**) cells are shown. Scale bar: 500 μm. **g** Numbers of osteocyte-like cells per trabecular bone area. The numbers of osteocyte-like cells in the trabecular bone (mean ± SD) are shown. The numbers of osteocyte-like cells are significantly increased by transplantation with BMSCs. $^*P < 0.05$

index in the 560 μg/10^7 cells group was significantly lower than that in the 560 μg/0 cells group at 4 weeks after surgery, and remained at the same low level for the rest of the experiment. These findings suggest that transplantation should be performed with BMSCs to inhibit *E. coli*-derived rhBMP-2-induced bone resorption.

Because the bone-inducing ability of rhBMP-2 is dose-dependent [32], BMSCs were transplanted at 10^7 and 10^5 cells in the present study. The regenerated bone width in the 140 μg/10^7 cells group increased to nearly the same level as those in the 560 μg rhBMP-2 with 10^5 and 0 cells groups. Moreover, the mechanical strength in the 140 μg/10^7 cells group did not differ significantly from those in the 560 μg with 10^7 and 10^5 cells groups. In addition, although the data are not shown, the maximum load at failure in the 560 μg/10^7 cells group did not differ significantly from that for intact canine ulnae. These findings suggest that BMSCs also had an effect according to the number of the transplanted cells.

The regenerated bone in the present study was confirmed to show a definite bone structure by histological examination. However, osteoclasts and osteoblasts, which are important for bone remodeling, were hardly observed. TGF-β promotes osteoclast apoptosis [35], and apoptotic osteoclasts are quickly removed by phagocytes [36]. Furthermore, rhBMP-2 promotes the differentiattion of BMSCs into osteoblasts [15]. Meanwhile, in their final phase of differentiation, osteoblasts become osteocytes [37]. In the present study, the histological examination was performed at only 12 weeks after transplantation once the experimental period had ended. Based on the above observations, it is suggested that osteoclasts and osteoblasts were not observed, though many osteocytes were observed. The number of osteocytes is an important factor that determines bone mass and strength [38] In the present study, the numbers of osteocyte-like cells in the histological examinations confirmed the results of the X-ray examination and mechanical testing.

Sciadini et al. [9] reported that bone-void structures, which may occur when the carrier is absorbed before being replaced by new bone, were present when high doses of rhBMP-2 were used. Seeherman et al. [34] also reported the appearance of transient bone resorption prior to bone formation in the X-ray and histological examinations. In the present study, bone-void structures were mostly found in the 560 μg/0 cells group, which also showed the highest non-uniformity index among all the experimental groups. However, the bone-void number and non-uniformity index of the bone mineral density appeared to be improved in both the 560 μg with 10^7 and 10^5 cells groups, although the bone-void numbers did not differ significantly between the groups (data not shown). Further studies are needed to determine the mechanism underlying the formation of bone-voids structures.

Conclusions

In the present study, implantation of *E. coli*-derived rhBMP-2 combined with BMSCs not only increased the amount of bone formation, but also stabilized the bone mineral density and reduced the non-uniformity. Therefore, the results of the present study suggest that transplantation of osteoprogenitor cells together with rhBMP-2 is important for reconstruction of large bone defects to achieve stable therapeutic outcomes. However, the histological examinations wre performed at only 12 weeks after transplantation. This time point is regarded as the period required for complete main regenerated bone formation, because no significant differences were observed in the trabecular areas among all samples (data not shown). Therefore, it is necessary to perform histological examination at several time point to evaluate t the process underlying the regenerated bone formation. In addition, osteoprogenitor cells such as BMSCs have the disadvantage of increased risk of infection because of the need for in vitro expansion and culture, and also require more complex surgical procedures. *E. coli*-derived rhBMP-2 promotes the differentiation of undifferentiated cells into osteoblasts [28]. This effect may be even larger for osteoprogenitor cell-rich bone marrow and cancellous bone than for BMSCs. Therefore, it may be possible to use other cells and avoid the risk imposed by in vitro culture. In future studies, the combined use of rhBMP-2 with autologous transplantable tissue should be investigated to further improve this technique for clinical application.

Acknowledgment
The authors thank Dr. Shigeyuki Wakitani of the Graduate School of Health and Sports Sciences, Mukogawa Women's University, Hyogo, Japan for assistance.

Authors' contributions
TI contributed to the study conception, data collection, data analysis, laboratory experiments, and drafting and writing of the manuscript. YH contributed to the study design, laboratory experiments, and manuscript preparation. HI contributed to the laboratory experiments and data collection. MS contributed to the laboratory experiments and data collection. KT contributed to the laboratory experiments. TY contributed to the data analysis. SS contributed to the data analysis. HA, YH, and MT supervised the study and carried out the manuscript editing. All authors read and approved the final manuscript.

Competing interests
Hiroyuki Irie and Michiko Sakamoto are employees of HOYA Technological Corporation. This employment had little effect on the present study. The other authors declare that they have no competing interests.

Consent for publication
Not applicable.

Author details
[1]Division of Veterinary Surgery, Nippon Veterinary and Life Science University, 1-7-1 Kyonan-cho, Musashino, Tokyo 180-8602, Japan. [2]HOYA Technosurgical Corporation, 1-1-110 Tsutsujigaoka, Akishima, Tokyo 196-0012, Japan. [3]Division of Animal and Clinical Regenerative Medicine, Kurashiki University of Science and Arts, 2640 Nishinoura, Tsurajima-machi, Kurashiki, Okayama 712-8505, Japan. [4]Division of Veterinary Anatomy, Nippon Veterinary and Life Science University, 1-7-1 Kyonan-cho, Musashino, Tokyo 180-8602, Japan.

References

1. Boyce AS, Reveal G, Scheid DK, Kaehr DM, Maar D, Watts M, et al. Canine investigation of rhBMP-2, autogenous bone graft, and rhBMP-2 with autogenous bone graft for the healing of a large segmental tibial defect. J Orthop Trauma. 2009;23:685–92.
2. Burkus JK, Heim SE, Gornet MF, Zdeblick TA. The effectiveness of rhBMP-2 in replacing autograft: an integrated analysis of three human spine studies. Orthopedics. 2004;27:723–8.
3. Govender S, Csimma C, Genant HK, Valentin-Opran A, Amit Y, Arbel R, Aro H, et al. Recombinant human bone morphogenetic protein-2 for treatment of open tibial fractures: a prospective, controlled, randomized study of four hundred and fifty patients. J Bone Joint Surg Am. 2002;84-A:2123–34.
4. Jones CB, Sabatino CT, Badura JM, Sietsema DL, Marotta JS. Improved healing efficacy in canine ulnar segmental defects with increasing recombinant human bone morphogenetic protein-2/allograft ratios. J Orthop Trauma. 2008;22:550–9.
5. Kirker-Head C, Karageorgiou V, Hofmann S, Fajardo R, Betz O, Merkle HP, et al. BMP-silk composite matrices heal critically sized femoral defects. Bone. 2007;41:247–55.
6. Musgrave DS, Bosch P, Ghivizzani S, Robbins PD, Evans CH, Huard J. Adenovirus-mediated direct gene therapy with bone morphogenetic protein-2 produces bone. Bone. 1999;24:541–7.
7. Ruhé PQ, Kroese-Deutman HC, Wolke JG, Spauwen PH, Jansen JA. Bone inductive properties of rhBMP-2 loaded porous calcium phosphate cement implants in cranial defects in rabbits. Biomaterials. 2004;25:2123–32.
8. Itoh T, Mochizuki M, Nishimura R, Matsunaga S, Kadosawa T, Kokubo S, et al. Repair of ulnar segmental defect by recombinant human bone morphogenetic protein-2 in dogs. J Vet Med Sci. 1998;60:451–8.
9. Sciadini MF, Johnson KD. Evaluation of recombinant human bone morphogenetic protein-2 as a bone-graft substitute in a canine segmental defect model. J Orthop Res. 2000;18:289–302.
10. Fischgrund JS, James SB, Chabot MC, Hankin R, Herkowitz HN, Wozney JM, et al. Augmentation of autograft using rhBMP-2 and different carrier media in the canine spinal fusion model. J Spinal Disord. 1997;10:467–72.
11. Ohyama T, Kubo Y, Iwata H, Taki W. Beta-tricalcium phosphate combined with recombinant human bone morphogenetic protein-2: a substitute for autograft, used for packing interbody fusion cages in the canine lumbar spine. Neurol Med Chir (Tokyo). 2004;44:234–40.
12. Arzi B, Verstraete FJ, Huey DJ, Cissell DD, Athanasiou KA. Regenerating mandibular bone using rhBMP-2: part 1-immediate reconstruction of segmental mandibulectomies. Vet Surg. 2015;44:403–9.
13. Verstraete FJ, Arzi B, Huey DJ, Huey DJ, Athanasiou KA. Regenerating mandibular bone using rhBMP–2: part 2-treatment of chronic, defect non-union fractures. Vet Surg. 2015;44:410–6.
14. Harada Y, Itoi T, Wakitani S, Irie H, Sakamoto M, Zhao D, et al. Effect of Escherichia coli produced recombinant human BMP-2 on the regeneration of segmental canine ulnar defects. J Bone Miner Metab. 2012;30:388–99.
15. Cheng H, Jiang W, Phillips FM, Haydon RC, Peng Y, Zhou L, et al. Osteogenic activity of the fourteen types of human bone morphogenetic proteins (BMPs). J Bone Joint Surg Am. 2003;85-A:1544–52.
16. Dennis JE, Caplan AI. Differentiation potential of conditionally immortalized

mesenchymal progenitor cells from adult marrow of a H-2Kb-tsA58 transgenic mouse. J Cell Physiol. 1996;167:523–38.
17. Jaiswal N, Haynesworth SE, Caplan AI, Bruder SP. Osteogenic differentiation of purified, culture-expanded human mesenchymal stem cells in vitro. J Cell Biochem. 1997;64:295–312.
18. Johnstone B, Hering TM, Caplan AI, Goldberg VM, Yoo JU. In vitro chondrogenesis of bone marrow-derived mesenchymal progenitor cells. Exp Cell Res. 1998;238:265–72.
19. Yoo JU, Barthel TS, Nishimura K, Solchaga L, Caplan AI, Goldberg VM, et al. The chondrogenic potential of human bone-marrow-derived mesenchymal progenitor cells. J Bone Joint Surg Am. 1998;80:1745–57.
20. Lieberman JR, Daluiski A, Stevenson S, Wu L, McAllister P, Lee YP, et al. The effect of regional gene therapy with bone morphogenetic protein-2-producing bone-marrow cells on the repair of segmental femoral defects in rats. J Bone Joint Surg Am. 1999;81:905–17.
21. Pittenger MF, Mackay AM, Beck SC, Jaiswal RK, Douglas R, Mosca JD, et al. Multilineage potential of adult human mesenchymal stem cells. Science. 1999;284:143–7.
22. Salkeld SL, Patron LP, Barrack RL, Cook SD. The effect of osteogenic protein-1 on the healing of segmental bone defects treated with autograft or allograft bone. J Bone Joint Surg Am. 2001;83-A:803–16.
23. Silva GV, Litovsky S, Assad JA, Sousa AL, Martin BJ, Vela D, et al. Mesenchymal stem cells differentiate into an endothelial phenotype, enhance vascular density, and improve heart function in a canine chronic ischemia model. Circulation. 2005;111:150–6.
24. Caplan AI. Mesenchymal stem cells. J Orthop Res. 1991;9:641–50.
25. Bruder SP, Kraus KH, Goldberg VM, Kadiyala S. The effect of implants loaded with autologous mesenchymal stem cells on the healing of canine segmental bone defects. J Bone Joint Surg Am. 1998;80:985–96.
26. Kadiyala S, Jaiswal N, Bruder SP. Culture-expanded, bone marrow-derived mesenchymal stem cells can regenerate a critical-sized segmental bone defect. Tissue Eng Part A. 1997;3:173–85.
27. Key JA. The effect of a local calcium depot on osteogenesis and healing of fractures. J Bone Joint Surg Am. 1934;16:176–84.
28. Yano K, Hoshino M, Ohta Y, Manaka T, Naka Y, Imai Y, et al. Osteoinductive capacity and heat stabirity of recombinant human bone morphogenetic protein-2 produced by Escherichia coli and dimerized by biochemical processing. J Bone Miner Metab. 2009;27:355–63.
29. Kadiyala S, Young RG, Thiede MA, Bruder SP. Culture expanded canine mesenchymal stem cells possess osteochondrogenic potential in vivo and in vitro. Cell Transplant. 1997;6:125–34.
30. Kokubo S, Fujimoto R, Yokota S, Fukushima S, Nozaki K, Takahashi K, et al. Bone regeneration by recombinant human bone morphogenetic protein-2 and a novel biodegradable carrier in a rabbit ulnar defect model. Biomaterials. 2003;24:1643–51.
31. Mankani MH, Kuznetsov SA, Avila NA, Kingman A, Robey PG. Bone formation in transplants of human bone marrow stromal cells and hydroxyapatite-tricalcium phosphate: prediction with quantitative CT in mice. Radiology. 2004;230:369–76.
32. Skillington J, Choy L, Derynck R. Bone morphogenetic protein and retinoic acid signaling cooperate to induce osteoblast differentiation of preadipocytes. J Cell Biol. 2002;159:135–46.
33. Valcourt U, Moustakas A. BMP signaling in osteogenesis, bone remodeling and repair. Eur J Trauma. 2005;31:464–79.
34. Seeherman HJ, Li XJ, Bouxsein ML, Wozney JM. rhBMP-2 induces transient bone resorption followed by bone formation in a nonhuman primate core-defect model. J Bone Joint Surg Am. 2010;92:411–26.
35. Manolagas SC. Birth and death of bone cells: basic regulatory mechanisms and implications for the pathogenesis and treatment of osteoporosis. Endocr Rev. 2000;21:115–37.
36. Hughes DE, Dai A, Tiffee JC, Li HH, Mundy GR, Boyce BF. Estrogen promotes apoptosis of murine osteoclasts mediated by TGF-beta. Nat Med. 1996;2:1132–6.
37. Palumbo C, Palazzini S, Marotti G. Osteocyte differentiation in the tibia of newborn rabbit: an ultrastructural study of the formation of cytoplasmic processes. Acta Anat (Basel). 1990;137:350–8.
38. Manolagas SC, Parfitt AM. What old means to bone. Trends Endocrinol Metab. 2010;21:369–74.

14

Scrapie incidence and *PRNP* polymorphisms: rare small ruminant breeds of Sicily with TSE protecting genetic reservoirs

Maria Vitale[1*], Sergio Migliore[1], Maria La Giglia[1], Placido Alberti[1], Vincenzo Di Marco Lo Presti[1] and Jan P. M. Langeveld[2]

Abstract

Background: Transmissible spongiform encephalopathies (TSE) are fatal neurodegenerative diseases of several mammalian species, including humans. In Italy, the active surveillance through rapid tests on brain stem from small ruminants started in 2002 on randomly selected samples of healthy slaughtered animals. Sampling number was proportionally related to the regional small ruminant population. Of the twenty Italian regions, Sicily has the second largest population of small ruminants which is mainly constituted by crossbreed animals (>70 %). Sicily contains also three native sheep breeds *Pinzirita, Comisana* and *Valle del Belice*. Native goat breeds are *Girgentana, Messinese, Argentata dell'Etna, Maltese* and *Rossa Mediterranea*. The polymorphisms of prion protein gene (*PRNP)* may influence disease susceptibility and breeding programs for genetic TSE resistance are being applied in sheep. Protective alleles have been recently reported for goats also. These differ from those in sheep and may allow breeding programs in the near future.

In this paper the data of active surveillance for scrapie control in general population of small ruminants in Sicily are reported together with the analysis on the polymorphism of *PRNP* in a number of Sicilian autochthonous breeds. The evaluation of the frequency of protective alleles is fundamental for the implementation of a TSE resistance breeding program.

Results: TSE surveillance in small ruminants in Sicily showed a of total fifty seven scrapie outbreaks from 1997 to 2014 involving mainly crossbreed animals. The *PRNP* polymorphism analysis in autochthonous breeds showed protective allele frequencies of 30–40 % ARR in sheep and 12–18 % K222 in three of the four goat breeds; these breeds are distributed over limited areas of the island.

Conclusion: The study on *PRNP* polymorphisms in Sicilian small ruminant population showed higher frequency of the protective alleles compared to most other European breeds. Our results suggest that *PRNP* genetic variety in Sicilian sheep and goats can be a resource for TSE resistance breeding programmes while maintaining the conservation of endangered breeds and valorisation of their typical food products.

Keywords: Scrapie surveillance, Autochthonous breeds, *PRNP* polymorphism, Breeding programs, TSE

* Correspondence: marvitus@yahoo.com
[1]Istituto Zooprofilattico Sperimentale of Sicily "A. Mirri", Palermo, Italy
Full list of author information is available at the end of the article

Background

Transmissible spongiform encephalopathies (TSE) are fatal neurodegenerative diseases known to affect several mammalian species, including humans and ruminants. TSEs in ruminants include scrapie in sheep and goats, bovine spongiform encephalopathy (BSE) in cows and chronic wasting disease (CWD) in cervids. Scrapie is not regarded as a human health risk, whereas BSE has been recognized as the cause of a new TSE in humans defined as variant Creutzfeldt-Jakob disease (vCJD) [1, 2].

The second largest Italian small ruminants population is present in Sicily with about 880 thousands sheep and 132 thousands goats reared in 11,416 farms [3]. A significant biodiversity is represented by three native dairy sheep breeds (*Comisana, Valle del Belice* and *Pinzirita*) and five native dairy goat breeds (*Girgentana, Messinese, Argentata dell'Etna, Maltese* and *Rossa Mediterranea* or *Derivata di Siria)*, in addition to other Italian breeds. These breeds have an important role in the production of high quality milk requested for typical dairy products.

Prion protein (PrP) is encoded by *PRNP* gene and is strongly conserved among mammals [4]. Mutations and polymorphisms of *PRNP* sequences may influence disease susceptibility through modified protein conformation. The PrP polymorphic forms are equally expressed, however in prion material the deposition of the polymorphic-variant PrP^{Sc} can differ between two allotypes in a heterozygous individual [5–7].

In various sheep breeds the level of risk for scrapie is associated with *PRNP* genotype [8] particularly at the three codons: 136 (alanine or valine; A, V), 154 (histidine or arginine; H, R), and 171 (glutamine, arginine or histidine; Q, R, H). *PRNP* haplotypes VRQ and ARQ are considered the most susceptible to classical scrapie, whereas the ARR allele has been linked to resistance [9, 10].

In goats the analysis on *PRNP* polymorphisms showed that some polymorphic variants can be protective for the disease but their prevalence in different breeds are still under investigation. The polymorphisms that might be related to TSE resistance are present at *PRNP* codon 222 with a lysine (K) instead of glutamine (Q) [11–16] and at codon 146 with a serine (S) or an aspartic acid (D) instead of asparagine (N) [17, 18]. Strong evidence by experimental challenges in goats, rodents had shown that with the K222 allele a high level of TSE-resistance can be reached even if present in heterozygous animals [19–22].

The active surveillance by rapid diagnosis in sheep and goats started in EU in 2002 on random sampled animals. Fallen and healthy slaughtered animals over 18 months of age were included for a total number of tests that has varied each year. In Italy from 2002 to 2014, 656 positive flocks were detected on a total 620,000 tested animals (Italian Reference Centre for Animal Encephalopathy, personal communication).

The overall results of TSE surveillance and *PRNP* polymorphisms studies in native small ruminant breeds of Sicily are reported in this paper to evaluate the biodiversity of *PRNP* gene related to TSE resistance in autochthonous breeds.

Methods

Rapid diagnosis test on regularly slaughtered animals

The data on TSE surveillance reported in the paper are referred to the routine activity on the slaughtered animals for TSE control under the regulation (EC) No 999/2001, laying down rules for the prevention, control and eradication of certain transmissible spongiform encephalopathies. Almost 102 thousand regularly slaughtered sheep and goats older than 18 months have been tested in Sicily from April 2002 to December of 2014 (Italian Reference Centre for Animal Encephalopathy, personal communication). The majority of tested animals were crossbreeds because pure breeds represent a very small percentage of the zootechnical patrimony in the island. Sampling was randomly performed each year at the abattoirs to reach the number required by the national surveillance plan. The number of tests was related to the regional population of sheep and goat. Rapid diagnosis test for TSE was performed through the years by either Western blot (The Prionics®-Check WESTERN), ELISA (TeSeE Purification and Detection Biorad), chemiluminescent Elisa (Enfer TSE ELISA –Abbott USA) or in more recent years by IDEXX EIA following manufacturer's instructions.

Sampling and molecular analysis for polymorphism studies in native breeds

Consent for the sampling was obtained from the animal's owners and blood collection was performed according to the principles of Good Clinical Practice (VICH GL9 GCP, 2000).

Sheep: analysis were performed on a total of 1,295 individuals of *Valle del Belice*, 1,341 *Comisana* and 84 *Pinzirita* sheep from several flocks in different Sicilian provinces. Some flocks were analysed under personal request of veterinarians and breeders some according to the first Sicilian regional plan for genetic resistance selection.

Goat: analysis were performed on 504 pure breed animals, specifically 179 *Girgentana*, 102 *Rossa Mediterranea*, 80 *Argentata dell'Etna* and 143 *Maltese* enrolled for the specific collaboration of goat breeders.

DNA extraction from blood samples for *PRNP* polymorphism analysis was performed with E.Z.N.A Tissue-DNA-kit (Omega®) and Biosprint® 96 One-For-All Vet kit (Qiagen®) according to the manufacturer's protocol.

Sheep genotyping was performed by reverse hybridization method using the Kit Ovine PrP Gene Test, from Nuclear Laser Medicine, following manufactures' instructions and by allelic discriminations by real-time PCR with TaqMan probes in Applied Byosystem 7700. A couple of TaqMan probes (with FAM and VIC) for each SNP were used in single PCR reaction for the codon 136, 154 and 171 respectively, involved in disease susceptibility. In the homozygous animals only FAM or VIC signal can be detected while in the heterozygous both signals are present.

The sequencing on the amplified coding sequence of goat PrP gene was performed by Kit BigDye Terminator v3.1 Cycle Sequencing and ABI prism 3130 genetic analyzer (Applied Biosystem).

Statistical analysis

Statistical analysis were performed using Chi-Square test (2x2 Contingency table). ARR allele was compared among the main two sheep breeds and K222 variant among the goat breeds with a significance level of $P \leq 0.05$. Fisher exact test was used for *Maltese* goat that showed a low K222 frequency (0.3 %)

Results

In a small ruminants population of 1,023,919 heads [3], 57 scrapie outbreaks had been detected up to the end of 2014; only one sheep and one goat were classified as atypical cases. Outbreaks involved 30 sheep flocks, 5 goat flocks and 22 mixed flocks of sheep and goats together which is a common farming situation in Sicily. During the active surveillance on a total of almost 102,000 tested animals, 50 scrapie outbreaks were detected with an incidence of 12.24 cases per 10,000 tested animals. The majority of scrapie positive sheep were crossbreeds of mixed genetic background (mostly Sicilian autochthonous plus *Sarda* sheep), while the autochthonous animals concerned one *Pinzirita*, one *Valle del Belice* and four *Comisana* outbreaks (Table 1). Genetic polymorphism analysis in sheep had shown that almost all TSE positive individuals were of ARQ/ARQ *PRNP* genotype which is the most frequent in classical scrapie cases in Italy; less than 2 % of positive animals had VRQ/ARQ and ARQ/AHQ genotypes. The analysis in Sicilian sheep breeds on a total of 1395 individuals of *Valle del Belice*, 1541 *Comisana* and 84 *Pinzirita* showed that the susceptible haplotype ARQ is present at almost 59, 48 and 59 % while the resistant ARR at 32.8, 40.4 and 33.3 % respectively (Table 2). We compared the ARR allele frequencies between the group of *Valle del Belice* and *Comisana* respectively using the Chi-Square test and the result was significant with a *p-value* of 0.010 and 0.023 in *Valle del Belice* and *Comisana* breeds respectively (Table 2). Statistical analysis in *Pinzirita* sheep was not carried out because the sample was not representative of the whole population, however *Pinzirita* genetic background is present in *Valle del Belice* which was derived from a crossing between *Pinzirita-Comisana* and *Sarda* sheep to increase milk production.

Table 1 Scrapie outbreaks reported in Sicily from 1997 to 2014[a]

year	# outbreaks	affected species	sheep breeds	goat breeds
1997	3	ovine-caprine	*Pinzirita* - crossbreed	*Argentata dell' Etna* - crossbreed
1998	1	ovine-caprine	*Comisana*	*Rossa Mediterranea*
1999	1	ovine	*Sarda*	
2000	2	ovine	*Bergamasca* - crossbreed	
2002	6	ovine-caprine	*Comisana* - crossbreed	*Rossa Mediterranea* - *Maltese* - crossbreed
2003	5	ovine-caprine	*Comisana* - *Pinzirita* -*Sarda* - crossbreed	crossbreed
2004	4	ovine-caprine	*Pinzirita* - crossbreed	crossbreed
2005	8	ovine-caprine	*Comisana* - crossbreed	*Rossa Mediterranea* - crossbreed
2006	7	ovine-caprine	*Valle del Belice* - crossbreed	*Rossa Mediterranea* - crossbreed
2007	7	ovine-caprine	*Comisana* - crossbreed	crossbreed
2008	1	ovine-caprine	crossbreed	crossbreed
2011	2	ovine-caprine	crossbreed	*Girgentana* - crossbreed
2012	6	ovine-caprine	*Sarda* - crossbreed	*Rossa Mediterranea* - crossbreed
2013	2	ovine	crossbreed	
2014	2	ovine	*Sarda* - crossbreed	

[a] Scrapie outbreaks were detected through passive surveillance (symptomatic animals) from 1997 to 2000 and through active surveillance by rapid diagnosis on stem-brains from 2002 to the end of 2014

The application of breeding programs in goats could also aid the ongoing EU efforts to full eradicate scrapie. The investigation into the relationships between caprine PRNP haplotypes and resistance to scrapie in goat breeds is important for the design of an effective breeding program. Our study on autochthonous goat breeds showed an 18.7 % frequency of the protective variant K222 in *Girgentana* [23], 12 % in *Rossa Mediterranea*, 16 % in *Argentata dell'Etna* and 0.3 % in *Maltese* (Table 3). Statistical analysis among goat breeds for the presence of K222 variant was performed with Chi-Square test considering each breed versus all goat samples. In *Maltese* goat which has a low K222 frequency we used Fisher exact test. The results were significant in *Girgentana* and *Maltese* breeds with a *p-value* of

Table 2 Haplotype frequencies of PRNP in Sicilian autochthonous sheep breeds[a]

PRNP codons			Sheep breeds		
136	**154**	**171**	***Valle del Belice (%)***	***Comisana (%)***	***Pinzirita (%)***
A	R	Q	58.9	47.8	59.2
A	R	**R**	**32.8**	**40.4**	**33.3**
	p-value		*(0.010)*	*(0.023)*	
A	R	**H**	0.8	2.8	-
A	**H**	Q	5.3	1.7	3.3
V	R	Q	2.2	7.3	4.2

[a] The analysis was performed on a total of 1395 individuals of *Valle del Belice*, 1541 *Comisana* and 84 *Pinzirita* sheep. The haplotypes are presented in decreasing frequency; in bold are the polymorphic variant amino acid versus wild type (ARQ). For ARR haplotype we performed statistical analysis using Chi Square test with a significant level of $p \leq 0.05$. In brackets the *p-value* results. Statistical analysis in *Pinzirita* was not performed

0.047 and 0.002 respectively. In contrast, in *Rossa Mediterranea* and *Argentata dell'Etna* a *p-values* of 0.933 and 0.306 were obtained respectively (Table 3).

Discussion

The results of passive and active surveillance had shown how 57 scrapie outbreaks have occurred in the period from 1997 to 2014 in Sicily. The disease probably became endemic in the island when an infected vaccine against *Mycoplasma agalactiae* was used in small ruminant flocks [24]. Scrapie is not regarded as a human health risk, but to reduce the risk of scrapie or BSE in sheep the EU decided to implement selection against susceptible *PRNP* alleles (Commission Regulation EC 999/2001 and Commission Decisions 2002/1003/EC3 and 2003/100/EC4). Since then, several member states established breeding programs to enrich for resistant alleles. In Sicily a regional public plan for genetic selection in sheep started in 2005 for pure breed animals and was extended to cross breed flocks with more than 200 animals in 2013. In addition, genotyping of several flocks had started in 2005 on voluntary basis particularly to manage scrapie outbreaks. A previous study on limited number of pure breed sheep flocks (*Valle del Belice* and *Comisana*) and cross breed animals from five outbreaks showed already a good level of ARR haplotype frequency [25]. The results of a more extended analysis on reproductive males and females and young animals from pure breed sheep flocks in different Sicilian provinces confirmed the high frequency of the resistant haplotypes (Table 2). It is widely recognized that stamping out in sheep is not an efficient strategy for TSEs eradication probably because the pathogenic prion protein is highly persisting in the environment and naïve animals can acquire the infection from the soil [26]. In contrast the selective breeding program is a good way to manage scrapie outbreaks and the best alternative to stamping out of animals which represents a great economic loss for the farmers and a serious threat of extinction for the endangered breeds [27, 28]. The application of breeding programs in goats could also aid the ongoing EU efforts to reduce the chance of scrapie in sheep populations since, goats may represent a possible scrapie reservoir for sheep. This would theoretically also apply if goats were positive for the zoonotic BSE strain [29–31]. In Europe, very few cases of goat scrapie had been recorded prior to 2002 but in Sicily the first clinical case in goat was reported in a mixed flock in 1997 and 27 outbreaks have been diagnosed with 9 including pure breed animals. Any breeding program should consider the endangered status of each goat population to preserve the genetic variability and the biodiversity also when dealing with disease control. For these reasons, the investigation into the relationships between caprine *PRNP* haplotypes and resistance to scrapie in goat breeds is important [11–17, 31]. With the K222 allele a high level of TSE-resistance can be reached even if present in heterozygous animals [19–22]. Except for *Maltese*, all other Sicilian goats presented K222 variant in frequency higher than most commercial breeds although more analysis are necessary for *Argentata dell'Etna* and *Rossa Mediterranea*.

Our results suggest that a breeding program to select for ARR haplotype in sheep and K222 resistant allele in goat is feasible in the autochthonous breeds of Sicily.

Small ruminants are bred worldwide, particularly in difficult and marginal geographical territories (mountains or dry areas) to which they are well adapted. The native breeds are usually confined but important in

Table 3 Allelic frequencies in Sicilian autochthonous goats breeds[a]

Allele	Girgentana (%)	*Rossa Mediterranea (%)*	*Argentata dell'Etna (%)*	*Maltese (%)*
37V	0.3	1.5	-	24.1
125V	-	-	1.3	-
137I	-	-	2.5	0.3
143R	3.8	2.5	-	0.7
151H	-	-	2.5	-
154H	7.6	7.4	13.8	5.6
168Q	18.4	3.4	2.5	-
222K *p-value*	18.7 *(0.047)*	12.7 *(0.933)*	16.3 *(0.306)*	0.3 *(0.002)*
240P	57.3	51.0	51.3	52.1

[a] The analysis was performed on 179 *Girgentana*, 102 *Rossa Mediterranea*, 80 *Argentata dell'Etna* and 143 *Maltese*. For the presence of K222 variant we used Chi-square test with a significant level of $p \leq 0.05$ in *Girgentana, Rossa Mediterranea* and *Argentata dell'Etna*. In *Maltese* we used Fisher exact test with a significance level of $P \leq 0.05$

low-income rural areas even in developed countries. The focus on increasing biosecurity and quality of local animal production can stimulate the breeding and protection of autochthonous animals through a revival of their economic value as suggested by FAO [32].

Conclusions

The high prevalence of the two TSE resistance related ARR haplotype and K222 allele present in Sicilian sheep and goat breeds respectively, shows how the genetic biodiversity could serve as a resource for the selection of resistance to disease, in our case for TSE eradication. It is very probable that enhancing the frequencies of resistant polymorphisms could be sufficient to reach a sufficiently high level of heterozygosis with the advantage to maintain both biodiversity and resistance. Genetic selection for resistance could assure the full eradication of scrapie in small ruminants. These results may increase interest in the breeding of Sicilian autochthonous breeds preserving the biodiversity on the island. Additionally the promotion of typical dairy and meat products with high quality and biosecurity from autochthonous animals might represent a driving force for the economy in rural areas.

Abbreviations

amino acid code, A, alanine; V, valine; R, arginine; Q, glutamine; H, histidine; K, lysine; S, serine; D, aspartic acid; N, asparagine; BSE, bovine spongiform encephalopathy; CWD, chronic wasting disease; DNA, deoxyribonucleic acid; ELISA, enzyme linked immunosorbent assay; EU, European Union; FAO, Food and Agriculture Organization; PCR, polymerase chain reaction; *PRNP*, prion protein gene; PrP, prion protein; PrPs, scrapie prion protein; TSE, transmissible spongiform encephalopathy; vCJD, vCreutzfeldt-Jakob disease

Acknowledgements

We thank the public veterinary services (ASP, aziende sanitarie provinciali) of all Sicilian provinces for the active support accomplished during TSE' surveillance. We thank also the precious collaboration of the farmers of the autochthonous small ruminant breeds.

Funding

This work is supported by EMIDA ERA-NET project: "GOAT-TSE-FREE and Ricerca finalizzata Code:RF-2010-2318525 to MV from Italian Ministry of Health. The funding source had no role in study design; in the collection, analysis and interpretation of data; in the writing of the report; and in the decision to submit the article for publication.

Authors' contributions

MV conceived and designed the proposal, participated in the coordination and management of the study. SM participated in sample collection, laboratory testing and drafting of the article, MLG and PA collected, tested and analyzed the data. VDMLP participated in sample collection and in the coordination of the study. JPML participated in the study design and the edition of article. All authors have read and approved the final manuscript.

Competing interest

The authors declare that they have no competing interests. The work is an original paper and is not under consideration in other journals.

Consent for publication

Not applicable.

Author details

[1]Istituto Zooprofilattico Sperimentale of Sicily "A. Mirri", Palermo, Italy. [2]Department of Infection Biology, Central Veterinary Institute of Wageningen UR, Lelystad, The Netherlands.

References

1. Will RG, Ironside JW, Zeidler, M, Cousens SN, Estibeiro K, Alperovitch A, Poser S, Pocchiari M, Hofman A, Smith PG. A new variant of Creutzfeldt-Jakob disease in the UK. Lancet. 1996;347:921–5.
2. Wadsworth JD, Collinge J. Update on human prion disease. Biochim Biophys Acta. 1997;1772(6):598–609.
3. Anagrafe Zootecnica - Banca Dati Nazionale - Istituto "G. Caporale" Teramo. 2014. http://statistiche.izs.it/portal/page?_pageid=73,12918&_dad=portal&_schema=PORTAL&op=view_rep&p_report=plet_rep_r1_ovi_capr_new&p_liv=R&p_sigla_liv=190 (accessed 10 Mar 2015).
4. Sakudo A, Xue G, Kawashita N, Ano Y, Takagi T, Shintani HY, Onodera T, Ikuta K. Structure of the prion protein and its gene: an analysis using bioinformatics and computer simulation. Curr Protein Pept Sci. 2010;11:166–79.
5. Jacobs JG, Bossers A, Rezaei H, van Keulen LJ, McCutcheon S, Sklaviadis T, Lantier I, Berthon P, Lantier F, et al. Proteinase K-resistant material in ARR/VRQ sheep brain affected with classical scrapie is composed mainly of VRQ prion protein. J Virol. 2011;85(23):12537–46.
6. Nicot S, Bencsik A, Migliore S, Canal D, Leboidre M, Agrimi U, Nonno R, Baron T. L-type bovine spongiform encephalopathy in genetically susceptible and resistant sheep: changes in prion strain or phenotypic plasticity of the disease-associated prion protein? J Infect Dis. 2014;209(6):950.
7. Langeveld JP, Jacobs JG, Hunter N, van Keulen LM, Lantier F, van Zijderveld FG, Bossers A. Prion-type dependent deposition of PRNP-allelic products in heterozygous 4 sheep. J Virol. 2016;90:805–12.
8. González L, Martin S, Begara-McGorum I, Hunter N, Houston F, Simmons M, Jeffrey M. Effects of agent strain and host genotype on PrP accumulation in the brain of sheep naturally and experimentally affected with scrapie. J Comp Pathol. 2002;126(1):17–29.
9. Belt P, Muileman IH, Schreuder BEC, Bos-de Ruijter J, Gielkens ALJ, Smits MA. Identification of five allelic variants of the sheep PrP gene and their association with natural scrapie. J Gen Virol. 1995;76:509–17.
10. Bossers A, Screuder BEC, Muileman IH, Belt PB, Smits MA. PrP genotype contributes to determining survival times of sheep with natural scrapie. J Gen Virol. 1996;77:2669–73.
11. Billinis C, Panagiotidis CH, Psychas V, Argyroudis S, Nicolaou A, Leontides S, Papadopoulos O, Sklaviadis T. Prion protein gene polymorphisms in natural goat scrapie. J Gen Virol. 2002;83:713–21.
12. Acutis PL, Bossers A, Priem J, Riina MV, Peletto S, Mazza M, Casalone C, Forloni G, Ru G, Caramelli M. Identification of prion protein gene polymorphisms in goats from Italian scrapie outbreaks. J Gen Virol. 2006;87:1029–33.
13. Vaccari G, Di Bari MA, Morelli L, Nonno R, Chiappini B, Antonucci G, Marcon S, Esposito E, Fazzi P, et al. Identification of an allelic variant of the goat PrP gene associated with resistance to scrapie. J Gen Virol. 2006;87:1395–402.
14. Barillet F, Mariat D, Amigues Y, Faugeras R, Caillat H, Moazami-Goudarzi K, Rupp R, Babilliot J M, Lacroux C, et al. Identification of seven haplotypes of the caprine PrP gene at codons 127, 142, 154, 211, 222 and 240 in French Alpine and Saanen breeds and their association with classical scrapie. J Gen Virol. 2009;90:769–76.
15. Bouzalas IG, Dovas CI, Banos G, Papanastasopoulou M, Kritas S, Oevermann A, Papakostaki D, Evangelia C, Papadopoulos O, et al. Caprine PRNP polymorphisms at codons 171, 211, 222 and 240 in a Greek herd and their association with classical scrapie. J Gen Virol. 2010;91(Pt 6):1629–34.

16. Corbière F, Perrin-Chauvineau C, Lacroux C, Costes P, Thomas M, Brémaud I, Martin S, Lugan S, Chartier C, et al. PrP-associated resistance to scrapie in five highly infected goat herds. J Gen Virol. 2013;94:241–5.
17. Papasavva-Stylianou P, Kleanthous M, Toumazos P, Mavrikiou P, Loucaides P. Novel polymorphisms at codons 146 and 151 in the prion protein gene of Cyprus goats, and their association with natural scrapie. Vet J. 2007;173:459–62.
18. Papasavva-Stylianou P, Windl O, Saunders G, Mavrikiou P, Toumazos P, Kakoyiannis C. PrP gene polymorphisms in Cyprus goats and their association with resistance or susceptibility to natural scrapie. Vet J. 2011; 187(2):245–50.
19. Bossers A, Andreoletti O, Goldmann W, Torres JM, Acin C, Groschup M, Acutis PL, Agrimi U, Sklaviadis T, et al. Improvement of goat TSE discriminative diagnosis and susceptibility based assessment. Final public report of EU project GoatBSE. FOOD-CT-2006-36353 of BSE infectivity in goat milk and meat; 2013. http://www.goatbse.eu/site/files/GoatBSE_final_activity_report_public.pdf.
20. Aguilar-Calvo P, Espinosa JC, Pintado B, Gutiérrez-Adán A, Alamillo E, Miranda A, Prieto I, Bossers A, Andreoletti O, Torres JM. Role of the goat K222-PrP(C) polymorphic variant in prion infection resistance. J Virol. 2014; 88(5):2670–6.
21. Lacroux C, Perrin-Chauvineau C, Corbière F, Aron N, Aguilar-Calvo P, Torres JM, Costes P, Brémaud I, Lugan S, Schelcher F, Barillet F, Andréoletti O. Genetic resistance to scrapie infection in experimentally challenged goats. J Virol. 2014;88(5):2406–13.
22. Aguilar-Calvo P, Fast C, Tauscher K, Espinosa JC, Groschup MH, Nadeem M, Goldmann W, Langeveld J, Bossers A, Andreoletti O, et al. Effect of Q211 and K222 PRNP polymorphic variants in the susceptibility of goats to oral infection with Goat-BSE. J Infect Dis. 2015;212:664–72.
23. Migliore S, Agnello S, Chiappini B, Vaccari G, Mignacca SA, Di Marco Lo Presti V, Di Domenico F, Vitale M. Biodiversity and selection for scrapie resistance in goats: genetic polymorphism in "Girgentana" breed in Sicily, Italy. Small Rum Res. 2015;125:137–41.
24. Bertolini S, Maurella C, Bona C, Ingravalle F, Desiato R, Baioni E, Chiavacci L, Caramelli M, Ru G. A relevant long-term impact of the circulation of a potentially contaminated vaccine on the distribution of scrapie in Italy. Results from a retrospective cohort study. Vet Res. 2012;43(1):63.
25. Van Kaam J, Finocchiaro R, Vitale M, Pinelli F, Scimonelli M, Vitale F, Portolano B, Oltenacu PA, Caracappa S. Prion protein gene frequencies in three Sicilian dairy sheep populations. Ital J Anim Sci. 2009;7:87–94.
26. Smith CB, Booth CJ, Pedersen JA. Fate of prions in soil: a review. J Environ Qual. 2011;40:449–61.
27. Melchior MB, Windig JJ, Hagenaars TJ, Bossers A, Davidse A, van Zijderveld FG. Eradication of scrapie with selective breeding: are we nearly there? BMC Vet Res. 2010;4(6):24.
28. Nodelijk G, van Roermund HJ, van Keulen LJ, Engel B, Vellema P, Hagenaars TJ. Breeding with resistant rams leads to rapid control of classical scrapie in affected sheep flocks. Vet Res. 2011;42:5.
29. Eloit M, Adjou K, Coulpier M, Fontaine JJ, Hamel R, Lilin T, Messiaen S, Andreoletti O, Baron T, et al. BSE agent signatures in a goat. Vet Rec. 2005; 156:523–4.
30. Jeffrey M, Martin S, González L, Foster J, Langeveld JP, van Zijderveld FG, Grassi J, Hunter N. Immunohistochemical features of PrP(d) accumulation in natural and experimental goat transmissible spongiform encephalopathies. J Comp Pathol. 2006;134(2–3):171–81.
31. Spiropoulos J, Lockey R, Sallis RE, Terry LA, Thorne L, Holder TM, Beck KE, Simmons MM. Isolation of prion with BSE properties from farmed goat. Emerg Infect Dis. 2011;17(12):2253–61.
32. FAO. Secondary Guidelines for Development of National Farm Genetic resource Management Plans: management of small populations at risk. Roma: FAO; 1998.

Estimation of the sensitivity and specificity of two serum ELISAs and one fecal qPCR for diagnosis of paratuberculosis in sub-clinically infected young-adult French sheep using latent class Bayesian modeling

Yoann Mathevon[1], Gilles Foucras[1], Rémy Falguières[2] and Fabien Corbiere[1*]

Abstract

Background: The objective was to evaluate the diagnostic accuracy of two serum ELISAs and one quantitative PCR on feces for the diagnosis of paratuberculosis in sub-clinically infected young-adult sheep. A cross-sectional study was performed to collect 1197 individual blood and fecal samples from 2- to 3-year-old sub-clinically infected ewes in 14 closed meat sheep flocks in France. Fecal excretion was determined using qPCR based on IS900 sequence detection, and serology was performed on serum samples using two commercial ELISAs. Data were analyzed in a 3-test multiple-population Bayesian latent class model accounting for potential dependence between the three tests fitted in OpenBUGS. Separate analyses were performed according to whether doubtful ELISA results were handled as positive or negative and based on two thresholds for fecal qPCR (Ct ≤ 42 or Ct ≤ 40).

Results: The best fit to the data was provided by accounting for a pairwise dependence between the two ELISAs on sensitivity and pairwise dependence between the three tests on specificity. Under this model, the estimated ELISA sensitivities were 17.4% (95% PCI: 10.6 – 25.9) and 17.9% (95% PCI 11.4 – 25.6), with estimated specificities of 94.8% (95% PCI: 93.1 – 96.3) and 94.0% (95% PCI: 92.2 – 95.7). Fecal qPCR demonstrated significantly higher sensitivity (47.5%; 95% PCI: 29.3 – 69.9) and specificity (99.0%; 95% PCI: 97.9 – 99.9) than the ELISAs. Assumptions regarding doubtful ELISA results and qPCR thresholds had only a slight impact on test accuracy estimates. Models not accounting for pairwise dependence between ELISA and fecal qPCR results yielded higher sensitivity and specificity estimates but always provided a worse fit to the data.

Conclusions: Although the overall sensitivity of serum ELISAs and fecal qPCR remains low, the higher diagnostic performances of fecal qPCR make it more suitable for paratuberculosis diagnosis in sub-clinically infected sheep. Our results also illustrate that all dependence structures should be investigated when evaluating diagnostic test accuracy and selection based on a rigorous statistical approach.

Keywords: Paratuberculosis, Sheep, Elisa, Fecal quantitative PCR, Sensitivity, Specificity, Bayesian latent class model

* Correspondence: f.corbiere@envt.fr
[1]IHAP, Ecole Nationale Vétérinaire de Toulouse, 23 chemin des Capelles, F-31076 Toulouse Cedex 3, France
Full list of author information is available at the end of the article

Background

Surveillance and control of paratuberculosis are largely hampered by the lack of sensitivity of available diagnostic tests, especially for the detection of sub-clinically infected (i.e., clinically healthy) animals. Historically, the evaluation of diagnostic test accuracy for the diagnosis of paratuberculosis has been based on cases confirmed by histopathological examination, fecal or tissue culture or repeated fecal culture for the detection of *Mycobacterium avium subsp. paratuberculosis* (MAP), the causative agent of paratuberculosis. However, due to the long and complex physiopathology of the disease, these cases do not include all latent cases of infection, generally leading to biased estimates of sensibility of diagnostic tests [1, 2].

In the last few decades, however, special attention has been given to the evaluation of diagnostic test accuracy in sub-clinically infected animals. Because of the unknown true disease status of the study subjects, due to the absence of a perfect reference test, latent class models have been increasingly used. These non-gold standard methods were first introduced by Hui and Walter (1980) [3] for 2 conditionally independent tests and two populations and were further extended to take account of conditional dependence between tests [2–6]. Bayesian modeling has been extensively developed to tackle non-identifiability issues that might arise in such models by incorporating prior knowledge of test performances [7, 8].

When erroneously assumed, the assumption of conditional independence between tests can seriously bias parameter estimations [9, 10]. Conditional dependence has been taken into account in most cases when evaluating two or more tests based on the same biological process (i.e., two fecal culture methods or two serological tests) for the diagnosis of paratuberculosis in cattle or in small ruminants [11–14]. Conversely, the a priori assumption of conditional independence between tests based on the identification of MAP (i.e., fecal culture, Ziehl-Neelsen stained fecal smear or fecal PCR) and those targeting the immune response (i.e., serum ELISA or AGID) has often been made [12, 15] but has been explicitly evaluated in only a few studies [16, 17].

One other assumption underlying latent class models is that the accuracy of tests is constant across all populations, or in other words, that the various infection stages among different populations are homogeneously distributed [2]. This assumption may, however, be difficult to stick to in practice, especially when sampling without controlling for factors that influence test accuracy [18]. For paratuberculosis, the increasing test sensitivity with the course of infection at the individual level would advocate for an age-specific evaluation of test accuracy [19]. This may lead to wide confidence or credible intervals of accuracy estimates, especially when prevalence is low and sample size is limited, as shown by simulation studies [20] and experience in field studies [16, 15]. Furthermore, a diagnostic test's sensitivity may also vary between species, age and possibly MAP strains [2], while its specificity may be influenced by the presence of environmental mycobacterial [21].

Fecal quantitative PCR (qPCR) has been widely developed in the last two decades as an alternative to fecal culture for the detection of animals. It is less time consuming, especially for the detection of S-strains (sheep strains) of MAP that grow slowly in vitro compared to C-strains (cattle strains) [22]. There is also growing evidence that fecal qPCR might be at least as sensitive as, or even more sensitive than, fecal culture [23, 24]. However, its analytical sensitivity depends on several factors, including sample quality, DNA extraction methods, DNA target and qPCR systems [25, 26]. Furthermore, from an epidemiological point of view, Bayesian latent class models have seldom been applied to evaluate the diagnostic accuracy of fecal PCR [12], and estimates for sheep are scarce [14].

In this context, it would be unwise to simply extrapolate already published estimates of diagnostic test accuracy to any situation without utmost caution. In this study, we used a latent class approach in a Bayesian framework to estimate the diagnostic accuracy of two serum ELISAs and one fecal qPCR for the diagnosis of paratuberculosis in sub-clinically infected young-adult meat sheep, focusing on a narrow age range. Special attention was paid to the possibility of conditional dependence between tests under evaluation.

Methods

Flock and animal selection

Fourteen meat flocks with a size ranging from 290 to 1400 adult ewes (median 610) were selected for the study. They all belonged to the same breeders' association located in the Lot administrative region of France. Inclusions criteria were (i) Causse du Lot purebred closed flocks with no introduction of replacement ewes for at least 4 years, (ii) history of positive serological results and/or of clinical cases of paratuberculosis, and (iii) no history of vaccination against paratuberculosis. Sampling was performed from March 2014 to March 2015, avoiding the month before and after lambing as well as the month after artificial insemination or mating. Although it has been shown that the sensitivity of serological testing may be enhanced in early and late lactation in cattle [15, 21], this sampling scheme was applied to fulfill breeders' requests to reduce animal stress. Only 2- to 3-year-old ewes were included, using their eartag as an indicator of their birth cohort. Individual ages at sampling were calculated based on birth date available from the French Systeme National d'Information Génétique (SNIG) database. Ewes showing obvious clinical signs of paratuberculosis, if any, were excluded because the target population was sub-clinically infected animals. If no feces could be retrieved intra-rectum at the time of sampling, animals were excluded and the next one fulfilling the inclusion criteria was substituted. Depending on flock size, the target sample size ranged between 60 and 150 ewes per flock.

Sample collection and handling

A handful of feces was sampled from the rectum of selected animals using single-use gloves without lubricant and was placed in an individually identified sterile plastic bag for transportation. In parallel, a five-milliliter blood sample was also collected from the jugular vein in vacuum tubes without anticoagulant (Vacutainer® System). Feces and blood samples were frozen at −20 °C prior to analysis. Animal handling was performed in compliance with the European Commission Directive 2010/63/EU. All farmers gave written consent for their animals to be used in this study.

Laboratory testing

Serological tests

Two commercial ELISA tests were applied to serum samples using an overnight incubation protocol following the manufacturer's instructions: ELISA A (ID Screen Paratuberculosis Indirect®, batch 602, IDVet, Montpellier, France) and ELISA B (IDEXX paratuberculosis screening® kit, batch 5074, IDEXX, Montpellier, France). Negative and positive controls provided by the manufacturers were included on each ELISA plate, and manufacturer's guidelines were strictly followed for interpretation of sample to positive (S/P) ratio results: for ELISA A serum, samples with S/*P* values <60%, between 60 and 70%, and ≥70% were considered negative, doubtful, and positive for MAP antibodies, respectively. For ELISA B, the negative and positive thresholds were 45% and 55%, respectively.

Fecal real-time PCR

First, fecal samples underwent a concentration procedure using the ADIAFILTER system (BioX, Rochefort, Belgium) following the manufacturer's instructions. Ten grams of feces were rehydrated overnight in 70 mL of bidistilled sterile water. The top 10 mL of the supernatant were then filtered and centrifuged using the ADIAFILTER® disposal. Pellets were then resuspended in 500 μL of bi-distilled water and mixed with 300 mg of 150-250 μm silica beads (Silibeads, Sigmund Lindner, Warmensteinach, Germany) for 30 s at 6800 rpm three times in a bead beater (Precellys 24®, Bertin Technologies, Montigny-le-Bretonneux, France). A magnetic bead-based DNA extraction was performed on a Kingfisher Flex® magnetic particle processor (Thermo Fisher Scientific, Courtaboeuf, France) following the NucleoMag 96 tissue protocol (Macherey-Nagel, Hoerdt, France), with addition of an extraction control (ADIAVET™ PARATB REAL TIME, BioX, Rochefort, Belgium) in each plate well. Samples were subjected to qPCR (ADIAVET™ PARATB REAL TIME, BioX, Rochefort, Belgium), following the manufacturer's instructions. Each sample was also tested for amplification of the internal control. Bi-distilled water and synthetic IS900 DNA provided in the amplification kit were used as negative and positive controls, respectively. Forty-five amplification cycles were performed on a LightCycler 480 (Roche Life Science, Meylan, France), and fluorescent signals were recorded in two channels, with FAM detecting IS900 and VIC detecting the extraction control. Due to the overlapping spectra of the two dyes, a color compensation step was applied. Raw fluorescence data were obtained from the LightCycler 480 and modeled using the qpcR package [27] in R software [28]. Cycle thresholds were determined using second derivative maximum (CpD2). According to the manufacturer's recommendations, samples that reached fluorescence with a cycle count (Ct) below 40 were considered positive. A higher threshold (Ct ≤ 42) was also considered. Indeed, careful examination of late fluorescence curves indicated that they were associated with low but unambiguously positive results up to 42 Ct, while non-specific amplification results could not be ruled out beyond this threshold.

All tests were performed blind for other test outcomes.

Target conditions

The purpose of this evaluation was to provide an accurate appraisal of sensitivity and specificity of two ELISAs and one fecal qPCR for the diagnosis of paratuberculosis in sub-clinically infected 2- to 3-year-old ewes. The target condition for this evaluation was MAP-infected animals that shed enough bacteria in their feces to potentially test positive on fecal PCR at the time of sampling, that mounted an antibody response towards MAP that could be detected by ELISA, or both. Following the Nielsen and Toft (2008) definition [29], this target condition included both infected and infectious animals but probably only few affected ones, as ewes showing obvious clinical signs of paratuberculosis were excluded on farms. Note that animals passively shedding MAP in their feces [30, 31] as a result of heavy environmental contamination were also included in our target conditions.

Statistical analysis

Separate analyses were performed for the four scenarios according to whether doubtful ELISA results were handled as positive or negative and on the choice of the positive cut-off for fecal qPCR (Ct ≤ 42 or Ct ≤ 40). Based on previous serological results, history of paratuberculosis clinical cases and judgment of practicing veterinarians and technicians supervising the flocks, flocks were grouped into 4 sub-populations according to the within-flock suspected prevalence of infection: very low (3 flocks, 287 sampled ewes), low (5 flocks, 299 sampled ewes), moderate to high (6 flocks, 447 sampled ewes) and very high (2 flocks, 164 samples ewes).

Model definition

We applied multiple populations Bayesian Latent Class models [32, 33] to estimate the diagnostic accuracy of the two ELISAs and the fecal qPCR in the absence of gold standard.

The models were defined following the approach by Dendikuri and Joseph (2001) [4] that uses a multinomial distribution to model the frequency of the 8 observed combinations of test outcomes. The simplest model assumes conditional independence between tests (i.e., given the true disease state of a sample, the outcome of one test does not have any influence on the probability of a positive or negative outcome in a second test). Under this assumption, the probability of a combination of test outcomes in a given population only depends on the true prevalence within this population and the sensitivities and specificities of diagnostic tests, which are assumed constant across all populations [3]. If T_i + denotes the event of a positive outcome for test i, $i = 1, \ldots, 3$, Se_i and Sp_i denote the sensitivity and specificity of test i, respectively, and π_j, the true prevalence in a given population j, $j = 1 \ldots 4$, then the probability of all three test being positive on a sample in this population is given by

$$P(T_1^+, T_2^+, T_3^+) = \pi_j Se_1 Se_2 Se_3 + (1-\pi_j)(1-Sp_1) \times (1-Sp_2)(1-Sp_3)$$

The probability of other combinations of test outcomes can be easily derived analogously. The assumption of conditional independence between tests may, however, not hold in practice and should be challenged against models allowing for the conditional dependence between tests [2]. We considered the approach proposed by Dendikuri and Joseph (2001) [4], where pairwise dependence of sensitivities and specificities of tests are explicitly modeled by covariance terms (*Covse* and *Covsp*). In the fully dependent case, the probability of all three tests being positive on a sample within population j is then given by

$$\begin{aligned} P(T_1^+, T_2^+, T_3^+) = {} & \pi_j(Se_1Se_2Se_3 + Covse_{23}Se_1 + Covse_{13}Se_2 \\ & + Covse_{12}Se_3 + Covse_{123}) + (1-\pi_j) \\ & ((1-Sp_1)(1-Sp_2)(1-Sp_3) + Covsp_{23} \\ & (1-Sp_1) + Covsp_{13}(1-Sp_2) + Covsp_{12} \\ & (1-Sp_3) - Covsp_{123}) \end{aligned}$$

Starting from the fully saturated model below, covariance terms were removed one-by-one following a stepwise backward selection procedure using the Deviance Information Criterion (DIC) as the selection criterion [34]. The DIC evaluates the model fit while penalizing the number of parameters, and it is generally accepted that models with smaller DIC are better supported by the data.

Comparing diagnostic test accuracies

The Bayesian posterior probability of difference (PPD) in sensitivity and specificity between tests was estimated using the Boolean step function in OpenBUGS [12, 16]. If PPD <0.05 or >0.95, we concluded that the sensitivities (or specificities) of two compared tests were significantly different.

Serial and parallel testing

The accuracy of serial and parallel testing for the combinations of one ELISA and fecal qPCR was finally evaluated. For two conditionally dependent tests, namely, Test 1 and Test 2, the sensitivity (Se_{ser}) and specificity (Sp_{ser}) of serial testing are given by

$$Se_{ser} = Se_1Se_2 + CovSe_{12}$$

$$Sp_{ser} = 1-((1-Sp_1)(1-Sp_2) + CovSp_{12}),$$

where $CovSe_{12}$ and $CovSp_{12}$ denote the covariance terms for the pairwise dependence of sensitivities and specificities, respectively.

Sensitivity (Se_{par}) and specificity (Sp_{par}) of parallel testing were given by

$$Se_{par} = 1-((1-Se_1)(1-Se_2) + CovSe_{12})$$

$$Sp_{par} = Sp_1Sp_2 + CovSp_{12}$$

Prior distributions

Uniform distributions in the range from 0 to 1 were used as priors for sensitivity and prevalence model parameters. Based on previous published estimates in sheep [16, 35–37], the specificity of ELISAs and fecal qPCR was set at 0.95, with 95% certainty to be greater than 0.80. The corresponding Beta distribution Beta (21.20, 2.06) was generated using the epi.betabuster function embedded in the epiR package in R software [38] and was used as prior distribution for all specificity parameters.

Constraints were defined for covariance terms so that each of the 8 probabilities of combinations of test outcomes was between 0 and 1 [4], and uniform distributions between the lower and upper constraint bounds were used as non-informative priors.

Implementation

Computations were performed with OpenBUGS [39] embedded in R software using the R2OpenBUGS package [40]. Posterior estimates for test sensitivity and specificity were generated using the Markov Chain Monte Carlo (MCMC) sampling method and the Gibbs algorithm. Three simulation chains of 200,000 iterations were run with different starting values, with the first 10,000 iterations discarded as the burn-in period. The chains were then thinned, taking every tenth sample to reduce autocorrelation among the samples. The convergence of the chains following the initial burn-in period was assessed visually by examining the traces, histories, Monte Carlo errors and the Gelman-Rubin diagnostic plots [41, 42]. The posterior distribution of each parameter was summarized using the mean and the 95% posterior credible interval (95% PCI). Analysis and graphing of the MCMC output were conducted using the coda package in R [43].

The aggregated data sets supporting the results of this article and the R2OpenBUGS code used are provided as additional files (Additional files 1 and 2).

Sensitivity analysis and model assumption checking

To assess the influence of prior information on the estimates of model parameters, poorly informative uniform distributions in the range of 0.5 to 1 were also considered for specificities. These truncated distributions were chosen to avoid convergence issues of single MCMC chains due to label switching [44].

To verify the assumption of constant test accuracy across all populations, we first excluded each of the 4 populations and subsequently each of the 14 flocks, one at a time, and re-ran all investigated models.

Results

Complete tests results were available for 1197 animals fulfilling the inclusion criteria, with a median sample size per flock of 89 (minimum 59, maximum 147). The median age at sampling was 2.5 years (lower quartile 2.3, upper quartile 2.7).

Test results

The cross-tabulated counts of the dichotomous outcome of the three tests are given in Table 1 for the 1197 sampled animals when assuming a fecal qPCR positive threshold of Ct ≤ 42. The proportion of concordant test results was greater between the two ELISAs (1137/1197 = 95%) than between fecal qPCR and ELISA A (1047/1137 = 87%) or ELISA B (1051/1197 = 88%). Both ELISAs yielded fewer positive test results (n = 85 for ELISA A, n = 93 for ELISA B) than fecal qPCR (n = 105).

Doubtful results were few for both ELISAs tests and significantly fewer for ELISA A (n = 8) compared to ELISA B (n = 23, Fisher's Exact test p = 0.0109). Setting the positive cut-off at Ct ≤ 42 for fecal qPCR, rather than Ct ≤ 40, yielded 32 more positive samples.

Model selection

Doubtful ELISA results and moving the positive cut-off from 40 to 42 for fecal qPCR had no influence on model selection. Based on DIC, the best fitting model (model 1) was the one with a pairwise dependence between ELISA A and ELISA B on sensitivity and pairwise dependence between the three tests on specificity (Table 2). This model always outperformed the one assuming a conditional independence between fecal qPCR and both ELISAs on sensitivity and specificity (model 2). The difference in the DIC of model 1 and model 2 was always greater than 12.5, suggesting that including covariance terms between the fecal qPCR and both ELISAs provides a better fit to the data, although this was only significant for specificity. As expected, the assumption of conditionally independent ELISAs was not supported by the data, as shown by the high DIC values of model 3 (Table 2).

Estimated accuracy of diagnostic tests

The posterior distributions for sensitivity and specificity of the three tests and prevalence are summarized in

Table 1 Cross-classified positive (+) and negative (−) results of two serum ELISAs and one fecal PCR in sub-populations 1 to 4 for sub-clinically infected 2- to 3-year-old French Causse du Lot sheep

ELISA A	ELISA B	Fecal qPCR	Subpop. 1	Subpop. 2	Subpop. 3	Subpop. 4	Total
+	+	+	0	2	5(4)	8 (5)	15 (11)
+	+	−	9 (7)	11 (7)	14 (14)	10 (6)	44 (34)
+	−	+	0	1	2	2	5 (5)
+	−	−	6 (7)	5 (8)	9 (6)	1 (6)	21 (27)
−	+	+	1	3	6 (4)	1	11 (9)
−	+	−	9 (5)	6 (4)	7 (6)	1	23 (16)
−	−	+	0	4(3)	37 (17)	33 (28)	74 (48)
−	−	−	262 (267)	267 (271)	367 (394)	108 (115)	1004 (1047)
	Total		287	299	447	164	1197

Doubtful ELISA and fecal qPCR Ct ≤ 42 results were treated as positive. When doubtful ELISA and fecal qPCR 40 ≤ Ct ≤ 42 results were treated as negative, counts are shown in brackets

Table 2 Bayesian Deviance Information Criterion (DIC) for model 1 to 3 under different scenarios

		Deviance Information Criterion		
Doubtful ELISA results	Fecal qPCR positive cut-off	Model 1[a]	Model 2[b]	Model 3[c]
Positive	Ct ≤ 42	120.4	134.2	227.9
Positive	Ct ≤ 40	114.3	130.1	197.5
Negative	Ct ≤ 42	115.6	128.2	222.1
Negative	Ct ≤ 40	114.3	127.5	194.5

[a]Models with pairwise dependence between ELISA A and ELISA B for sensitivity and pairwise dependence between the three tests for specificity
[b]Models with pairwise dependence between ELISA A and ELISA B for sensitivity and specificity and assuming conditional independence of fecal qPCR
[c]Models assuming fully conditional independence between the three tests

Table 3 in form-of-point estimates (mean) and 95% Bayesian posterior density credible intervals (95% PCI). For comparison purposes, the results from model 2 and model 3 are also shown. The estimated sensitivity and specificity were similar for ELISA A and ELISA B (Se ≈ 17%, PPD = 0.121; Sp ≈ 95%, PPD = 0.401) (Table 3, model 1). The fecal qPCR was found to be more sensitive (47.5%) and specific (99.0%) than ELISA tests, with PPD > 0.999 and posterior 95% credible interval excluding zero. Under the assumption of complete independence between the fecal qPCR and both ELISA tests (model 2), higher estimated sensitivities were obtained, especially for fecal qPCR (56.3%), without substantial changes for estimated specificities. The fully conditional independent model (model 3) yielded unrealistic significantly higher estimated sensitivity and specificity for ELISA A (Se = 70.0%, Sp = 98.7%) and ELISA B (Se = 80.0%, Sp = 98.9%) than for fecal qPCR (Se = 31.3%, Sp = 93.2%).

From model 1, ELISA A and ELISA B appeared positively correlated for sensitivity and specificity (Covse median of 0.108 and 95% PCI between 0.068 and 0.153; Covsp median 0.029 and 95% PCI between 0.018 and 0.033). No evidence of correlation was found between ELISAs and fecal qPCR for sensitivity. In model 1, covariance terms for specificity between the fecal qPCR and ELISA A (Covsp median 0.001 and 95% PCI between 0.0009 and 0.00529) and ELISA B (Covsp median 0.00472 and 95% PCI between 0.00029 and 0.01179) were very small, although significantly different from 0.

No substantial differences in estimated sensitivity and specificity were observed when analyzing the three other datasets (Table 4). Treating doubtful ELISA results as negative mostly induced a slightly lower estimated sensitivity of ELISA B (14.7%), which was expected from the larger number of doubtful results obtained with this test compared to ELISA A. Similarly, changing the positive cut-off for fecal qPCR from Ct ≤ 42 to Ct ≤ 40 yielded a slightly lower estimated sensitivity for fecal qPCR

Table 3 Mean and 95% posterior credible intervals (PCI) for the sensitivity (Se) and specificity (Sp) of two serum ELISAs and on fecal qPCR and true prevalence (Ps) of MAP in sub-populations 1 to 4

		Mean (95% PCI)		
		Model 1[a]	Model 2[b]	Model 3[c]
DIC		120.4	134.2	227.9
ELISA A	Se	17.9 (11.4; 25.6)	19.7 (13.1; 27.3)	70.0 (56.0; 85.6)
	Sp	94.8 (93.1; 96.3)	95.0 (93.4; 96.5)	98.7 (97.4; 99.9)
ELISA B	Se	17.4 (10.6; 25.9)	23.2 (15.8; 31.5)	80.0 (63.7; 95.3)
	Sp	94.0 (92.2; 95.7)	94.8 (93.2; 96.4)	98.9 (97.5; 99.9)
Fecal qPCR	Se	47.5 (29.3; 69.9)	56.3 (36.9; 77.3)	31.3 (21.8; 41.9)
	Sp	99.0 (97.9; 99.7)	99.4 (98.4; 99.9)	93.2 (91.6; 94.7)
Sub-pop. 1	P1	0.01 (0.0; 0.03)	1.2 (0.1; 3.8)	6.6 (3.1; 11.0)
Sub-pop. 2	P2	5.4 (1.6; 11.5)	6.2 (2.5; 11.9)	8.1 (4.7; 12.3)
Sub-pop. 3	P3	21.7 (13.1; 34.5)	19.2 (12.1; 29.4)	8.4 (5.2; 12.3)
Sub-pop. 4	P4	57.3 (35.4; 88.8)	47.2 (31.0; 70.4)	15.5 (9.7; 22.6)
$\Delta_{\text{ELISA A - ELISA B}}$	Se	0.5 (−5.6; 5.9)	−3.5 (−9.9; 2.5)	−10.0 (−28.8; 9.3)
	Sp	0.8 (−0.8; 2.4)	0.2 (−1.2; 1.5)	−0.2 (−1.9; 1.5)
$\Delta_{\text{Fecal PCR - ELISA A}}$	Se	29.6 (13.7; 50.9)	36.7 (18.6; 57.9)	−38.8 (−56.4; −22.4)
	Sp	4.2 (2.5; 6.0)	4.4 (2.6; 6.2)	−5.5 (−7.4; −3.7)
$\Delta_{\text{Fecal PCR - ELISA B}}$	Se	30.1 (14.5; 50.8)	33.1 (16.0; 53.4)	−48.8 (−66.4; −30.8)
	Sp	5.0 (3.4; 6.7)	4.6 (2.8; 6.4)	−5.7 (−7.7; −3.8)

Doubtful ELISA and fecal qPCR Ct ≤ 42 results were treated as positive
[a]Models with pairwise dependence between ELISA A and ELISA B for sensitivity and pairwise dependence between the three tests for specificity
[b]Models with pairwise dependence between ELISA A and ELISA B for sensitivity and specificity and assuming conditional independence of fecal qPCR
[c]Models assuming fully conditional independence between the three tests

Table 4 Mean and 95% posterior credible intervals (PCI) for the sensitivity (Se) and specificity (Sp) of two serum ELISAs and one fecal qPCR, depending on different scenarios

Dataset		Mean (95% PCI)	
		Se	Sp
Doubtful ELISA results as negative, fecal qPCR cut-off Ct ≤ 42	ELISA A	17.3 (11.0; 24.8)	95.3 (93.7; 96.7)
	ELISA B	14.7 (8.5; 22.4)	95.6 (94.0; 97.0)
	Fecal qPCR	50.9 (31.3; 73.3)	99.2 (98.2; 99.8)
Doubtful ELISA results as positive, fecal qPCR cut-off Ct ≤ 40	ELISA A	21.0 (12.8; 30.8)	94.8 (93.1; 96.3)
	ELISA B	20.0 (11.9; 30.2)	94.0 (92.2; 95.6)
	Fecal qPCR	40.7 (23.5; 63.2)	99.0 (98.0; 99.7)
Doubtful ELISA results as negative, fecal qPCR cut-off Ct ≤ 40	ELISA A	21.2 (12.9; 31.0)	95.3 (93.7; 96.7)
	ELISA B	17.4 (9.5; 27.5)	95.5 (94.0; 96.9)
	Fecal qPCR	45.8 (26.2; 69.3)	99.2 (98.2; 99.8)

Estimates were obtained with model 1

(40.7%) and slightly higher estimated sensitivity for ELISA A (21.0%) and ELISA B (20.0%). In any case, the estimated specificity of the three tests remained mostly unchanged.

Serial and parallel testing

Serial and parallel testing were evaluated for model 1 (Table 5). For both ELISA and fecal qPCR combinations, serial testing was associated with a slight increase in specificity but a strong drop in sensitivity to below 9%. The use of ELISA and fecal qPCR in parallel testing led to an increased estimated sensitivity compared to fecal qPCR alone, though at the price of a loss of specificity.

Sensitivity analysis and model assumption checking

The use of poorly informative prior distributions for specificities and resampling subpopulations or flocks did not yield any substantial change of the parameter estimates. This suggests a very weak influence of prior distributions on estimation and that the assumption of constant sensitivities and specificities was not unreasonable. Furthermore, model selection based on DIC remained unchanged, strengthening our findings regarding the conditional dependence between test results.

Table 5 Mean and 95% posterior credible intervals (PCI) for the sensitivity (Se) and specificity (Sp) of serial and parallel testing using one serum ELISA and the fecal PCR

		Mean (95% PCI)	
		ELISA A – Fecal qPCR	ELISA B – Fecal qPCR
Serial testing	Se_{ser}	8.7 (3.8; 15.8)	8.5 (3.5; 16.0)
	Sp_{ser}	99.8 (99.3 – 100.0)	99.3 (98.5; 99.9)
Parallel testing	Se_{par}	56.6 (38.8;76.1)	55.8 (37.4; 75.9)
	Sp_{par}	93.8 (91.8; 95.6)	93.1 (90.7; 95.1)

Estimates were obtained with model 1, with doubtful ELISA results and fecal qPCR Ct ≤ 42 treated as positive

Discussion

We used a Bayesian latent class approach to estimate the diagnostic accuracy of two serum ELISAs and one fecal qPCR for the detection of 2- to 3-year-old subclinically infected sheep. This evaluation follows the standards for the reporting of diagnosis accuracy for paratuberculosis [1] that were recently extended to Bayesian latent class models [2].

Latent class models are highly sensitive to assumptions made regarding the conditional dependence between tests [10]. We found that treating all three tests as conditionally independent (model 3) led to biased results, with strongly overestimated sensitivities for both ELISAs. This finding is supported by the high DIC value obtained for this model and was already emphasized by simulation studies [20]. In the same way, we found that the assumption of conditional independence between fecal qPCR and ELISAs (model 2) was not supported by the data. Although the conditional independence between fecal culture and ELISA may hold [16, 17], to our knowledge, there is no available study evaluating the conditional dependence between fecal qPCR and ELISA. Indeed, the a priori assumption of conditional independence is made in most cases but not formally tested [12, 15]. In our study, covariance terms between fecal qPCR and ELISAs were only significant in the specificity part of the model and were considerably less than the one found between the two ELISAs. However, based on DIC values, models that accounted for this dependence were unambiguously favored and led to estimates that were moderately lower than those obtained under the conditional independence assumption. These findings may or may not apply to evaluations of other commercial ELISAs and PCRs, depending on the antigens used and gene targets, respectively. In some instances, moreover, the dependence between tests may be of minimal importance, especially if the individual estimates (i.e., specificity) are close to one [2]. However, our results suggest that, when possible, models accounting for all dependence of sensitivities and specificities should be evaluated first and possibly simplified based on a rigorous selection process. Complete saturated models may, however, not be identifiable (i.e., with the number of parameters greater than the degrees of freedom permitted by the data), allowing only restrained covariance structures to be evaluated [44].

One other assumption underlying latent class models is that the various infection stages among the different populations are homogeneously distributed [2]. Our study was based on animals belonging to a narrow age range (2 to 3 years), which, to our point of view, offers several advantages. First, it might have lessened the selection biases related to a non-homogenous sampling across the different infection stages among populations, since an age representative sample of animals might be difficult to achieve in practice. In large herds/flocks where only partial sampling is often applied due to cost constraints, focusing on specific age cohorts may also allow for an easier and more robust comparison of prevalence estimates between herds/flocks. Finally, at the herd/flock level, a narrow age range may facilitate year-over-year comparison of results. The drawback of such an approach is that our results may be strongly linked to our study population and should be carefully extrapolated to other situations.

As both ELISA and fecal qPCR provide a continuous range of result values, the classification of samples as positive or negative results in a loss of information [45] and in inconclusive test results (in our case, doubtful ELISA results and characteristic amplification curves with Ct > 40 for fecal qPCR according to the manufacturer's recommended positive threshold). As they may have a strong influence on accuracy estimates [46], inconclusive results were classified either as positive or negative in separate analyses following standards for reporting of diagnosis accuracy studies. However, because there were only a few, doubtful ELISA results did not cause any considerable differences in the summaries of test performances. In the same way, choosing a Ct ≤ 42 rather than Ct ≤ 40 threshold for the fecal qPCR did not lead to a dramatic change in sensitivity estimates. These changes were of the order of magnitude as those observed between statistical models 1 and 2.

Point estimates of both ELISA sensitivities obtained in our study (14 - 21%) are similar to or slightly lower than those obtained in other studies for the detection of subclinically infected sheep reviewed in Nielsen and Toft (2008) [29]. ELISA B was recently applied on serum and milk in Greek dairy sheep and yielded higher sensitivity estimates (46-49%) [47]. The reasons for these discrepancies are not known but could be related to the age structure of study samples, breed differences or possibly regional MAP strain variations. Conversely, our specificity estimates (94-96%) were in concordance with those found in already mentioned studies in sheep [16, 35–37] and support the idea that ELISA is far from being perfectly specific.

Fecal qPCR has the potential to be a rapid and sensitive method of MAP diagnosis, especially in sheep in which fecal cultures performed poorly. We found that fecal qPCR had higher diagnostic accuracy than ELISA, with sensitivity estimates close to those obtained by Baumann et al. [14] in sheep when using the Ct ≤ 40 cut-off for positive results. Moving the cut-off up to Ct ≤ 42 was associated with slightly enhanced sensitivity estimates with almost no change in specificity estimates. While the specificity of fecal qPCR was very high, it was not absolute at the Ct ≤ 42 or Ct ≤ 40 cut-off. An even more conservative value (i.e., Ct ≤ 38) was also evaluated without improvement of specificity estimates (results not shown). Although the specificity of the IS900 target for the detection of MAP is of concern, as other mycobacteria with IS900-like sequences have been described [48], considerable improvements have been made in PCR probe and primer designs in recent years [49, 50], and this hypothesis is currently unlikely. However, other targets exclusive to MAP, such as the hspx gene [51], have shown non-perfect specificity for the detection of infectious animals when evaluated in Bayesian latent class models [14]. Rather, this might reflect the potential of pass through of orally ingested organisms by uninfected animals [30, 31] or the small yet existent possibility of cross-contamination of samples during collection or laboratory processing. The multi-copy presence of the IS900 target in the MAP genome (14-18 copies) might conversely provide higher analytical sensitivity compared to some specific alternative targets (f57, ISMAP02, hspx) that are only present in six or fewer copies [52, 53]. Moreover, 10.0 g of feces were processed for the qPCR detection, lowering the possibility of missing MAP aggregates [54]. Nevertheless, as stated in our results, the epidemiological sensitivity of fecal qPCR, even based on the IS900 target, remains low in 2- to 3-year-old subclinically infected sheep (40-50%). This might reflect the low number of infected animals that shed MAP in their feces within this age cohort, or that intermittent shedding prevented their detection at the time of sampling, or both.

Our specificity estimates for ELISAs and qPCR are based on data collected in flocks suspected or known to be infected by MAP. Therefore, they may not reflect those that would have been obtained in truly paratuberculosis-free flocks, in which they could be expected to be higher [55]. However, the large-scale application of an imperfectly specific test (even with specificity as high as 99.5%) is questionable for detection purposes, as it would lead to numerous false positive results in paratuberculosis-free flocks that would require further investigation. Conversely, this lack of specificity may have fewer adverse impacts on infected flock monitoring programs, as the positive predictive value of tests will be higher, and no confirmatory testing will generally be requested [56].

Finally, the estimated sensitivity of fecal qPCR had wide credible intervals. In latent class model analysis, reasons responsible for such findings are low true values of diagnostic test accuracy, low true prevalence, small sample size, small difference in prevalence between sub-populations, lack of global identifiability of the model, or parameter estimates close to 0.5 [20, 44, 57]. Although a large number of sheep were sampled, the estimated true prevalence was rather low in two out of four sub-populations (0.8% and 5.4%, respectively), and therefore, the sensitivity estimates were based on a limited number of positive results. This is also illustrated by the very narrow intervals for fecal qPCR sensitivity estimates provided by multiplying the original data by ten (11,970 animals) (results not shown).

The serial use of fecal qPCR for the confirmation of ELISA-positive individuals allows for an almost perfect specificity, especially for ELISA A (99.8%). Serial testing was, however, associated with a very low global sensitivity, meaning that the true infectious status of an ELISA-positive individual that would be subsequently tested as qPCR-negative in feces would remain uncertain. The interferon-gamma release assay provides a positive response earlier in the course of the disease than fecal culture [58] and would therefore be advised in such cases. However, this assay also requires careful interpretation, as it cannot distinguish between infected and exposed animals [59]. As shown in Table 5, the diagnostic accuracy at the individual level could be enhanced by the use of serum ELISA and fecal qPCR in parallel testing. This reflects the fact that fecal shedding of MAP and the humoral response are poorly correlated and that parallel testing might target different individuals. This is also stated by the non-significant covariance terms for sensitivity between fecal qPCR and serum ELISAs in our Bayesian latent class model and is in accordance with experimental infection results indicating that some persistently shedding sheep may develop clinical disease in the absence of an antibody response [60]. The use of tests in combination, however, substantially adds to the cost of control, which may or may not be acceptable to sheep owners. Moreover, the higher cost of individual fecal qPCR (approximately 35 euros or 39 USD) compared to serum ELISA (approximately 6 euros or 7 USD) limits its use at a large scale in France.

Conclusions

An accurate appraisal of diagnostic test accuracy is of critical importance for a better evaluation of paratuberculosis control programs. In this study, we showed that the assumption of conditional independence between fecal qPCR and serum ELISA was not supported by the data and that accounting for this dependence provided slightly different accuracy estimates. Fecal qPCR demonstrated a higher sensitivity and specificity than serum ELISA, but the overall sensitivity of both diagnostic approaches remains low in 2- to 3-year-old sub-clinically infected animals. These findings advocate for more frequent testing of animals in a longitudinal follow-up scenario. Studies are in progress to evaluate the consequence of these estimated diagnostic test accuracy for surveillance programs at the flock level.

Additional files

Additional file 1: R code for Bayesian Latent Class models. Bayesian Latent Class Models (model 1 to 3) that were used in this study. (DOCX 25 kb)

Additional file 2: Aggregated data set. Aggregated diagnostic test results for the 4 sub-populations, given whether doubtful ELISA results were handled as positive or negative and based on two thresholds for fecal qPCR. (DOCX 15 kb)

Abbreviations

CovSe: covariance term on sensitivity; CovSp: covariance term on specificity; CpD2: second derivative maximum; Ct: cycle threshold; DIC: deviance information criterion; MAP: Mycobacterium avium spp. paratuberculosis; MCMC: Markov Chain Monte Carlo; PCI: Bayesian posterior credible interval; PPD: Bayesian posterior probability of difference; qPCR: quantitative polymerase chain reaction; S/P: sample-to-positive ratio; Se: sensitivity; Se_{par}: sensitivity of parallel testing; Se_{ser}: sensitivity of serial testing; SNIG: Systeme National d'Information Génétique; Sp: specificity; Sp_{par}: specificity of parallel testing; Sp_{ser}: specificity of serial testing

Acknowledgements

The authors thank all farmers, farm technicians and veterinary practitioners and students for their involvement in and dedication to this study.

Funding

This study was funded by the INRA GISA Metaprogram PICSAR and Region Midi-Pyrénées (PAROVLOT program). The lead author received a PhD grant from both funding bodies. The funding bodies did not have any direct role in the study design or sample collection.

Authors' contributions

YM, FC and GF developed and designed the study and participated in the animal sampling. YM carried out the laboratory analysis. YM and FC carried out the data analysis. YM, FC and GF drafted the initial manuscript. RF provided additional assistance in coordination of the study and animal sampling. All authors read and approved the final manuscript.

Consent for publication

Not applicable.

Competing interests

The authors declare that they have no competing interests.

Author details

[1]IHAP, Ecole Nationale Vétérinaire de Toulouse, 23 chemin des Capelles, F-31076 Toulouse Cedex 3, France. [2]CAPEL Ovilot, 237 avenue Pierre Semard, 46000 Cahors, France.

References

1. Gardner IA, Nielsen SS, Whittington RJ, Collins MT, Bakker D, Harris B, et al. Consensus-based reporting standards for diagnostic test accuracy studies for paratuberculosis in ruminants. Prev Vet Med. 2011;101:18–34.
2. Kostoulas P, Nielsen SS, Branscum AJ, Johnson WO, Dendukuri N, Dhand NK, et al. STARD-BLCM: standards for the reporting of diagnostic accuracy studies that use Bayesian latent class models. Prev Vet Med. 2017;138:37–47.

3. Hui SL, Walter SD. Estimating the error rates of diagnostic tests. Biometrics. 1980;36:167–71.
4. Dendukuri N, Joseph L. Bayesian approaches to modeling the conditional dependence between multiple diagnostic tests. Biometrics. 2001;57:158–67.
5. Georgiadis MP, Johnson WO, Gardner IA, Singh R. Correlation-adjusted estimation of sensitivity and specificity of two diagnostic tests. J R Stat Soc Series B Stat Methodol. 2003;52:63–76.
6. Berkvens D, Speybroeck N, Praet N, Adel A, Lesaffre E. Estimating disease prevalence in a Bayesian framework using probabilistic constraints. Epidemiology. 2006;17:145–53.
7. Johnson WO, Gastwirth JL, Pearson LM. Screening without a "gold standard": the Hui-Walter paradigm revisited. Am J Epidemiol. 2001;153:921–4.
8. Branscum AJ, Gardner IA, Johnson WO. Estimation of diagnostic-test sensitivity and specificity through Bayesian modeling. Prev Vet Med. 2005;68:145–63.
9. Vacek PM. The effect of conditional dependence on the evaluation of diagnostic tests. Biometrics. 1985;41:959–68.
10. Gardner IA, Stryhn H, Lind P, Collins MT. Conditional dependence between tests affects the diagnosis and surveillance of animal diseases. Prev Vet Med. 2000;45:107–22.
11. Kostoulas P, Leontides L, Billinis C, Florou M. Application of a semi-dependent latent model in the Bayesian estimation of the sensitivity and specificity of two faecal culture methods for diagnosis of paratuberculosis in sub-clinically infected Greek dairy sheep and goats. Prev Vet Med. 2006;76:121–34.
12. Wells SJ, Collins MT, Faaberg KS, Wees C, Tavornpanich S, Petrini KR, et al. Evaluation of a rapid fecal PCR test for detection of Mycobacterium Avium subsp. paratuberculosis in dairy cattle. Clin Vaccine Immunol. 2006;13:1125–30.
13. Angelidou E, Kostoulas P, Leontides L. Bayesian validation of a serum and milk ELISA for antibodies against Mycobacterium Avium subspecies paratuberculosis in Greek dairy goats across lactation. J Dairy Sci. 2014;97:819–28.
14. Bauman CA, Jones-Bitton A, Jansen J, Kelton D, Menzies P. Evaluation of fecal culture and fecal RT-PCR to detect Mycobacterium Avium Ssp. paratuberculosis fecal shedding in dairy goats and dairy sheep using latent class Bayesian modeling. BMC Vet Res. 2016;12:212.
15. Norton S, Johnson WO, Jones G, Heuer C. Evaluation of diagnostic tests for Johne's disease (Mycobacterium Avium subspecies paratuberculosis) in New Zealand dairy cows. J Vet Diagn Investig. 2010;22:341–51.
16. Kostoulas P, Leontides L, Enoe C, Billinis C, Florou M, Sofia M. Bayesian estimation of sensitivity and specificity of serum ELISA and faecal culture for diagnosis of paratuberculosis in Greek dairy sheep and goats. Prev Vet Med. 2006;76:56–73.
17. Weber MF, Verhoeff J, van Schaik G, van Maanen C. Evaluation of Ziehl-Neelsen stained faecal smear and ELISA as tools for surveillance of clinical paratuberculosis in cattle in the Netherlands. Prev Vet Med. 2009;92:256–66.
18. Bermingham ML, Handel IG, Glass EJ, Woolliams JA, de Clare Bronsvoort BM, McBride SH, et al. Hui and Walter's latent-class model extended to estimate diagnostic test properties from surveillance data: a latent model for latent data. Sci Rep. 2015;5:11861.
19. Nielsen SS, Toft N. Age-specific characteristics of ELISA and fecal culture for purpose-specific testing for paratuberculosis. J Dairy Sci. 2006;89:569–79.
20. Toft N, Jorgensen E, Hojsgaard S. Diagnosing diagnostic tests: evaluating the assumptions underlying the estimation of sensitivity and specificity in the absence of a gold standard. Prev Vet Med. 2005;68:19–33.
21. Nielsen SS, Gronbaek C, Agger JF, Houe H. Maximum-likelihood estimation of sensitivity and specificity of ELISAs and faecal culture for diagnosis of paratuberculosis. Prev Vet Med. 2002;53:191–204.
22. Stevenson K. Genetic diversity of Mycobacterium Avium subspecies paratuberculosis and the influence of strain type on infection and pathogenesis: a review. Vet Res. 2015;46:64.
23. Kawaji S, Begg DJ, Plain KM, Whittington RJ. A longitudinal study to evaluate the diagnostic potential of a direct faecal quantitative PCR test for Johne's disease in sheep. Vet Microbiol. 2011;148:35–44.
24. Laurin EL, Chaffer M, McClure JT, McKenna SL, Keefe GP. The association of detection method, season, and lactation stage on identification of fecal shedding in Mycobacterium Avium Ssp. paratuberculosis infectious dairy cows. J Dairy Sci. 2015;98:211–20.
25. Timms VJ, Mitchell HM, Neilan BA. Optimisation of DNA extraction and validation of PCR assays to detect Mycobacterium Avium subsp. paratuberculosis. J Microbiol Methods. 2015;112:99–103.
26. Fock-Chow-Tho D, Topp E, Ibeagha-Awemu EA, Bissonnette N. Comparison of commercial DNA extraction kits and quantitative PCR systems for better sensitivity in detecting the causative agent of paratuberculosis in dairy cow fecal samples. J Dairy Sci. 2017;100:572–81.
27. Spiess AN. qpcR: Modelling and analysis of real-time PCR data. R package version 1.4-0. [https://cran.r-project.org/web/packages/qpcR/index.html]. 2014. Accessed 31 July 2016.
28. R Core Team. R: A language and environment for statistical computing. R Foundation for Statistical Computing, Vienna, Austria [https://www.R-project.org/]. Accessed 31 Jul 2016.
29. Nielsen SS, Toft N. Ante mortem diagnosis of paratuberculosis: a review of accuracies of ELISA, interferon-gamma assay and faecal culture techniques. Vet Microbiol. 2008;129:217–35.
30. Sweeney RW, Whitlock RH, Hamir AN, Rosenberger AE, Herr SA. Isolation of mycobacterium paratuberculosis after oral inoculation in uninfected cattle. Am J Vet Res. 1992;53:1312–4.
31. Moloney BJ, Whittington RJ. Cross species transmission of ovine Johne's disease from sheep to cattle: an estimate of prevalence in exposed susceptible cattle. Aust Vet J. 2008;86:117–23.
32. Joseph L, Gyorkos TW, Coupal L. Bayesian estimation of disease prevalence and the parameters of diagnostic tests in the absence of a gold standard. Am J Epidemiol. 1995;141:263–72.
33. Enoe C, Georgiadis MP, Johnson WO. Estimation of sensitivity and specificity of diagnostic tests and disease prevalence when the true disease state is unknown. Prev Vet Med. 2000;45:61–81.
34. Spiegelhalter DJ, Best NG, Carlin BP, Van Der Linde A. Bayesian measures of model complexity and fit. J R Stat Soc Series B Stat Methodol. 2002;64:583–639.
35. Hope A, Kluver P, Jones S, Condron R. Sensitivity and specificity of two serological tests for the detection of ovine paratuberculosis. Aust Vet J. 2000;78:850–6.
36. Sergeant ES, Marshall DJ, Eamens GJ, Kearns C, Whittington RJ. Evaluation of an absorbed ELISA and an agar-gel immuno-diffusion test for ovine paratuberculosis in sheep in Australia. Prev Vet Med. 2003;61:235–48.
37. Gumber S, Eamens G, Whittington RJ. Evaluation of a Pourquier ELISA kit in relation to agar gel immunodiffusion (AGID) test for assessment of the humoral immune response in sheep and goats with and without mycobacterium paratuberculosis infection. Vet Microbiol. 2006;115:91–101.
38. Stevenson M. EpiR : Tools for the analysis of epidemiological data (Version 0.9-79) [https://cran.r-project.org/web/packages/epiR/index.html]. 2016. Accessed 31 July 2016.
39. Lunn D, Spiegelhalter D, Thomas A, Best N. The BUGS project: Evolution, critique and future directions. Stat Med. 2009;28:3049–67.
40. Sturtz S, Ligges U, Gelman A. R2WinBUGS: a package for running WinBUGS from R. J Stat Softw. 2005;12:1–16.
41. Brooks SP, Gelman A. General methods for monitoring convergence of iterative simulations. J Comput Graph Stat. 1998;7:434–55.
42. Gelman A, Rubin DB. Inference from iterative simulation using multiple sequences. Stat Sci. 1992:457-72.
43. Plummer M, Best N, Cowles K, Vines K. Coda: convergence diagnosis and output analysis for MCMC. R News. 2006;6(1):7–11.
44. Jones G, Johnson WO, Hanson TE, Christensen R. Identifiability of models for multiple diagnostic testing in the absence of a gold standard. Biometrics. 2010;66:855–63.
45. Nielsen SS, Toft N, Jorgensen E, Bibby BM. Bayesian mixture models for within-herd prevalence estimates of bovine paratuberculosis based on a continuous ELISA response. Prev Vet Med. 2007;81:290–305.
46. Shinkins B, Thompson M, Mallett S, Perera R. Diagnostic accuracy studies: how to report and analyse inconclusive test results. BMJ. 2013;346:f2778.
47. Angelidou E, Kostoulas P, Leontides L. Bayesian estimation of sensitivity and specificity of a commercial serum/milk ELISA against the Mycobacterium Avium subsp. Paratuberculosis (MAP) antibody response for each lactation stage in Greek dairy sheep. Prev Vet Med. 2016;124:102–5.
48. Englund S, Bolske G, Johansson KE. An IS900-like sequence found in a mycobacterium sp. other than Mycobacterium Avium subsp. paratuberculosis. FEMS Microbiol Lett. 2002;209:267–71.
49. Kawaji S, Taylor DL, Mori Y, Whittington RJ. Detection of Mycobacterium Avium subsp. paratuberculosis in ovine faeces by direct quantitative PCR has similar or greater sensitivity compared to radiometric culture. Vet Microbiol. 2007;125:36–48.
50. Plain KM, Marsh IB, Waldron AM, Galea F, Whittington AM, Saunders VF, et al. High-throughput direct fecal PCR assay for detection of Mycobacterium Avium subsp. paratuberculosis in sheep and cattle. J Clin Microbiol. 2014;52:745–57.
51. Ellingson JL, Bolin CA, Stabel JR. Identification of a gene unique to Mycobacterium Avium subspecies paratuberculosis and application to diagnosis of paratuberculosis. Mol Cell Probes. 1998;12:133–42.

52. Li L, Bannantine JP, Zhang Q, Amonsin A, May BJ, Alt D, et al. The complete genome sequence of Mycobacterium Avium subspecies paratuberculosis. Proc Natl Acad Sci U S A. 2005;102:12344–9.
53. Mobius P, Hotzel H, Rassbach A, Kohler H. Comparison of 13 single-round and nested PCR assays targeting IS900, ISMav2, f57 and locus 255 for detection of Mycobacterium Avium subsp. paratuberculosis. Vet Microbiol. 2008;126:324–33.
54. Christopher-Hennings J, Dammen MA, Weeks SR, Epperson WB, Singh SN, Steinlicht GL, et al. Comparison of two DNA extractions and nested PCR, real-time PCR, a new commercial PCR assay, and bacterial culture for detection of Mycobacterium Avium subsp. paratuberculosis in bovine feces. J Vet Diagn Investig. 2003;15:87–93.
55. Brenner H, Gefeller O. Variation of sensitivity, specificity, likelihood ratios and predictive values with disease prevalence. Stat Med. 1997;16:981–91.
56. Thrusfield M. Veterinary epidemiology. Third ed. USA: Wiley-Blackwell; 2007. p. 305–30.
57. Georgiadis MP, Johnson WO, Gardner IA. Sample size determination for estimation of the accuracy of two conditionally independent tests in the absence of a gold standard. Prev Vet Med. 2005;71:1–10.
58. Huda A, Jungersen G, Lind P. Longitudinal study of interferon-gamma, serum antibody and milk antibody responses in cattle infected with Mycobacterium Avium subsp. paratuberculosis. Vet Microbiol. 2004;104:43–53.
59. Mortier RA, Barkema HW, De Buck J. Susceptibility to and diagnosis of Mycobacterium Avium subspecies paratuberculosis infection in dairy calves: a review. Prev Vet Med. 2015;121:189–98.
60. Stewart DJ, Vaughan JA, Stiles PL, Noske PJ, Tizard ML, Prowse SJ, et al. A long-term study in merino sheep experimentally infected with Mycobacterium Avium subsp. paratuberculosis: clinical disease, faecal culture and immunological studies. Vet Microbiol. 2004;104:165–78.

16

Magnetic resonance features of the feline hippocampus in epileptic and non-epileptic cats

Anne Christine Claßen[1*], Sibylle Kneissl[2], Johann Lang[3], Alexander Tichy[4] and Akos Pakozdy[5]

Abstract

Background: Hippocampal necrosis in cats has been reported to be associated with epileptic seizures. Magnetic resonance imaging (MRI) features of temporal lobe (TL) abnormalities in epileptic cats have been described but MR images from epileptic and non-epileptic individuals have not yet been systematically compared. TL abnormalities are highly variable in shape, size and signal, and therefore may lead to varying evaluations by different specialists. The aim of this study was to investigate whether there were differences in the appearance of the TL between epileptic and non-epileptic cats, and whether there were any relationships between TL abnormalities and seizure semiologies or other clinical findings. We also investigated interobserver agreement among three specialists.

Methods: The MR images of 46 cats were reviewed independently by three observers, who were blinded to patient data, examination findings and the review of the other observers. Images were evaluated using a multiparametric scoring system developed for this study. Mann–Whitney U-tests and chi-square were used to analyse the differences between observers' evaluations. The kappa coefficient (k) and Fleiss' kappa coefficient were used to quantify interobserver agreement.

Results: The overall interobserver agreement was moderate to good (k =0.405 to 0.615). The MR scores between epileptic and non-epileptic cats did not differ significantly. However, there was a significant difference between the MR scores of epileptic cats with and without orofacial involvement according to all three observers. Likewise, MR scores of cats with cluster seizures were higher than those of cats without clusters.

Conclusion: Cats presenting with recurrent epileptic seizures with orofacial involvement are more likely to have hippocampal pathologies, which suggests that TL abnormalities are not merely unspecific epileptic findings, but are associated with a certain type of epilepsy. TL signal alterations are more likely to be detected on FLAIR sequences. In contrast to severe changes in the TL which were described similarly among specialists, mild TL abnormalities may be difficult to interpret, thus leading to different assessments among observers.

Keywords: Feline temporal lobe epilepsy, Orofacial automatism, Orofacial involvement, Magnetic resonance imaging, Epileptic seizure, Hippocampal necrosis, Hippocampal sclerosis, Interobserver agreement, Cluster seizures, Status epilepticus

* Correspondence: anne-classen@gmx.de
A part of this study was presented as a poster at the 2014 Annual Meeting of the European College of Veterinary Neurology in Madrid, Spain
[1]Small Animal Veterinary Hospital Stommeln, D 50259 Pulheim, Germany
Full list of author information is available at the end of the article

Background

Over the past two decades, several case reports on feline hippocampal necrosis (HN) have been published in Europe, Asia, and the United States [1–9], indicating that necrosis of the hippocampus and piriform lobe associated with the appearance of epileptic seizures in feline patients is a worldwide phenomenon. Magnetic resonance imaging (MRI) is routinely used in human epileptic patients [10–12], and hippocampal sclerosis (HS) has been identified as the single most frequently detected feature of mesial temporal lobe (TL) epilepsy in humans [11].

In cats, MRI is also the method of choice for antemortem detection of intracranial pathologies, including hippocampal changes. However, there has not been a systematic comparison of MR images of TLs in healthy and epileptic cats, and little is known about the accuracy of this diagnostic modality or the potential subjectivity of the observers' assessments. Thus, it remains unclear whether changes in the hippocampal size and signal are always associated with the occurrence of epileptic seizures or whether they can also be present in non-epileptic patients.

The aims of this retrospective, multi-observer study were to examine whether there was a difference in the TL signal between epileptic and non-epileptic cats and whether an abnormal MR signal was related to seizure semiology or other clinical findings in epileptic patients. In addition, the degree of agreement among three independent observers was assessed. We hypothesised that marked hippocampal signal alterations in MRI would be associated with the occurrence of epileptic seizures in feline patients. Cats suffering from TL seizures (including orofacial automatisms) were expected to be diagnosed with hippocampal lesions more often than cats suffering from non-temporal epileptic seizures of different aetiologies. We also expected good agreement among specialists in identifying signal alterations, and that fluid-attenuated inversion recovery (FLAIR) sequences would be superior to other MR sequences in detecting variations in TL signal intensity.

Methods

Medical records of cats housed at the University of Veterinary Medicine, Vienna, between August 2011 and May 2013 were searched for animals that underwent high field-MRI (Magnetom Espree, 1.5 Tesla, Siemens Healthcare, Erlangen, Germany). Inclusion criteria were availability of at least one transverse T1-weighted scan, one post-contrast T1 turbo spin-echo (T1C), one FLAIR, and either one transverse T2 or 3D sagittal T2-weighted scan. A series of subtracted pre- and post-contrast images was found for most cases. Imaging studies that met the inclusion criteria were selected independently by A.C., who was not actively involved in the review process. All patients were anonymised by assigning a randomised patient number.

The images were independently evaluated by one neurologist (AP, DECVN) and two radiologists (SK, non-certified; JL, DECVDI). Each of the three observers had more than 10 years of experience in MRI interpretation. The observers were blinded to patient data and history, examination findings, and the review of the other two observers.

Observers recorded their evaluations on the TL signal using an itemised form. The multiparametric scoring system consisted of two subdivisions (Code I, II Table 1). Code I classified the signal intensity of the hippocampi in relation to the paramedian grey matter; the normal hippocampal signal intensity was considered to be slightly hyperintense on FLAIR and T2-weighted images compared to the paramedian grey matter. Code II consisted of signal intensity, signal shape, and contrast enhancement as parameters, which were combined into a total score (overall assessment); this code was recently used to describe MR images in dogs [13] and was modified for this study.

Statistical analyses

The statistical analyses were performed using IBM SPSS v. 20 (SPSS Inc., Chicago, IL, USA).

A Mann–Whitney *U*-test was used to analyse the differences in TL MR morphology between patients grouped by history, that is, evidence of epileptic seizures, status epilepticus (SE), cluster seizures (CS), orofacial involvement (OI), and number of epileptic seizures prior to MRI. Status epilepticus was defined as seizures of more than thirty minutes duration or repeated seizures without full recovery whereas cluster seizures were determined as more than one seizure within 24 h.

The weighted kappa coefficient (k) was used to quantify pairwise agreement between observers. A value of 1.0 implied complete agreement and 0.0 indicated a level of agreement expected by chance alone (categories were: 0.0–0.2 poor agreement; 0.21–0.40 fair agreement; 0.41–0.60 moderate agreement; 0.61–0.80 good agreement; 0.81–1.0 excellent agreement). Fleiss' kappa coefficient for multiple raters was also calculated to estimate the overall agreement among the three observers. For all statistical tests, $p < 0.05$ was considered significant.

An additional system was introduced to compare the individual overall assessments of each observer. A four-point gap between scores was considered poor agreement, three points indicated fair agreement, two points showed moderate agreement, and a one point difference indicated good agreement. The agreement was considered perfect if the observers rated the images with the same score.

Table 1 Scoring scheme used according to codes I and II

Score	Code I	Code II	
1	Normal	Definitely normal	Normal TL signal, shape and no contrast enhancement
2	Questionable	Probably normal	Slightly increased/decreased TL signal
3	Moderately increased or decreased signal intensity	Equivocal	Distinctly increased/decreased TL signal
4	Severely increased or decreased signal intensity	Probably abnormal	Distinctly increased/decreased TL signal and abnormal shape
5	-	Definitely abnormal	Abnormal TL signal, shape and contrast enhancement

Code I - Hippocampal signal intensity
Code II - Overall TL signal and shape characteristics

Results

MR images of 46 cats were included in the study. Twenty-five cats (54.3 %) were females (22 spayed and three intact) and 21 (45.7 %) were males (20 neutered and one intact). The mean age of the cats was 7 years (range 3 months to 15 years), and the breeds represented were European shorthair ($n = 32$), domestic shorthair ($n = 8$), and one of each of the following breeds: Persian, Norwegian forest cat, Maine Coon, Devon rex, European longhair, and Chartreux.

The indication for brain MRI was epileptic seizures in 27 cases (58.7 %) and other neurological disorders in 19 (41.3 %) cats. Nineteen epileptic cats (41.3 %) showed CS and seven (15.2 %) had experienced at least one SE. Fifteen cats (32.6 %) presented epileptic seizures with OI. Of these, eight (17.4 %) had 1–5 seizures, five (10.9 %) had 6–10, five (10.9 %) had 11–25, and eight (17.4 %) had > 25 epileptic fits prior to undergoing MRI. In one case (2.2 %), it was not possible to clarify how many seizures the animal had experienced prior to MRI because it was owned by an animal shelter.

Four of the nineteen non-epileptic patients presented with tetraparesis (8.7 %), three presented with vestibular dysfunction (6.5 %), and two cats with each of circling (4.3 %), obsessive walking (4.3 %), aggression (4.3 %), or anisocoria (4.3 %). One cat each was examined because of hemiparesis (2.2 %), collapse (2.2 %), behavioural changes other than aggression (2.2 %), and for medical evaluation of cerebellar rigidity (2.2 %). MRI of the non-epileptic patients revealed intracranial neoplasia (31,6 %), unremarkable MRI scan (31,6 %), extracranial neoplasia (21,1 %), internal otitis (10,5 %) and ear polyp (5,3 %).

Using the additional system of testing agreement by comparing the magnitude difference between scores, the overall agreement was perfect among three observers in 52.2 % of cases and perfect to good (i.e., maximum difference of one point between scores) in 67.4 % cases. In 17.4 % of cases the overall agreement was fair to poor. The overall interobserver agreement (Code II) ranged from k = 0.405 to 0.615. Of all comparisons between observers, observers A and B had the best agreement, with a k value of 0.615. All interobserver analyses resulted in 0.8 > k >0.4, which is considered to be moderate to good agreement. Fleiss' kappa was 0.493, which also implies a moderate agreement among all three observers.

Table 2 lists the mean MR scores (regarding the overall assessment, Code II) for TL MR morphology for patients with different histories. For statistical analysis rating distributions were compared using chi-square test. The rating distribution did not differ between epileptic and non-epileptic cats (observers A $p = 0.27$, B $p = 0.283$, C $p = 0.528$; overall $p = 0.111$).

The MR images of cats that had a history of epileptic seizures with OI were rated with mean Code II scores of 3.2 (observer A), 2.9 (observer B), and 3.4 (observer C). The rating distribution of epileptic cats with OI differed significantly from epileptic cats without OI (observer A: $p < 0.001$; observer B:, $p = 0.002$; observer C:, $p = 0.027$, overall $p = 0.001$) and from the non-epileptic cats (observer A:, $p = 0.009$; observer B:, $p = 0.071$; observer C: $p = 0.228$, overall: $p = 0.001$).

The TL MR morphologies of epileptic cats with at least one SE were rated significantly higher than those that had never experienced SE only by observers A (observer A: $p = 0.016$; observer B: $p = 0.067$; observer C:

Table 2 Mean MR scores (Code II) from observers A, B, and C for patients with different histories. For statistical analysis chi-squared comparison of rating distribution was used

	Observer		
Patient History	A	B	C
Epileptic cats	2.3	2.1	2.5
Nonepileptic cats	1.4	1.6	1.8
Epileptic cats without orofacial involvement	1.1	1.2	1.4
Epileptic cats with orofacial involvement	3.2	2.9	3.4
Epileptic cats with status epilepticus	3.3	3.1	3.3
Epileptic cats without status epilepticus	1.7	1.6	2.1
Epileptic cats with cluster seizures	2.6	2.3	3.2
Epileptic cats without cluster seizures	1.4	1.5	1.6
Cats with 1–5 seizures prior to MRI	1.9	1.8	1.4
Cats with 6–10 seizures prior to MRI	1.0	1.0	1.3
Cats with 11–25 seizures prior to MRI	2.8	2.3	4.2
Cats with >25 seizures prior to MRI	2.9	2.8	3.1

$p = 0.376$, overall: $p = 0.001$). In addition, all observers rated the images of cats with a history of CS with a significantly higher Code II score than cats with no history of CS (observer A: $p = 0.012$; observer B: $p = 0.076$; observer C: $p = 0.0028$; overall $p < 0.001$ Fig. 1).

There was a tendency that with an increasing number of seizures the TL abnormalities were more severe, however the difference was not significant. Significant and nearly significant was the difference regarding Code II scores given for images of the subgroup of epileptic cats that had 11–25/more than 25 seizures compared to non-epileptic cats (A: $p = 0.066/0.083$, B: $p = 0.23/0.096$, C: 0.092/0.321, overall 0.009/0.051).

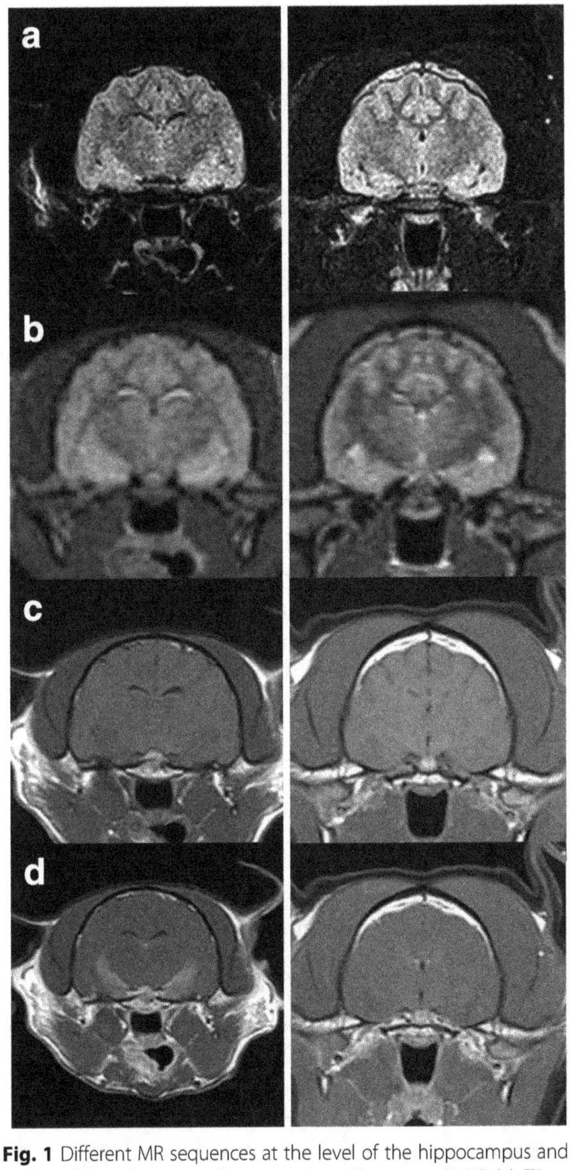

Fig. 1 Different MR sequences at the level of the hippocampus and piriform lobe of two cats for comparison. Transverse FLAIR (**a**), T2-weighted (**b**), pre- (**c**) and post-contrast (**d**) T1-weighted images at the level of the hippocampus and piriform lobe in a 9-year-old male Maine Coon with reported seizures with orofacial involvement (*left*) and 3-year-old female neutered European Shorthair Cat suffering from epileptic seizures without orofacial automatisms (*right*). The MR overall assessment (Code II) was considered definitely abnormal (score 5) by all three observers in the former and definitely normal (score 1) in the latter case

Table 3 lists the mean Code I scores for the hippocampal signal intensity changes seen on the five MR sequences evaluated. Higher Code I scores (scores range from 1–4 points) illustrate greater signal changes of the hippocampal signal. The mean of Code I scoring points given for T2 images was 1.5 (observer A), 1.7 (observer B), and 1.8 (observer C), which referred to a normal to questionable signal intensity of the hippocampi. The mean Code I scores given for the FLAIR images were 2.0 (observer A), 1.7 (observer B), and 1.9 (observer C). These results referred to a normal to questionable signal intensity (observers B and C) or questionable signal intensity (observer A). The signal intensity of native T1-weighted images was given a mean score of 1.4 (observer A), 1.5 (observer B), and 1.0 (observer C). These results referred to a normal (observer C) or normal to questionable signal intensity (observers A and B). The T1-weighted images after intravenous contrast application were given mean Code I scores of 1.6 (observer A), 1.4 (observer B), and 1.6 (observer C), all normal to questionable signal intensities. Finally, the subtracted pre- and post-contrast images were given mean scores of 1.4 (observer A), 1.4 (observer B), and 1.7 (observer C), all normal to questionable signal intensities.

Discussion

As a group, MR images of the TL of cats suffering from any kind of epileptic seizure did not differ significantly from those of cats without epileptic disorders. However when stratified according to seizure semiology, or

Table 3 Comparison of MR assessment of signal change (Code I) using different sequences

	Observer A				Observer B				Observer C			
SP	1	2	3	4	1	2	3	4	1	2	3	4
T2	35	2	8	1	30	3	8	4	22	11	10	1
	76.1	4.3	17.4	2.2	66.7	6.7	17.8	8.9	50.0	25.0	22.7	2.3
FLAIR	24	2	15	5	30	3	7	4	21	10	11	2
	52.2	4.3	32.6	10.9	68.2	6.8	15.9	9.1	47.7	22.7	25.0	4.5
T1	38	0	5	2	32	4	8	1	43	0	1	0
	84.4	0.0	11.1	4.4	71.1	8.9	17.8	2.2	97.7	0.0	2.3	0.0
T1C	35	0	6	5	37	0	3	4	30	4	6	4
	76.1	0.0	13.0	10.9	84.1	0.0	6.8	9.1	68.2	9.1	13.6	9.1
SUB	35	0.0	3	4	35	2	1	4	27	1	6	4
	83.3	0.0	7.1	9.5	83.3	4.8	2.4	9.5	71.1	2.6	15.8	10.5

SP: MR scoring points, where 1 = normal signal, 2 = questionable, 3 = slightly increased or decreased, and 4 = severely increased or decreased. Table shows counts in first row and percentages in second row

occurrence of CS or SE, MR images of the TL of cats with a history of epileptic seizures with OI, or cats with CS or SE, differed significantly from epileptic cats that did not, and from non-epileptic cats.

Previous studies have suggested that alterations in the feline TL visible on MR images were caused by various underlying conditions, including astrogliosis, oedema, hypoxia, idiopathic HN and HS, inflammation, intracranial infection, ischemia, malformation and neoplastic conditions [1–9]. A potential toxin or infectious agent cannot be ruled out, nor can genetic predisposition or febrile seizures early in life, as described in human medicine [14]. The hippocampus is also known to have a very low seizure threshold compared to other parts of the brain and is therefore more susceptible to active participation in a post-discharge evoked by a different part of the brain, or even to become an epileptic focus itself [15]. Since the initial histological description of HS in humans, there has been debate about whether HS is a nonspecific result of a primary epileptogenic lesion restricted to the hippocampus, whether it is caused by damage to the cells due to the spread of epileptic discharges to this area, or even whether it develops due to other causes [11]. There is evidence that HN and HS in children is multi-causal [16]; the same can be reasonably assumed for feline patients. At present it is not possible to distinguish the underlying cause of a TL abnormality by diagnostic imaging alone, even if repeated scans could help to differentiate between reversible and irreversible lesions.

Changes in the TL MR morphology seem to be rare in non-epileptic cats and occur much more frequently in epileptic cats with OI compared to other cats. Therefore, we suspect that OI in epileptic cats is not only a specific epileptic phenomenon for feline temporal lobe epilepsy (TLE), in line with early experimental studies [17], but is also significantly associated with temporal lobe changes detected in MR images.

As expected, the images of cats with a history of CS or SE were given significantly higher MR scores (however not by all three observers) compared to the images of cats that had never suffered CS or SE. These groups also included cats presenting OI, since the majority of the cats with OI also had CS or SE.

SE and CS likely cause more severe damage to neurons compared to infrequent short seizures due to the long period in which neurons are exposed to synchronous electric activity [18]. Previous studies have shown that the hippocampus, in particular, tends to develop irreversible MRI-detectable pathologies after convulsive SE [19]. However, we did not evaluate the time span between the last observed epileptic event and the day of diagnostic imaging. Therefore, it is possible that even if there was acute damage to the neurons of the TL, this damage could have been reversible and there may have been sufficient time for the cells to reorganise before the images were taken. This aspect has never been investigated in cats but should be taken into account in further studies as early postictal MRI abnormalities can also be both causes and consequences of seizure [18].

We expected that signal alterations in the hippocampal area would be detected more frequently in cats that experienced a higher number of seizures prior to MRI. Indeed, there was such a tendency but differences in ratings were only significant between non-epileptic patients and patients with 11–25 or more than 25 seizures prior to MRI. These results may indicate that a certain number of a specific kind of seizure is necessary to cause visible MRI changes. Similarly, recent studies in rats showed that hippocampal volume loss was not correlated with seizure frequency [20]. Since the certain number of seizures our subjects had experienced could only be estimated in some cases, these data must be interpreted with caution. Moreover, because the number of postictal days prior to imaging is unknown, MR abnormalities could also be caused by reversible oedema.

In our study, FLAIR sequences were rated with the highest scores. Because the signal of intraventricular cerebrospinal fluid is suppressed, the FLAIR sequence for periventricular lesions is more conspicuous than T2-weighted sequences. T2-weighted sequences were only slightly inferior to FLAIR sequences in detecting alterations of the TL signal, consistent with earlier results [21, 22]. T1C-weighted images were ranked third, and pre-contrast T1-weighted images were ranked fourth. This leads to the conclusion that only lesions that show contrast enhancement are reasonably detectable on T1-weighted images. In human medicine, the gold standard scan protocol includes high-resolution T2-weighted images, with or without inverting the contrast. MR techniques such as hippocampal volume measurements, T2 relaxometry, MR spectroscopy and diffusion tensor imaging of the hippocampus are sometimes used in human medicine [23]. These dedicated techniques are not yet routinely available in veterinary medicine and MR volumetry and diffusion tensor imaging were only performed on few cats experimentally [24, 25]. The hippocampal volume was significantly reduced unilaterally in one study in familial strain of spontaneous epileptic cats in comparison with a healthy control group [24], but this aspect was not investigated by our study.

In this study, there was moderate-good interobserver agreement among specialists, although the overall agreement was perfect among the three observers in 52.2 % of cases and perfect to moderate in 82.6 % of all cases. There were many factors influencing the assessment of images in this blind study. Because the hippocampal signal was not measured objectively in this study, MRI interpretation was associated with considerable subjectivity, although this aspect has not been explicitly discussed in veterinary medicine. Opinions differ in clinical practice regarding what constitutes a normal TL signal, and this discrepancy may result in markedly different assessments among observers [26]. Because the hippocampus contains more grey matter than surrounding parts of the brain [27], mild T2 hyperintensity should be considered normal, but no standard value can be given. Although all three observers involved in this study were expert in neuroimaging, they had diverse backgrounds and different numbers of years' experience in this specific field of diagnostic imaging, which could have led to different interpretations of the lesion anatomic location, pattern, mass effect, and contrast medium uptake. This discrepancy may also be explained, at least in part, by the tendency of some practitioners to score as uncertain for equivocal patients, whereas others prefer to commit to a diagnosis. Because of partial volume averaging it also may be difficult to distinguish whether the hyperintense signal arises from the hippocampus or the lateral ventricle and in some cases there were intracranial masses present, which displaced the hippocampal tissue and may have interfered with the MR signal of this region. If this was the case, some observers refused to evaluate the specific images. We conclude that subjectivity of the assessments is also a factor that may lead to discrepant evaluations and thus must not be underestimated.

This study had several limitations. First, it was a descriptive study of the agreement among three observers. Because it did not take the final diagnosis into account (most of the patients are still alive and only few histopathologic examinations have been performed yet), no conclusion could be made to the comparability of the radiographic and pathohistologic assessments. Second, the observers had no knowledge of the patients' histories or physical and neurological examinations and could not contextualise the images. Third, we can not rule out for sure, that patients presenting with altered mentation or behavioral changes were suffering from non-convulsive status epilepticus and were misclassified as non-epileptics. Fourth, although the images were all taken at the same institution, some variability in positioning and MR sequence availability were noted. Fifth, our observers had little specific training in using the scoring system provided and it is possible that this also had an effect on the scoring. Finally, because there was no follow-up imaging, observers could not differentiate between reversible and irreversible changes of the affected side. However, such differentiation is likely relevant but this issue was investigated in cats only experimentally [28]. Volumetry could be helpful as hippocampal size might increase in oedema and decreases in sclerosis. The recently published recommendation on a veterinary epilepsy-specific MRI protocol by the International Veterinary Epilepsy Task Force also emphasised the importance of the evaluation of the hippocampi. At least visual assessment should be carried out including size, symmetry, atrophy and signal changes, however volumetric measurement may be meaningful in the future [29].

Conclusions

Temporal lobe epilepsy with hippocampal sclerosis is well researched in human medicine, and there is strong evidence that TLE with HS may also be common in cats. Feline patients presenting with recurrent epileptic seizures with orofacial involvement or cluster seizures/status epilepticus are more likely to have hippocampal pathologies that are detectable by MRI and especially on FLAIR sequences. Changes in temporal lobe signal intensity (especially T2 hyperintensity) are more pronounced in cats suffering from TLE than in cats with any other kind of epileptic disorders and are therefore most likely specific pathophysiologic phenomena of this condition. However, non-specific consequence from status epilepticus or cluster seizures may play a role.

Mild hippocampal signal alterations may be difficult to interpret and lead to different assessments among observers, in contrast to severe changes, which are described in a similar way by different specialists.

Abbreviations

CS, cluster seizures; FLAIR, fluid attenuated inversion recovery; HN, hippocampal necrosis; HS, hippocampal sclerosis; MRI, magnetic resonance imaging; OI, orofacial involvement; SE, status epilepticus; SUB, subtracted pre- and post-contrast images; T, Tesla (unit of the magnetic field); T1, T1-weighted image; T1C, post-contrast T1-weighted image; T2, T2-weighted image; TL, temporal lobe; TLE, temporal lobe epilepsy

Acknowledgements

We thank Sabine Dengg, RT, who acquired and anonymized the MR images.

Funding

The study was funded by the vice-rectorship for research and international relations of the University of Veterinary Medicine Vienna.

Authors' contributions

AC helped with anonymizing the MR images, was involved in the data interpretation, wrote the initial draft and contributed substantially to the writing of the final manuscript. AP developed the initial concept, was involved in research planning, clinical work-up, MR analysis, data interpretation and manuscript revision. SK contributed to the acquisition and analysis of the MR images, was involved in revising the manuscript, and provided the images for the figures. JL contributed to the analysis of the MR images, data interpretation and revision of the manuscript. AT helped with the data interpretation, did the statistical evaluation and was involved in the revision of the manuscript. All authors read and approved the final version of the manuscript.

Competing interests

The authors declare that they do not have any competing interests.

Consent for publication

Not applicable.

Author details

[1]Small Animal Veterinary Hospital Stommeln, D 50259 Pulheim, Germany. [2]Clinical Unit of Diagnostic Imaging, University of Veterinary Medicine, A 1210 Vienna, Austria. [3]Division of Clinical Radiology, Vetsuisse Faculty, University of Bern, CH 3012 Bern, Switzerland. [4]Department of Biomedical Sciences, University of Veterinary Medicine, A 1210 Vienna, Austria. [5]Clinic for Internal Medicine, University of Veterinary Medicine, A 1210 Vienna, Austria.

References

1. Fatzer R, Gandini G, Jaggy A, Doherr M, Vandevelde M. Necrosis of hippocampus and piriform lobe in 38 domestic cats with seizures: a retrospective study on clinical and pathologic findings. J Vet Intern Med. 2000;14:100–4.
2. Schmied O, Scharf G, Hilbe M, Michal U, Tomsa K, Steffen F. Magnetic resonance imaging of feline hippocampal necrosis. Vet Radiol Ultrasound. 2008;49(4):343–9.
3. Schriefl S, Steinberg TA, Matiasek K, Ossig A, Fenske N, Fischer A. Etiologic classification of seizures, signalment, clinical signs, and outcome in cats with seizure disorders: 91 cases (2000–2004). J Am Vet Med Assoc. 2008;233(10):1591–7.
4. Pakozdy A, Gruber A, Kneissl S, Leschnik M, Halasz P, Thalhammer JG. Complex partial cluster seizures in cats with orofacial involvement. J Feline Med Surg. 2011;13(10):687–93.
5. Mariony-Henry K, Monteiro R, Behr S. Complex partial orofacial seizures in English cats. Vet Rec. 2012;170:471.
6. Vanhaesebrouck AE, Posch B, Baker S, Plessas IN, Palmer AC, Constantino-Casas F. Temporal lobe epilepsy in a cat with pyriform lobe oligodendroglioma and hippocampal necrosis. J Feline Med Surg. 2012;4(12):932–7.
7. Gelberg HB. Diagnostic exercise: sudden behavior change in a cat. Vet Pathol. 2013;50:1156–7.
8. Tamura M, Hasegawa D, Uchida K, Kuwabara T, Mizoguchi S, Ochi N, et al. Feline anaplastic oligodendroglioma: long-term remission through radiation therapy and chemotherapy. J Feline Med Surg. 2013;15(12):1137–40.
9. Wagner E, Rosati M, Molin J, Foitzig U, Wahle AM, Fischer A, et al. Hippocampal sclerosis in feline epilepsy. Brain Pathol. 2014. doi: 10. 1111/bpa.12147
10. Grant R, Hadley DM, Condon B, Doyle D, Patterson J, Bone I, et al. Magnetic resonance imaging in the management of resistant focal epilepsy: pathological case report and experience of 12 cases. J Neurol Neurosurg Psychiatry. 1987;50(11):1529–32.
11. Wieser HG. Mesial temporal lobe epilepsy with hippocampal sclerosis. Epilepsia. 2004;45(6):695–714.
12. Mitsueda-Ono T, Ikeda A, Sawamoto N, Aso T, Hanakawa T, Kinoshita M, et al. Internal structural changes in the hippocampus observed on 3-Tesla MRI in patients with mesial temporal lobe epilepsy. Intern Med. 2013;52(8):877–85.
13. Keenihan EK, Summers BA, David FH, Lamb CR. Canine meningeal disease: associations between magnetic resonance imaging signs and histologic findings. Vet Radiol Ultrasound. 2013;54(5):504–15.
14. Kasperaviciute D, Catarino CB, Matarin M, Leu C, Novy J, Tostevin A, et al. Epilepsy, hippocampal sclerosis and febrile seizures linked by common genetic variation around SCN1A. Brain. 2013;136(10):3140–50.
15. Delgado JMR, Sevillano M. Evolution of repeated hippocampal seizures in the cat. Electroenceph Clin Neurophys. 1961;13:722–33.
16. Yoong M, Martinos MM, Chin RF, Clark CA, Scott RC. Hippocampal volume loss following childhood convulsive status epilepticus is not limited to prolonged febrile seizures. Epilepsia. 2013;54(12):2108–15.
17. Sato M. Hippocampal Seizure and Secondary Epileptogenesis in the "Kindled" Cat Preparations. Psychiatry Clin Neurosci. 1975;29(3):239–50.
18. Cianfoni A, Caulo M, Cerasec A, Della Marca G, Falcone C, Di Lella GM, et al. Seizure- induced brain lesions: a wide spectrum of variably reversible MRI abnormalities. Eur J Radiol. 2013;82(11):1964–72.
19. Kim JA, Chung JI, Yoon PH, Kim DI, Chung TS, Kim EJ, et al. Transient MR signal changes in patients with generalized tonicoclonic seizure or status epilepticus: periictal diffusion-weighted imaging. Am J Neuroradiol. 2001; 22(6):1149–60.
20. Polli RS, Malheiros JM, Dos Santos R, Hamani C, Longo BM, Tannús A, et al. Changes in hippocampal volume are correlated with cell loss but not with seizure frequency in two chronic models of temporal lobe epilepsy. Front Neurol. 2014;5:111.
21. Beningni L, Lamb CR. Comparison of fluid-attenuated inversion recovery and T2-weighted magnetic resonance images in dogs and cats with suspected brain disease. Vet Radiol Ultrasound. 2005;46:287–92.
22. Cherubini GB, Platt SR, Howson S, Baines E, Brodbelt DC, Dennis R. Comparison of magnetic resonance imaging sequences in dogs with multi-focal intracranial disease. J Small Anim Pract. 2008;49:634–40.
23. Deblaere K, Achten E. Structural magnetic resonance imaging in epilepsy. Eur Radiol. 2008;18(1):119–29.
24. Mizoguchi S, Hasegawa D, Kuwabara T, Hamamoto Y, Ogawa F, Fujiwara A, Matsuki N, Fujita M. Magnetic resonance volumetry of the hippocampus in familial spontaneous epileptic cats. Epilepsy Research. 2014;108:1940–1944.
25. Takahashi E, Dai G, Wang R, Ohki K, Rosen GD, Galaburda AM, Grant PE, Wedeen VJ. Development of cerebral fiber pathways in cats revealed by diffusion spectrum imaging. Neuroimage. 2010;49:1231–40.
26. Coan AC, Kubota B, Bergo FP, Campos BM, Cendes F. 3T MRI quantification of hippocampal volume and signal in mesial temporal lobe epilepsy improves detection of hippocampal sclerosis. American Journal of Neuroradioly. 2014;35:77–83.
27. Winkler C, Potter A. An anatomical guide to experimental research on the cat's brain. Amsterdam: W. Versluys; 1914.
28. Tanaka S, Tanaka T, Kondo S, Hori T, Fukuda H, Yonemasu Y, et al. Magnetic Resonance Imaging in Kainic Acid-induced Limbic Seizure Status in Cats. Neurol Med Chir. 1993;33(5):285–9.
29. Rusbridge C, Long S, Jovanovik J, Milne M, Berendt M, Bhatti SF, De Risio L, Farqhuar RG, Fischer A, Matiasek K, Muñana K, Patterson EE, Pakozdy A, Penderis J, Platt S, et al. International Veterinary Epilepsy Task Force recommendations for a veterinary epilepsy-specific MRI protocol. BMC Vet Res. 2015;11(1):194.

Salivary pH, calcium, phosphorus and selected enzymes in healthy dogs

Ilaria Iacopetti, Anna Perazzi*, Tamara Badon, Silvia Bedin, Barbara Contiero and Rebecca Ricci

Abstract

Background: Saliva in dogs, as in humans, is a complex fluid secreted by different salivary glands in the oral cavity to protect the oral mucosa and teeth. The use of saliva as a substitute for blood in diagnosing and prognosticating disease in humans is widely accepted. Salivary biochemistry has also been used as a marker for periodontal disease in humans. No studies have as yet investigated the relation between salivary biochemistry and periodontal disease in dogs, however; neither has the salivary composition of healthy dogs with no oral disease been assessed. The purpose of this study was to obtain an overview on pH distribution and a set of salivary biochemical analytes (calcium, phosphorus, lactate dehydrogenase, lysozyme and amylase) commonly related to oral health in humans in a subset population of healthy young dogs with no periodontal disease or previous oral disease. Data were analyzed to gather salivary reference ranges for pH and each parameter and to assess a possible correlation between salivary and serum analytes.

Results: Twenty-nine adult client-owned dogs were recruited for the study. Lactate dehydrogenase and lysozyme showed higher concentrations in saliva than in serum, whereas amylase showed the contrary. Salivary biochemistry values did not differ between males and females or between non-neutered and neutered individuals. No significant correlations between salivary and serum calcium, phosphorus, lactate dehydrogenase, amylase and lysozyme were identified in this study. Data allowed intervals for the salivary pH and other analytes investigated to be obtained from healthy dogs with healthy oral conditions.

Conclusions: These preliminary data can contribute to enlarge our understanding of the functional role of saliva and its relation to oral health in dogs.

Keywords: Saliva, Biochemistry, Healthy dog

Background

Saliva is a fluid mostly secreted from different salivary glands present in the oral cavity [1–3]. It contains a complex mixture of electrolytes and proteins with different biological roles in digestion, host defense, lubrication, and maintenance of oral and general health [1, 3, 4].

In human medicine, many researchers have used sialochemistry to diagnose systemic illnesses and monitor general patient health, and also as a disease risk indicator, demonstrating a close link between oral and systemic health [5]. There are compelling reasons to use saliva as a diagnostic fluid also in veterinary medicine. The greatest advantage is the method's non-invasiveness: saliva is easily collectable from different animal species [6, 7]. In dogs, saliva samples have been mainly used for cortisol determination, avoiding the stress created by venipucture for blood collection [8], and also for IgGs measurement [9], rabies virus antigen detection [10], drug monitoring [11], and CRP quantification [1].

Some studies conducted on humans have identified different salivary biomarkers for oral health status, such as lactate dehydrogenase [12–14], mucin and amylase [4, 15], Il-1ß, MMP-8 and MMP-8/TIMP-1 ratios [16], lactoferrin [17, 18] lysozyme [19], and TNF-alpha [20]. These authors demonstrated that these analytes generally increase in proportion to periodontal disease in humans. Although

* Correspondence: anna.perazzi@gmail.com
Department of Animal Medicine, Production and Health, University of Padua, Legnaro (Padua), Italy

periodontal disease is the most widespread oral disease in dogs, no studies have investigated the relationship between salivary biochemistry and the degree of severity of periodontal disease in this species [21]. Moreover, little is known on the salivary composition of healthy dogs with no oral disease.

Based on the limited literature available, the primary aim of this pilot study was to evaluate salivary pH and certain salivary analytes relevant to oral health, such as amylase, lactate dehydrogenase (LDH), lysozyme, calcium (Ca), and phosphorus (P) in healthy adult dogs with no oral disease. As these analytes have previously never been reported in literature, with exception of alpha-amylase, our results will eventually provide preliminary data to obtain salivary reference intervals. It is worth noting that as observed for certain analytes in humans, such as cortisol and adiponectin, saliva is a proven and accepted alternative to serum analysis in veterinary medicine [6]. A second objective is to assess whether parameter concentrations in saliva correlate with those found in serum.

Methods

Dogs

Adult client-owned dogs of different breeds and both sexes were recruited from patients of the Veterinary Teaching Hospital of the University of Padua. In order to be included in the study, dogs had to be young (less than 2 years old) and healthy on the basis of general physical examination, regularly vaccinated, and not to have received any antibacterial or anti-inflammatory medication for at least 6 months. Further inclusion criteria were no signs of oral pathology (grade 0 according to the classification of periodontal disease of the *American Veterinary Dental College*) [22] and no history of either oral disease or periodontal therapy, and dogs had to have been fed dry commercial food (kibbles). The study was approved by the Animal Welfare Committee of the University of Padua (authorization number n°#71/ 2015). The owner's written consent was obtained before the dog was enrolled in the study.

Saliva and blood collection

Both saliva and blood samples were obtained from all animals in the morning by the same examiner at the Veterinary Teaching Hospital of the University of Padua. In order to collect serum and saliva samples properly, dogs were prohibited from eating 12 h prior to sampling; furthermore, water was removed at least 1 h previously, as recommended by the manufacturer of the collection device. The oral cavity was thoroughly inspected to confirm the absence of any sign of oral pathology before saliva collection. Two dental cotton rolls[1] were used, one at a time. Each one was inserted in the dog's oral cavity using disposable gloves and pushed up to the molar teeth to make the dog chew for 1 min. Each cotton roll was immediately placed back in its own tube and centrifuged. After saliva collection, 6 ml of blood were taken by venipuncture from the cephalic vein of each dog using 22G needles and placed into evacuated plastic tubes containing either a coagulation accelerator or EDTA for biochemical and hematological analysis, respectively.

Saliva and blood analysis

Saliva and blood samples were analyzed at the Clinical Diagnostic Laboratory of the Department of Animal Medicine Production and Health of the University of Padua.

Salivette® tubes were centrifuged[2] for 2 min at 1000 g. After centrifugation, the two saliva samples obtained from each dog were pooled together in order to obtain a single sample of at least 300 μl of saliva. A visual quality assessment of hemolysis was assigned (using score 0 for no presence of blood to score 3 for severe presence of blood) to each saliva sample. Salivary pH was measured on each sample using litmus paper[3]. Saliva analysis, conducted using a BT1500 automated chemistry analyzer[4], included the quantification of amylase, LDH, lysozyme, Ca, and P. The calibration of the equipment was the same used for blood.

The EDTA blood samples were analyzed using ADVIA 120 Hematology Systems – Siemens Healthcare[5] equipped with Veterinary Software version 3.18.0-MS. A blood smear was performed for each sample to confirm the ADVIA data. The hematological analytes analyzed in this study included packed cell volume (PCV), platelet count (PLT), and leukocyte count (WBC), as well as the relative and absolute numbers of neutrophils, lymphocytes, monocytes, eosinophils, basophils, and large unstained cells (LUC) counts, and values for MPV, large platelet count, and platelet clumps (aggregates).

For serum biochemical analysis, coagulated samples were centrifuged (Labofuge 400, Heraeus Holding, Hanau, Germany) at 1750 g for 10 min at room temperature; serum was separated and immediately analyzed using a BT1500 automated chemistry analyzer. The analytes analyzed were: magnesium, alkaline phosphatase, aspartate aminotransferase, alanine aminotransferase, gamma-glutamyltransferase, LDH, creatinine, urea, total protein, globulins, cholesterol, triglycerides, glucose, and creatine kinase. Further, the analytes quantified in saliva were also measured in the serum. On board of the chemistry analyzer, Gesan reagents[6] were used for all tests, except for lysozyme, for which the commercial kits[7] , calibrated to manufacturer indications were used.

Statistical analysis

The analytes analyzed in blood and saliva (amylase, LDH, lysozyme, Ca and P) were submitted to PROC UNIVARIATE (SAS V.9.1, SAS Institute Inc., Cary, North Carolina, USA) to test the normality of their distribution (Shapiro Wilk test ≥0.90), and all analytes that did not match the normal hypothesis were log-transformed. All normally distributed analytes were analyzed by a linear model with fixed effects of sex, sterilization, interaction between sex and sterilization (PROC GLM, SAS V.9.1, SAS Institute Inc., Cary, North Carolina, USA). Non-normally distributed analytes were analyzed by non-parametric analysis (Mann-Whitney *U*-test). Spearman's test (PROC CORR, SAS V.9.1, SAS Institute Inc., Cary, North Carolina, USA) was used to assess the correlation between the analytes quantified in serum and saliva.

Reference intervals (lower and upper limits) of the salivary analytes measured in the study population were calculated on the basis of the recommendations for the determination of reference intervals in species of veterinary interest issued by the American Society for Veterinary Clinical Pathology (2011) using commercially available statistical MedCalc software[8]. In this analysis, the Robust method was adopted for the non-normally distributed salivary analytes, whereas the normal distribution method was used for the others. The Tukey method was used to identify suspected outliers, which were then excluded from analysis.

Results

Twenty-nine (29) adult client-owned dogs met the inclusion criteria and were recruited for the study: 13 males (5 neutered) and 16 females (8 neutered), with a mean age of 18.2 months (range, 10 to 24) and a mean body weight of 16.5 kg (range, 6 to 42.8 kg). The breed population included 18 mixed breed dogs, 4 Flat Coat Retrievers, 2 Whippets, 1 American Staffordshire Terrier, 1 Breton, 1 Great Dane, 1 German Shepherd and 1 Basenji. All dogs had a complete set of teeth with periodontal disease grade 0 and no history of oral disease or periodontal therapy. Hematological and biochemical analyses revealed that the study population's values were within the reference range (data not shown). All samples yielded a sufficient amount of saliva and could be used for analysis; none was discarded due to blood presence. The salivary pH and biochemistry values, as well as the same analytes measured in serum (mean ± DS, minimum, maximum and median), are shown in Table 1.

Some biochemistry analytes appear to be concentrated quite differently in saliva compared to serum: LDH and lysozyme are 18 and 9 times more concentrated in saliva, respectively, whereas amylase is 25 times less concentrated in saliva (Table 1); Ca and P presented a slightly higher concentration in serum than saliva (1.4 and 1.3 times, respectively). No significant effects of gender and reproductive state were detected for either saliva or serum analytes (Table 2).

No significant correlations were found between salivary and serum Ca, P, LDH, amylase and lysozyme in this study ($p > 0.05$). The reference intervals for the salivary analytes measured in the 29 selected dogs, as well as the method used for their determination, are reported in Table 3.

Discussion

Saliva is a unique clear fluid, composed of electrolytes, immunoglobulins, proteins and enzymes mostly secreted from different salivary glands [3]. The basic role of saliva is to protect the oral mucosa and teeth through lubrication, buffering and clearance action, and antibacterial and antiviral activity, and is also involved in taste and digestion [3]. Its protective effect has prompted several studies on the characteristics (composition and pH) of human saliva in an attempt to establish a relationship with periodontal disease [2, 4, 23].

Despite the fact that periodontal disease is the most widespread oral disease in dogs, only very limited study on saliva composition and oral health biomarkers in particular has been conducted in veterinary medicine to date. To the authors' knowledge, only one study has examined salivary pH and the concentration of certain minerals (e.g. Ca, P, Na and K) in healthy dogs, even if they play pivotal roles in tooth de/remineralization and calculus formation [7].

Table 1 Salivary and serum biochemistry values and salivary pH measured in the study population

Parameter	N	Mean (±DS)	Min	Max	Median	%95 CI for the mean
Saliva						
Ca mg/dl	29	7.48 ± 1,74	4.83	12	7.38	6.82–8.14
P mg/dl	29	3.57 ± 1,68	1.3	8.4	3.2	2.3–4.21
LDH UI/L	28	2394.9 ± 1669,5	341.2	7230.3	2013.1	1747.5–3042.2
Amylase UI/L	26	27.15 ± 19,18	6.25	95.66	25.48	19.40–34.90
Lysozyme mg/L	29	3.17 ± 4,08	0.25	20.03	1.77	1.61–4.72
pH	29	7.93 ± 0,46	7	9	8	7.76–8.10
Serum						
Ca mg/dl	28	10.35 ± 0,44	9.56	11.60	10.38	10.18–10.52
P mg/dl	28	4.67 ± 1,04	2.18	6.86	4.92	4.26–5.07
LDH UI/L	28	132.52 ± 79,71	43.65	362.38	106.24	101.61–163.43
Amylase UI/L	28	698.21 ± 223,29	325.34	1229.99	640.57	611.63–784.79
Lysozyme mg/L	28	0.36 ± 0,17	0.11	0.78	0.34	0.29–0.43

Min: lower identified value; Max: higher identified value

Table 2 Means ± SE of serum and salivary biochemical analytes distributed according to gender and reproductive state

Parameter	Females	Males	Neutered	Non-neutered
Saliva				
Ca mg/dl	7.23 ± 0.36	8.00 ± 0.41	8.03 ± 0.42	7.20 ± 0.37
P mg/dl	3.38 ± 0.40	3.70 ± 0.45	3.37 ± 0.46	3.70 ± 0.40
LDH UI/L	2088.87 ± 1.22	1645.17 ± 1.27	1974.64 ± 1.26	1740.33 ± 1.24
Amylase UI/L	19.32 ± 1.19	24.72 ± 1.22	20.49 ± 1.22	23.31 ± 1.20
Lysozyme mg/L	1.88 ± 1.31	1.88 ± 1.36	2.81 ± 1.36	1.25 ± 1.31
Serum				
Ca mg/dl	10.45 ± 0.11	10.21 ± 0.14	10.41 ± 0.14	10.25 ± 0.11
P mg/dl	4.69 ± 0.24	4.77 ± 0.30	4.99 ± 0.31	4.47 ± 0.25
LDH UI/L	105.27 ± 1.16	130.01 ± 1.21	118.10 ± 1.21	115.89 ± 1.17
Amylase UI/L	657.90 ± 1.10	733.86 ± 1.12	624.19 ± 1.12	773.49 ± 1.10
Lysozyme mg/L	0.31 ± 1.11	0.34 ± 1.18	0.31 ± 1.18	0.34 ± 1.11

The primary aim of this study was therefore to evaluate a set of salivary biochemical analytes relevant to oral health such as amylase, LDH, and lysozyme, as well as calcium, phosphorus, and salivary pH in a population of healthy young adult dogs with no periodontal disease or history of oral disease. The objective was to obtain reference values for the biochemistry of saliva associated with oral health, given that none are as yet available in literature for this species. Differences between gender and reproductive state were also investigated, as well as correlations with the concentrations of the same analytes in serum.

In our study, average dog saliva pH was found to be slightly more acidic than as reported by Lavy et al. [7] (pH 8.53 ± 0.34, range 8.50–8.65), and we observed a wider range of values in the population tested (7–9, median 8). As in humans, it is reasonable to think that many factors affect oral pH in dogs. This lower average pH value than that obtained by Lavy et al. [7] could also be explained by different oral health conditions in the two populations investigated. Lavy et al. [7] did not provide any information on the oral health condition of the dogs included in his study, however, and therefore, whether some individuals included in his study suffered from periodontal disease or whether this may have affected salivary biochemistry or pH is unknown. Gender-related differences in saliva pH and biochemical profile have recently been observed in human medicine [24]. Female subjects have smaller salivary glands, and this may contribute to these differences. In our study, however, no significant differences between male and female dogs were detected, neither were any differences identified between non-neutered and neutered individuals. Further, we cannot exclude that canine breeds may affect salivary pH and future studies should focus on this topic, as this was not the aim of the present one. It is well known that salivary calcium and phosphate concentrations are involved in maintaining the balance between demineralization and remineralization [7, 25]. This makes them good candidates for the monitoring of oral health.

In our study, salivary concentrations of Ca (7.48 mg/dl) and P (3.57 mg/dl) were respectively lower and higher than the values reported by Lavy et al. [7] (Ca: 11.6 mg/dl; P: 1.3 mg/dl). More studies should be addressed to quantifying mineral concentrations in canine saliva, taking different breeds and ages, and different feeding management and oral conditions into consideration.

Lactate dehydrogenase (LDH) is a ubiquitous enzyme that plays a key role in the clinical diagnosis of many disease processes [13, 14, 26]. As it is released in the extracellular environment after cellular lysis, it represents a marker of tissue breakdown and cell death [27]. LDH activity has been therefore quantified in whole saliva and shown to be a reliable diagnostic marker of periodontal disease in humans

Table 3 Reference intervals (lower and upper limits) of the salivary analytes measured in the study population based on the 90% CI of the mean (*P* values were calculated by the D'Agostino Pearson test; n SO: number of suspected outliers, detected by the Tukey method)

Analyte	P	n SO	Outliers	n dogs	Lower limit	Upper limit	Method
Ca mg/dl	0.03	2	11.99; 12	27	4.51	9.85	Robust
P mg/dl	0.014	1	8.4	28	0.15	6.27	Robust
LDH UI/L	0.005	3	33.8; 819.46; 7230	25	0	4025	Robust
Amylase UI/L	<0.001	1	95.66	25	0	52.05	Robust
Lysozyme mg/L	<0.001	2	12.21; 20.03	27	0	5.8	Robust
pH	0,09	0		29	7.03	8.82	Based on normal distribution

[12, 23, 26]. In the study by De la Peña et al., [12] human patients with healthy periodontium showed significantly lower salivary LDH activity than those with periodontal disease (mean: 1107 vs 1930 UI/L, respectively). In our study, canine patients with healthy periodontium showed a salivary LDH activity comparable to that shown by De la Peña et al. [12] in human patients with periodontal disease (mean: 1930 UI/L). In humans, higher levels of salivary LDH have been attributed to cell death and tissue breakdown in the oral mucosa, and the study of salivary LDH isoenzyme patterns by De la Peña and colleagues indicates that the exfoliated cells of the oral epithelium are the major source of salivary LDH. [12, 26] It is therefore possible that the high LDH values observed in the healthy dog population in our study are the consequence of a para-physiologic increased cellular turnover linked to ethologic characteristics of this species. Dogs use their mouth not only to eat food but also as a means of social interaction with other animals and objects, and this increases the possibilities of oral mucosal lesions. Furthermore, De la Peña et al., [12] reported higher concentrations of LDH in females than in males, which were in accordance with previous studies in humans [28], whereas, as previously stated, no gender effect was detected in our canine population.

Lysozyme is an antibacterial enzyme, which is present in all body fluids, including saliva. In the oral cavity, lysozyme is secreted from major and minor salivary glands, gingival crevicular fluid, and salivary leukocytes [2, 23, 29]. It appears to play an important role in controlling microbial overgrowth, reducing the number of bacteria in the dental biofilm, decreasing colonization, and modifying bacterial metabolism [5, 30, 31]. The mean salivary concentration of lysozyme in our study (3.17 mg/L) was much lower than the level reported by Felizardo et al. [30] in healthy humans (41.74 to 93.86 mg/L).

α -Amylase is a family of proteins, consisting of several isoforms that differ in charge and glycosylation. It is secreted mainly by the parotid glands. This enzyme is considered a good indicator of properly functioning salivary glands [5]. Traditionally, this salivary enzyme was thought only to initiate the digestion of starch in the oral cavity, being responsible for the breaking down of high molecular weight carbohydrates to lower molecular weight sugars. In a study by Chauncey et al. on metabolic processes occurring within mammalian salivary glands, it was shown that dog's parotid fluid is devoid of α-amylase activity and only traces were found in its submaxillary saliva. [32] This can be explained by the fact that dogs chew food very roughly, thus they do not need to initiate the digestion of starch in the mouth. However, in a recent study by Sousa-Pereira et al., a characterization of saliva in different mammal species was performed using a proteomic approach and α-amylase was detected in dogs' saliva, which might reflect the natural selection related to digestion efficacy and food recognition. [33] Furthermore, Contreras-Aguilar et al. recently confirmed the existence of α -amylase in canine saliva and demonstrated that this enzyme can be measured by a spectrophotometric assay and that increases after a sympathetic activation. [34] From studies carried out in humans [4], it is now well-known that α-amylase is involved in the non-immunological defence mechanism of the oral cavity, and that salivary glands respond to the disease by increasing the protective potential of saliva and reducing the rate of secretion after the resolution of the inflammatory process. That study showed that people with no periodontitis have an average α -amylase activity of 93.90 U/ml [4], which is much higher than the mean value detected in the healthy canine population investigated in our study (27,15 U/L).

Saliva is a hypotonic fluid compared to plasma, and some components are found in lower, higher or similar concentration. [35] The measurement of selected analytes in saliva is a proven and accepted alternative to serum analysis in human medicine, and some analytes such as cortisol and adiponectin have been shown to correlate well with the blood concentration in dogs [6]. In our study, however, none of the analytes measured in saliva correlated with those measured in serum. Moreover, the higher LDH and lysozyme concentration in saliva compared to serum may be related to the species and be linked to the dogs' increased need for oral mucosal defence. Contrarily, the lower salivary α -amylase concentration compared to serum, although potentially involved in the non-immunological defence of the oral cavity, may reflect the negligible need of this enzyme in saliva to digest starch.

Finally, the low number of subjects used in this study may represent a limitation of the reference interval calculation and these results should be confirmed in the future with a larger number of dogs.

Conclusion

Using a population of young healthy dogs with no signs of oral disease to gather reference intervals for salivary biochemical analytes related to periodontal disease in humans may be an important step forward in enlarging our understanding of saliva's functional role and relation to oral health in dogs. This study provides an overview of salivary composition with regard to certain biochemical analytes. No significant correlations between salivary and serum calcium, phosphorus, LDH, amylase and lysozyme were identified in this study. Conversely, LDH and lysozyme showed higher concentrations in saliva than in serum, whereas amylase was more concentrated in serum. Due to the paucity of information available in literature, however, further investigations on canine salivary biochemistry are recommended to confirm the results observed in this preliminary study and to investigate other analytes with possible associations to oral disease.

Endnotes

[1]Salivette®, Sarstedt AG & Co, Nümbrecht, Germany

[2]Labofuge 400, Heraeus Holding, Hanau, Germany

[3]Carlo Erba Reagenti – Gruppo Montedison, Milano, Italy.

[4]BT1500 automated chemistry analyzer, Biotecnica, Rome, Italy.

[5]ADVIA 120 Hematology Systems, Siemens Healthcare, Milan, Italy.

[6]Gesan Production s.r.l., Campobello di Mazara, Italy.

[7]PKL, Paramedical s.r.l., Faiano, Italy.

[8]MedCalc for Windows, version 12.5, MedCalc Software, Ostend, Belgium.

Abbreviations

Ca: calcium; CRP: c reactive protein; EDTA: ethylenediaminetetraacetic acid; IgGs: immunoglobulins; Il-1ß: Interleukin; K: potassium; LDH: lactate dehydrogenase; LUC: large unstained cells; MMP: matrix metalloproteinase; MPV: mean platelet volume; Na: sodium; P: phosphorous; PCV: packed cell volume; PLT: platelets; TIMP-1: Tissue Inhibitor of Metalloproteinase; TNF-alpha: tumor necrosis factor alpha; WBC: white blood cells

Acknowledgements

Not applicable.

Funding

No specific funding was received for this study.

Authors' contributions

AP and II conceived this study, participated in its design and coordination, and helped to draft the manuscript. RR made significant contributions to conception and design and provided final approval of the version to be published. TB and SB carried out laboratory analysis. BC performed statistical analysis. All authors have read and approved the final version of this manuscript.

Consent for publication

Not applicable.

Competing interests

The authors declare that they have no competing interests.

References

1. Parra MD, Tecles F, Martinez-Subiela S, Ceron JJ. Creactive protein measurement in canine saliva. J Vet Diagn Investig. 2005;17:139–44.
2. Schenkels LCPM, Veerman ECI, Nieuw Amerongen AV. Biochemical composition of human saliva in relation to other mucosal fluids. Crit Rev Oral Biol Med. 1995;6:161–75.
3. Krasteva A, Kisselova A. Salivary acute phase proteins as biomarker in oral and systemic disease. In: Veas F, editor. Acute phase proteins as early non-specific biomarkers of human and veterinary diseases. InTech Europe; 2011. p. 69–88.
4. Sanchez GA, Miozza VA, Delgado A, Busch L. Relationship between salivary mucin or amylase and the periodontal status. Oral Dis. 2013;19:585–91.
5. De Almeida PdV, Gregio AMT, Machado MAN, de Lima AS, Azevedo LR. Saliva composition and functions: a comprehensive review. J Cont Dent Pract. 2008;9:1–11.
6. Tvarijonaviciute A, Carillo-Sanchez JD, Garcia-Martinez JD, Tecles F, Martinez-Subiela S, German AJ, Ceron JJ. Measurement of salivary adiponectin concentrations in dogs. Vet Clin Path. 2014;43:416–21.
7. Lavy E, Goldberger D, Friedman M, Steinberg D. pH values and mineral content of saliva in different breeds of dogs. IJVM. 2012;67:244–8.
8. Wenger-Riggenbach B, Boretti FS, Quante S, Schellenberg S, Reusch CE, Sieber-Ruckstuhl NS. Salivary cortisol concentrations in healthy dogs and dogs with hypercortisolism. J Vet Intern Med. 2010;24:551–6.
9. German AJ, Hall EJ, Day MJ. Measurement of IgG, IgM and IgA concentrations in canine serum, saliva, tears and bile. Vet Immunol Immunopathol. 1998;64:107–21.
10. Kasempimolporn S, Saengseesom W, Lumlertdacha B, Sitprija V. Detection of rabies virus antigen in dog saliva using a latex agglutination test. J Clin Microbiol. 2000;38:3098–9.
11. Dunnett M, Littleford A, Lees P. Phenobarbitone concen- trations in the hair, saliva and plasma of eight epilectic dogs. Vet Rec. 2002;150:718–24.
12. De La Peña VA, Dios PD, Sierra RT. Relationship between lactate dehydrogenase activity in saliva and oral health status. Arch Oral Biol. 2007;52:911–5.
13. Malicka B, Skoskiewicz-Malinowska K, Kaczmarek U. Salivary lactate dehydrogenase and aminotransferases in diabetic patients. Medicine. 2016;95:47.
14. Nagao Y, Kawahigashi Y, Sata M. Association of Periodontal Diseases and Liver Fibrosis in patients with HCV and/or HBV infection. Hepat Mon. 2014; 14(12):e23264.
15. Kejriwal S, Bhandary R, Thomas B, Kumari S. Estimation of levels of salivary mucin, amylase and total protein in gingivitis and chronic periodontitis patients. J Clin Diagn Res. 2014 Oct;8(10):ZC56–60.
16. Rathnayake N, Åkerman S, Klinge B, Lundegren N, Jansson H, Tryselius Y, Sorsa T, Gustafsson A. Salivary biomarkers of oral health - a cross-sectional study. J Clin Periodontol. 2013;40:140–7.
17. Glimvall P, Wickstrçm C, Jansson H. Elevated levels of salivary lactoferrin, a marker for chronic periodontitis? J Periodont Res. 2012;47:655–60.
18. Yadav N, Lamba AK, Thakur A, Faraz F, Tandon S, Pahwa P. Effect of periodontal therapy on lactoferrin levels in gingival crevicular fluid. Aust Dent J. 2014 Sep;59(3):314–20.
19. Younes R, Yousfi M, Ghorra C, Khalife S, Igondjo-Tchen-Changotade S, Willig C, Senni K, Charpiot P, Naaman N, Godeau G. The defensive role of lysozyme in human gingiva in inflammatory periodontal disease. J Periodont Res. 2009;44:578–87.
20. Khosravi R, Ka K, Huang T, Khalili S, Nguyen BH, Nicolau B, Tran SD. Tumor necrosis factor- α and interleukin-6: potential interorgan inflammatory mediators contributing to destructive periodontal disease in obesity or metabolic syndrome. Mediat Inflamm. 2013;2013:728987.
21. Marshall MD, Wallis CV, Milella L, Colyer A, Tweedie AD, Harris SA. Longitudinal assessment of periodontal disease in 52 miniature schnauzers. BMC Vet Res. 2014;10:166.
22. Marretta SM, Leesman M, Burgess-Cassler A. McClure GDJr., Buelow M, Finn M. Pilot evaluation of a novel test strip for the assessment of dissolved thiol levels, as an indicator of canine gingival health and periodontal status. Can Vet J. 2012;53:1260–5.
23. Malathi K, Usha R, Sable D. Salivary enzymes-a diagnostic marker for periodontal disease. IJSR. 2013;2:68–80.
24. Prodan A, Brand HS, Ligtenberg AJM, Imangaliyev S, Tsivtsivadze E, van der Weijden GA, Crielaard W, Keijser BJF, Veerman ECI. Interindividual variation, correlations, and sex-related differences in the salivary biochemistry of young healthy adults. Interindividual variation, correlations, and sex-related differences in the salivary biochemistry of young healthy adults. Eur J Oral Sci. 2015;123:149–57.
25. Shahrabi MA, Nikfarjam JA, Alikhani AA, Akhoundi NB, Ashtiani MC, Seraj BA. Comparison of salivary calcium, phosphate, and alkaline phosphatase in children with severe, moderate caries, and caries free in Tehran's kindergartens. J Indian Soc Pedod Prevent Dent. 2008;7:74–8.
26. Kavyashree Lokesh K. Jayanthi lactate dehydrogenase: an enzymatic biomarker in oral health and disease. IJCDMR. 2015:1–3.
27. Gandolfo S, Pentenero M, Broccoletti R, Pagano M, Carrozzo M, Scully C. Toluidine blue uptake in potentially malignant oral lesions *in vivo*: clinical and histological assessment. Oral Oncol. 2006;42:89–95.
28. Tietz NW, Wekstein DR, Shuey DF, Brauer GAA. Two-year longitudinal reference range study for selected serum enzymes in a population more than 60 years of age. J Am Geriatr Soc. 1984;32:563–70.

29. Moslemi M, Sattari M, Kooshki F, Fotuhi F, Modarresi N, Sadrabad ZK, Shadkar MS. Relationship of salivary lactoferrin and lysozyme concentrations with early childhood caries. J dent res dent Clin Dent Prospect. 2015;9:109–14.
30. Felizardo KR, Gonçalves RB, Schwarcz WD, Poli-Frederico RC, Maciel SM, de Andrade FB. An evaluation of the expression profiles of salivary proteins lactoferrin and lysozyme and their association with caries experience and activity. Rev Odonto Ciênc 2010; 25:344–349.
31. Perera S, Uddin M, Hayes JA. Salivary lysozyme: a noninvasive marker for the study of the effects of stress on natural immunity. Int J Behav Med. 1997;4:170–8.
32. Chauncey HH, Henriques BL, Tanzer JM. Comparative enzyme activity of saliva from the sheep, hog, dog, rabbit, rat, and human. Arch Oral Biol. 1963;8:615–27.
33. De Sousa-Pereira P, Cova M, Abrantes J, Ferreira R, Trindade F, Barros A, Gomes P, Colac B, Amado F, Esteves PJ, Vitorino R. Cross-species comparison of mammalian saliva using an LC–MALDI based proteomic approach. Proteomics. 2015;15:1598–607.
34. Contreras-Aguilar MD, Tecles F, Martínez-Subiela S, Escribano D, Bernal LJ, Cerón JJ. Detection and measurement of alpha-amylase in canine saliva and changes after an experimentally induced sympathetic activation. 2017. BMC Vet Res. 2017;13(1):266.
35. Nunes LA, Mussavira S, Bindhu OS. Clinical and diagnostic utility of saliva as a non-invasive diagnostic fluid: a systematic review. Biochem Med. 2015; 25(2):177–92.

18

A preliminary survey of major diseases of ruminants and management practices in Western Tigray province, northern Ethiopia

Getachew Mebrahtu Welay[1*], Dawit Gebremichael Tedla[1], Gebreyohans Gebru Teklu[1], Shishay Kahsay Weldearegay[1], Mearg Belay Shibeshi[2], Haftom Hadush Kidane[3], Berhe Beyene Gebrezgiabher[4] and Teklehaymanot Huluf Abraha[5]

Abstract

Background: Despite the highest population, the productivity of Ethiopian livestock is low, and the direct contribution to the national economy is limited. Poor genetic potential, shortage of feed in quantity and quality, poor health care and management practices are the main contributors to low productivity and production. Data on animal disease and management practices are not in place, in this regard; we estimate the burden of animal health ailments and management practices in ruminants via simple cross-sectional study design in randomly selected peasant associations in western Tigray of northern Ethiopia.

Results: A preliminary disease survey in ruminants and their management practices comprising of cattle, sheep and goats was undertaken to evaluate the existence, burden of ruminant diseases and management practices. A total of 121 randomly selected household respondents of Maikhadrah and Bakhar (26.2%), Dansha (19.7%), Adi-Hirdi (18.0%), Adi-Remets and Inda-Selassie (36.1%) sub-districts were inspected throughout the study period. Most (81%) of farmers feed their animals on free grazing in the open environment travelling from highlands and midlands to lowlands in search of adequate feed (different species of grasses) and crop residues during the wet season up to the beginning of the dry season. Majority of farmers (43.8%) had veterinary access from governmental veterinary officers. Thirty-four (33.9%) of the respondents got veterinary access from illegal drug dealers in mini shops or market. Among the major disease constraints identified; Tick infestation (89.3%), lice infestation (68.6%) mange mite infestation (77.7%) lumpy skin disease (LSD) (42.1%), trypanasomiasis (62.8%) bovine pasteurellosis (52.1) mastitis (13.2%), sheep and goat pox (15.7), abortion (19.0%), dystocia (24.8%), retained fetal membrane (25.6%), prolapsed uterus (13.2%) delayed heat period (38.8%) were most endemic ailments directly affecting livestock production and farmers livelihood.

Conclusion: In conclusion management practices in livestock production is poor to a large extent. Burden and endemicity of livestock diseases are substantially higher. The data obtained could be the source of facts for planners in animal health service delivery system in this sub region.

Keywords: Disease survey, Management practices, Ruminants, Western Tigray, Northern Ethiopia

* Correspondence: getachewmebrahtu27@gmail.com
[1]Department Animal Sciences, College of Agriculture, Aksum University, P.O .Box: 314, Shire Campus, Shire, Ethiopia
Full list of author information is available at the end of the article

Background

Among all the livestock that constitute Ethiopian farm animals, ruminants comprising of cattle, sheep and goats are among the main source of draft power (cattle), wealth accumulation purposes and income generation [1]. Sheep and goat play an important economic role in the overall production system of large and small scale farmers, where most shoat production is for wool, leather and meat production [2].

Ethiopia is endowed with the largest livestock population of an estimated 53.4 million cattle 55.2% are female and 44.8% are males) 23.6 million sheep and 18.6 million goats [3] distributed within the different agro-ecological zones of the nation; about 99% of cattle populations are of local Zebu breed. The remaining 1% of exotic breeds is kept mainly for dairy production in urban and peri-urban areas to fulfill local market milk consumption demands.

Literatures indicate that livestock production and productivity are hindered by poor nutritional value both in quantity and quality, poor livestock husbandry practices, animal health ailments and husbandry constraints [4]. The aforementioned constraints result in subsistence-oriented livestock industry in Africa in general and in Ethiopia in particular [5]. Constraints arising from epidemics and pandemics of animal diseases have been contributed to increased livestock morbidity and mortality too. Consequently; this resulted in reduced livestock production and productivity [6–8].

Livestock husbandry practices are extensively managed on free grazing range/extensive system, specifically in the central part of Ethiopia where crop farming dominates the agricultural practices and with farmers keeping an average of 5 to 15 cows/shoats/household (HH) under the free range system, the animals move about freely to feed on forages/grasses, which are abundantly available during the raining season. Hardly are the animals provided supplementary feeds (personal observation) and despite poorly designed housing shelter is provide by their owners around their home stead areas to protect from predators [9].

In Ethiopia, where livestock agriculture is merely practiced; cattle are raised in an extensive way in small-holder production systems. As a result of extensive livestock production, productivity is hindered by losses due to animal health problems of which; anthrax, blackleg, lumpy skin disease (LSD),trypanosomiasis and other major health problems experienced are parasites, with liver fluke being the major internal parasites,followed by ticks and biting flies. Animal health is recognized to be significant source of production losses such as low weight gain, draught, fertility and lactation performances (Personal observation) [1, 10]. In terms of disease prevention and control, farmers are not fully aware/ hardly take up to veterinary vaccination and treatment center to the affected ruminants as they considered health management as too expensive and distance due to topographical problems to veterinary delivery services; soon after owners are forced taking/treat their animals to ethno-veterinary treatments personally rather than affording modern veterinary medication [11]. Farmers have used traditional medicines and practices to treat their animals for different kinds of livestock diseases alleviation [7].

Major animal health constraints and efficient livestock husbandry practices are yet to be identified and developed respectively. Therefore; the aim of this scenario was to recognize livestock ailments and management practices for further investigation and as decision-making tool for livestock agriculture development. Based on literatures and personal observations from need assessments, it is possible to hypothesize that the management practices in livestock agriculture is poorly practiced resulting in high densities of livestock disease burden.

Methods

Description of study design and setting

A cross-sectional study design was conducted in Western Zone of Tigray, Northern Ethiopia. This area is bordered by Sudan and Eritrea in the west and north respectively and Amhara regional state in the South. The study area includes three districts; Tsegede and Welkayte being highland agro ecological characteristics and lowland characteristics in Kafta-Humera. Six peasant associations were randomly selected per each districts identified as Adi-remets, Adi-hirdi, Inda-selassie, Dansha, Baekhar and Maikhadrah [Fig. 1].

Western Tigray (Humera) positioned at an elevation of 600 m above sea level; is characterized by a very harsh environment with an annual temperature ranging from 27 to 45 °C and rainfall ranges from 900 mm^3 to 1800 mm^3 per annum. Humera is one of Ethiopia's most fertile agricultural zones, with large-scale farming of cash crops such as sesame, maize, cotton, okra, and sorghum [12]. Agriculture is predominantly practiced next to crop agriculture. Local and Begait breeds of cattle, goats and sheep to which a study have been under taken are extensively reared in this sub region (District Agricultural and Rural Development office).

Data collection method

Simple random sampling technique was applied after dividing districts in to peasant associations and then at household level via multistage sampling procedure. Overall 121 randomly selected respondents comprising of household (HH) farmers, agricultural development agents (ADA) and veterinarians were involved during face to face interview. Structured and semi-structured

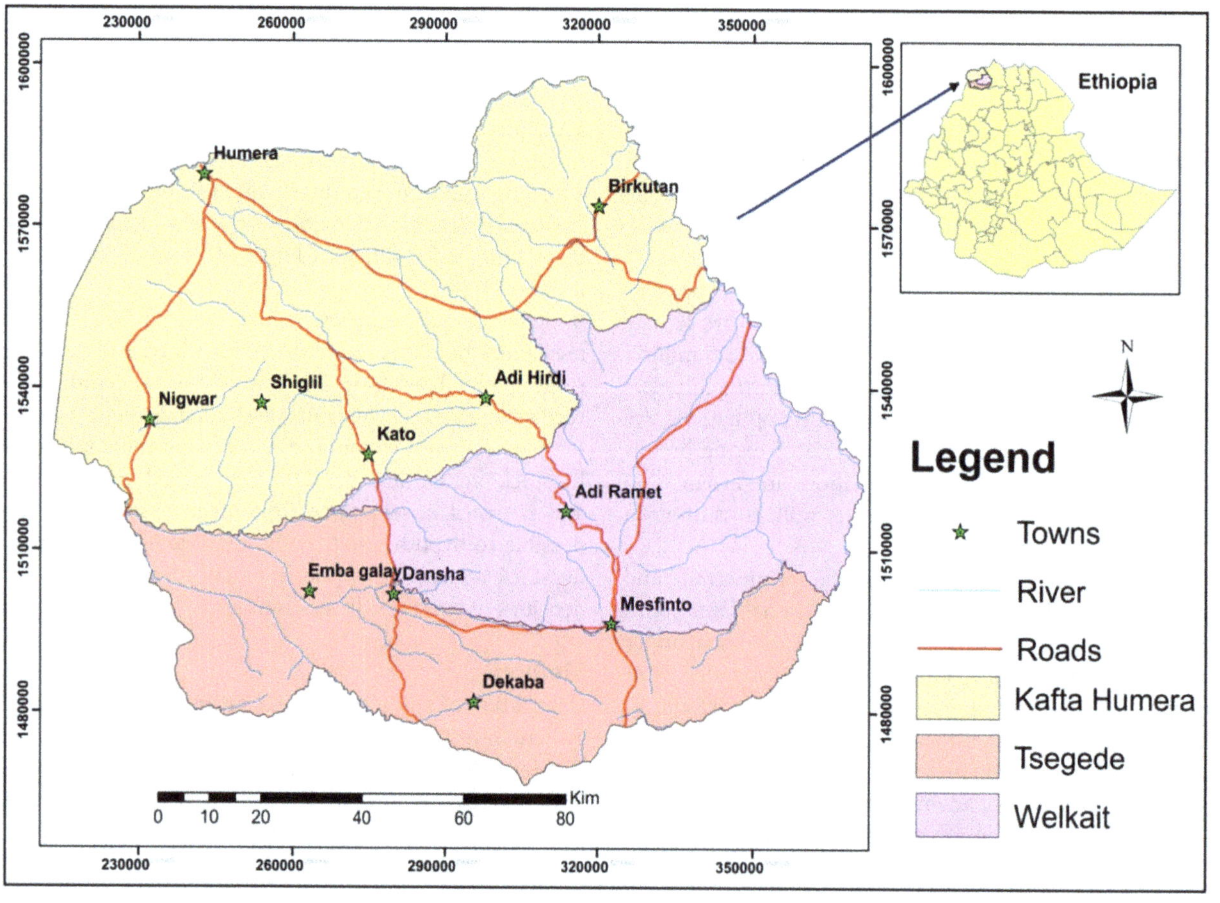

Fig. 1 Geographical location of western Tigray province showing the three study districts

questionnaire comprising of both qualitative and quantitative data was deliberately developed for this study [Additional file 1] and administered to respondents through *Tigrigna* regional language (farmers) and finally translated in to *English* during data entry and analysis soon after collection of raw data. The questionnaire was pre-tested before administration to the interviewees. Farmers have responded to different animal diseases as they recognize via their grass rooted knowledge of vernacular /local names of different diseases affecting their cattle, sheep and goats on the basis of different disease symptoms and pathognomonic signs. However, animal health personnel's (Vets and para-vets) from respected veterinary officers were involved during house to house visits to boost further disease classification and identification on the basis of physical examination.

Data management and statistical analysis

Raw data were entered, edited, checked and managed in to Microsoft Excel Spread Sheet Access. Data organization, summarization and analyses were performed after coding and rechecking, in SPSS Statistics for Windows, Version 20.0.(Armonk, NY:IBM Corp).Simple descriptive analysis was generated (means and proportions, counts and percentage summary statistics. and tests of significance for difference in means and proportions were estimated at 95% confidence interval and 5% (0.05) level of significance was considered as cut point.

Results

Housing and feeding system

The mean average number of cattle, sheep and goats per household were 15.58, 11.11 and 13.94 in that order. Mean age at first calving for cattle, sheep and goats was 55.82, 12.03 and 12.37 months respectively. House design for cattle was poorly designed non concrete/natural earthen floor open air around homestead (58%) whereas non concrete fenced with stone wall and wood wall near homestead (45%) housing design was practiced for small ruminants to protect from predators. Most (81%) of farmers feed their animals free grazing from the open environment travelling from highlands and midlands to lowlands in search of adequate feed (different species of grasses) and crop residues during the wet season up to the beginning of the dry season (Table 1).

Table 1 Management practices and veterinary delivery services in ruminants, Western Zone of Tigray, Northern Ethiopia (2015–2016)

Management characteristics and practices	Agro ecology		
	Lowland count (%)	Midland count (%)	Highland count (%)
Housing (cattle)			
Open air at grazing areas	24 (42.9)	–	1 (2.6)
Open air around home stead	20 (35.7)	21 (80.8)	29 (74.4)
Fenced	11 (19.6)	3 (11.5)	7 (17.9)
Corrugated iron with stone wall	–	–	–
Thatched roof with mad wall	1 (1.8)	2 (7.7)	2 (5.1)
Housing (Shoats)			
Open air at grazing areas	6 (10.7)	–	–
Open air around home stead	5 (8.9)	2 (7.7)	1 (2.6)
Fenced	19 (33.9)	14 (53.8)	22 (56.4)
Corrugated iron with stone wall	–	–	–
Thatched roof with mad wall	6 (10.7)	2 (7.7)	1 (2.6)
Sesame seed cake	2 (3.6)	–	–
Feeding system/supplementation	2 (3.6)	2 (7.7)	3 (7.7)
Sesame seed cake	2 (3.6)	–	–
Improved forage	2 (3.6)	2 (7.7)	3 (7.7)
Free grazing	38 (67.9)	24 (92.3)	36 (92.3)
Sorghum seed coat	12 (21.4)	–	–
Sesame seed coat	2 (3.6)	–	–
Veterinary service for ruminants when get sick			
Take to clinic	25 (44.6)	12 (46.2)	12 (35.9)
Treat personally with modern medicine	12 (21.4)	1 (3.8)	–
Take to traditional healer	6 (10.7)	4 (15.4)	7 (17.9)
Use personally traditional medicine	12 (21.4)	3 (11.5)	7 (17.9)
Take to clinic & Use personally traditional medicine	1 (1.8)	4 (15.4)	5 (12.8)
Take to clinic & Treat personally with modern medicine	–	2 (7.7)	6 (15.4)
Slaughter	–	–	–
Access to veterinary service			
Governmental veterinary clinic	25 (44.6)	10 (38.5)	18 (46.2)
Private veterinary clinic	7 (12.5)	1 (3.8)	–
Shop or market	17 (30.4)	9 (34.6)	15 (38.5)
Governmental and private	4 (7.1)	5 (19.2)	3 (7.7)
Governmental and shop or market	2 (3.6)	1 (3.8)	3 (7.7)
Governmental, private and shop or market	1 (1.8)	–	–
Distance to nearest veterinary service			
< 1 km	3 (5.6)	1 (3.8)	2 (5.1)
1–5 km	23 (42.6)	8 (30.8)	7 (17.9)
6–10 km	14 (25.9)	7 (26.9)	13 (33.3)
> 10 km	14 (25.9)	10 (38.5)	17 (43.6)
Reasons for loss of ruminants			
Predators	5 (8.9)	–	1 (2.6)
Disease incidents	39 (39.6)	15 (57.7)	20 (51.3)

Table 1 Management practices and veterinary delivery services in ruminants, Western Zone of Tigray, Northern Ethiopia (2015–2016) *(Continued)*

Management characteristics and practices	Agro ecology		
	Lowland count (%)	Midland count (%)	Highland count (%)
Poisoning	–	1 (3.8)	4 (10.3)
Drought	4 (7.1)	1 (3.8)	–
Disease and drought	5 (8.9)	7 (26.9)	13 (33.3)
Disease and predator	–	2 (7.7)	1 (2.6)

Access of veterinary service delivery

Majority of farmers (43.8%) had access for services from governmental veterinary officers. Thirty-four (33.9%) of the respondents got veterinary access from illegal drug dealers in mini shops or market. Nearly 7 % of farmers (6.6%) sought veterinary diagnosis and medication from private veterinary drug venders. In terms of disease prevention and control over their ruminant animals, farmers are not fully aware of taking/hardly take up to veterinary vaccination and treatment centers due to beyond their cost affordability, traditional beliefs that awaiting the sick animal for self-recovery; taking to traditional healer or long distance reasons. The nearest distance to veterinary service delivery center ranges from one kilometer (5%) to beyond ten kilometers (34.5%). Forty two percent of respondents (42.1%) could afford the cost for vaccination and treatment; nearly 10 % of the farmers (10.7%) treat personally with modern medicine; 14 % (14%) of them take their sick animal to traditional healers and 18 % of the respondents (18.2%) treated their sick ruminants personally from traditional and herbal medicines.

Main factors for livestock losses and diseases of ruminants

Livestock diseases are significant challenges to the livestock production sub-sector in Ethiopia. Main risk factors for livestock losses in the study sub-region were disease (61.2%), predators (5%), drought (4.1%), poisoning/grass toxicosis (4.1%) and theft (2.5%). Morbidity rates of cattle, sheep and goats were determined as 8, 12.5, and 15.5% in that order. Ninety one percent of all ailments identified were communicable diseases consisting of bacterial, viral, protozoal and parasitic infections.

The major ruminant disease constraints limiting livestock production in the study setting were lumpy skin disease (LSD) (42.1%), trypanasomiasis (62.8%) bovine pasteurellosis (52.1) mastitis (13.2%), sheep and goat pox (15.7%) foot rot (11.7%). Among the reproductive disorders; abortion (19.0%), dystocia (24.8%), retained fetal membrane (25.6%), uterine prolapsed (13.2%) delayed heat period/prolonged anestrous (38.8%) were the ailments identified. Grass toxicosis (21.5%), bloat (18.2%) and hyena byte (8.3%) were among the non-communicable ailments and injuries identified. Parasitic diseases of ticks (89.3%), lice (68.6%) and mange mite (77.7%) infestation were among the devastating health problems in livestock production system. Detail burden and frequency of endemic diseases are reported in agro ecological zone wise in (Table 2).

Discussions

This is the first survey narrating in livestock disease distribution and management practices ever undertaken in the field of animal production system. The study also describes the veterinary service delivery system in this sub-region western Tigray of Ethiopia.

Our study findings show a remarkable poor livestock management system and high disease burden. Breeding performance in our local breeds of cattle is very low, characterized by delayed age at first calving. Descriptive analysis show that the mean age at first calving for all ruminants is too long; this dalliance is due to the attribute of poor livestock management and handling practices from local livestock breeders and high incidence of animal diseases. Poor fertility and low genetic potential are contributing factors too [13]. There is a significant difference in mean age at first calving among the lowland, midland and highland across geographical locations. Mean time to first calving in lowlands is a lesser amount as compared to highland and midland ecological locations owing to high availability of feed from agricultural byproducts and grasses.

Livestock breeders are accustomed to feed their livestock free grazing type of feeding system from the locally available feed combinations of grasses, crop residues and crop aftermath. Livestock feeding system is characterized by inadequate provision of concentrate supplementation during the dry seasons when feeds are scarce. This arises from the fact that farmers prefer large number of ruminants in quantity that cannot afford feed and water at zero grazing level. This could be a leading grass rooted cause of low livestock production, productivity and susceptibility to abundant disease ailments [14, 15].

From the study, most frequently, it was observed that the major causes of livestock losses were due to disease, predators, drought, grass toxicosis and theft. This finding is lower in proportion in comparison to previous reports [14, 16]. In majority of farmers, large ruminants

Table 2 A preliminary survey of major diseases of ruminants Western Zone of Tigray, Northern Ethiopia (2015–2016)

Disease characteristics	Vernacular names	Agro ecology			Ethno-veterinary medicine Practices
		Lowland count (%)	Midland count (%)	Highland count (%)	
Tick infestation	Kurdid	53 (94.6)	21 (80.8)	34 (87.2)	Topical lotion with kerosene, picking manually
Lice infestation	Kumal, Kunchi-gobay	35 (62.5)	18 (69.2)	30 (76.9)	Washing with ash
Flea infestation	Kunchi	36 (64.3)	8 (30.8)	9 (23.1)	Dipping in ponds Cutting, shearing, clipping the fur
Biting Flies	Nihbay, Karma	35 (62.5)	10 (38.5)	7 (17.9)	-
Biting Birds	Chirna'e	12 (21.4)	—	—	Chasing from the back, Look after the back of their cattle against biting birds.
Mange mites	Abek, Shuhur, Juri, Hafew	43 (76.8)	23 (88.5)	28 (71.8)	Salt + butter (topical lotion)
Fasciolosis	Kaba				
Sheep Kid	Kimanjer	11 (19.6)	—	6 (15.4)	
LSD	Enfurur, Kubkubta, Togtogta, Shlimiye	27 (48.2)	10 (38.5)	15 (38.5)	Coffee ceremonial practices, smoking
GIT parasitosis	Wesfat, Gondera	29 (51.8)	13 (50.0)	13 (33.3)	Drenching with sagla (leaf)
Trypanosomosis	Silim	50 (89.3)	18 (69.2)	8 (20.5)	
Grass toxicosis	Afel, Efel, Maget	5 (8.9)	5 (19.2)	16 (41.0)	Drenching with yoghurt, Drenching with yoghurt, detergent and sesame oil.
Ovine pasteurellosis	Mieta, Bueta	19 (33.9)	3 (11.5)	3 (7.7)	Incision at facial artery
Caprine-pasteurollosis	Mieta, Bueta	23 (41.1)	10 (38.5)	11 (28.2)	Incision at facial artery
Bovine- pasteurellosis	Yelam-geta, Halafiyien, Hangofta, Shuwta, Kofa	27 (48.2)	15 (57.7)	21 (53.8)	Incision, Cauterization, Withholding water for 2–3 days
Anthrax	Megerem, Nefri	14 (25.0)	8 (30.8)	8 (20.5)	Cauterization
Lungworm	Se'al	2 (3.6)	6 (23.1)	5 (12.8)	-
Arthritis	Kirtimat	4 (7.3)	2 (7.7)	1 (2.6)	Incising,cauterization
Ascites	Himam-kebdi, Wel'e	0 (0.0)	5 (19.2)	8 (20.5)	Cauterization
Shoat pox	Infurur, Shilime	12 (21.4)	2 (7.7)	5 (12.5)	Smoking, coffee ceremonial
Paramphistomiasis	Keyahti-hasaku	6 (10.6)	-	5 (12.8)	-
Rabies	Himam-Ebudkelbi	-	6 (23.1)	4 (10.3)	Drinking whey (for humans)
Delayed heat period	Awra-gedib	3 (5.4)	15 (57.7)	29 (74.4)	-
Leech infestation	Alekti	-	-	4 (10.3)	Nasal drenching with tobacco leaf
Foreign bodies	Lastic	1 (1.8)	3 (11.5)	2 (5.1)	-
Blackleg	Weke'e	9 (16.1)	3 (11.5)	3 (7.7)	Drenching with shenfa'e,cauterization
Bovine Tuberculosis	Menkersa, Zigag	11 (19.6)	-	-	Cauterization,dusting.
Parafilariasis		-	-	4 (10.3)	Lotion with honey
Listroiosis	Azurit	-	-	2 (5.1)	
Actinobacilosis	Tokiba	5 (8.9)	-	5 (12.8)	Topical lotion with Butter +Charcoal
Brucellosis	Aber'e	3 (5.4)	5 (19.2)	1 (2.6)	-
Foot rot	Finfin, Hinkasse	8 (16.3)	-	3 (11.5)	Salting
Dermatophilosis	Urit	2 (3.6)	-	2 (5.1)	-
Cow mastitis	Himam-Tub	13 (23.2)	-	2 (5.1)	Cauterization
Contagious Bovine pleuropneumonia (CBPP)	Weke'e–samba, Samba-michi	11 (20.0)	-	5 (12.8)	-
Orf	Kafay	11 (30.6)	4 (25.0)	3 (12.5)	Water (H_2O) + Salt (NaCl)
Pest petis des ruminants (PPR)	Wetetie, Kur	12 (32.4)	4 (25.0)	3 (13.0)	-

Table 2 A preliminary survey of major diseases of ruminants Western Zone of Tigray, Northern Ethiopia (2015–2016) *(Continued)*

Disease characteristics	Vernacular names	Agro ecology			Ethno-veterinary medicine Practices
		Lowland count (%)	Midland count (%)	Highland count (%)	
Abortion	Chinga'fe, Aber'e	17 (30.4)	3 (11.5)	3 (7.7)	–
Contagious caprinepleuro pneumonia	Sanabu'e Samba-michi	3 (7.9)	–	2 (8.0)	–
Dystocia	Himam-Hirsi	25 (44.6)	2 (7.7)	3 (7.7)	Manual removal
Cysticercosis	Koso	–	–	1 (2.6)	–
Hydatidosis	–	2 (3.6)	–	1 (2.6)	–
Tunga-penetrans	Mojeliye	3 (5.4)	–	1 (2.6)	Manual removal, salting
Retained fetal membrane	Meskab	22 (39.3)	4 (15.4)	5 (12.8)	Local plant medicine+H_2O (drenched)
Uterine prolapsed	Mahtsen Miglbat	11 (19.6)	3 (11.5)	2 (5.1)	Manual intervention
Bloat	Menfahti	3 (5.4)	5 (19.2)	14 (35.9)	Drenching local malt, food oil, caticala/uozo and red peppers(powder), Puncturing(rumen)
Malignant tumor	Mandaeti	1 (1.8)	1 (3.8)	0 (0.0)	–
Phimosis	–	1 (1.8)	2 (7.7)	0 (0.0)	–
Paraphimosis	–	1 (1.8)	1 (3.8)	1 (2.6)	–
Actinomycosis	Zigag	6 (10.7)	2 (7.7)	1 (2.6)	Puncturing, Cauterization
Abscess	Hibat	4 (7.1)	2 (7.7)	2 (5.1)	Incising, cauterization
Metritits	Raksi-mahtsen	9 (16.1)	–	–	–
Thelaziasis	Hasaka-Ayeni	2 (3.6)	3 (11.5)	1 (2.6)	Manual drawing out
Bottle Jaw	–	1 (1.8)	–	3 (7.7)	–
Hyena bite	Zibe'e, Arawit	4 (7.1)	4 (15.4)	2 (5.1)	Slaughtering
Warts/skin cancers	Tuba-adgi	2 (3.6)	5 (19.2)	–	Cauterization, burning

are housed in poorly designed pens around homestead or at grazing areas in the open environment where feed and water are accessible as the farmers travelling via their family labor along with their cattle due to limited grazing areas from highlands and midlands to lowlands in search of adequate feed with different species of grasses and crop residues during the wet season up to the beginning of the dry season.

Greater parts of farmers have been getting access to veterinary services from governmental animal health centers. Although most farmers have got access from the aforementioned governmental institution, their intention to use private veterinary services and local traditional medicines is in a very demand. Thirty-four percent of the respondents got veterinary services from black market and illegal drug dealers in mini shops. Nearly 7 % of farmers sought veterinary diagnosis and medication from private veterinary clinic/pharmacy which is lower than a report from Kagira and Kanyariin Kisumu municipality of Kenya [15]. This constraint is due to the fact that the allocation of veterinary service delivery system is low; the quota is one veterinary clinic per three peasant associations. In terms of disease prevention and control over their ruminant animals, farmers are not fully aware of taking/rarely take up to veterinary vaccination and treatment centers due to different challenges; traditional beliefs that awaiting the sick animal for self-recovery; unable to afford medicines, taking to traditional healer, treat their animals personally or due to long distance to veterinary service delivery centers [14, 17].

During face to face interview, quantitative data were triangulated with qualitative data why most farmers are not taking their animals to veterinary service center prefer taking to other options. Their reply was the following statements;

"I am too busy to take my patient animals because of crop agricultural works during sawing to harvest."

" Outpatient treatment follow up due to long distance is tedious"

"Traditional medicines are more effective than modern medicines".

"Animal health practitioners do not inject the patient animal at site of swelling but in the intramuscular muscle".

This is because farmers prefer their ruminants get injected at the site of swelling to intramuscular injection; considering as if it were rapid treatment response.

Ethno-veterinary medicine deals with people's knowledge, skills, methods, practices and beliefs about the care of their animals [11, 18]. Farmers in various regions of the world still use ethno-veterinary medicines and practices to treat and alleviate infectious and non infectious ailments [9, 11]. Ethno veterinary medicines and practices often provide cheaper options than comparable modern drugs. Furthermore, ethno-veterinary medicine lends itself easily to local adaptation and application [18].

In this regard; our finding indicate that majority of livestock breeders use ethno-medicines and traditional practices like what farmers in various parts of the world do despite most breeders in this locality could afford the cost for vaccination and treatment. From this analysis nearly 10 % of the farmers treat personally with modern medicine; 14 % of them take their sick animal to traditional healers and 18 % of the respondents treated their sick ruminants personally from traditional practices and herbal medicines. These figures verify that Livestock owners could not rely on veterinary services only for control and prevention of various important livestock diseases; they need to develop socially acceptable and effective remedies from reasonably inexpensive sources that can complement modern medicines. The indigenous knowledge of Ethno veterinary medicine provides such an opportunity for livestock health care practices which are cheap and locally available than pharmacotherapy. We found Farmers can prepare and use homemade remedies without any expenditure [19, 20].

Among these number of infectious ailments reported in this current study; ectoparasitic infestation were found inflicting severe damages in ruminants [7]. This attribute is because of poor livestock handling practices; animals are freely grazing mixed with other non accaracide treated ruminants in rangelands and pastures [15]. Livestock owners seldom use modern anti-parasitic formulations; diazinon and accaracides and management practices to treat their cattle and shoats to treat against arthropod parasites (personal observation). Bacterial and viral infections are highly reported in our settings. This is more probably due to the fact that our study region is bordered by transboundry livestock disease prone ecological regions of Sudan, Eritrea and Amhara regional state in the West, North and South in that order [19]. In the context of our findings, livestock infections and infestations were being found as global livestock diseases important to the poor in line with the 2016 report of Office International Des Epizootics (OIE) [21].

Limitations

The study relies on participants' response rates, as a consequence; there might be under and/or over estimation of reporting in disease prevalence. Therefore, the estimated prevalence may not exactly show the exact burden of each disease in the study settings. Moreover, self report of ruminant diseases by farmers was used during major disease surveillances. Hence, recall bias could have been existed.

Conclusions

In conclusion the distribution of livestock diseases is substantially higher. Management practices in livestock production are poorly practiced. This is a greatest threat for livestock production and productivity. More fundamentally, investment in animal infections and infestations control and management practice strategies is necessary to reduce the multiple impacts of livestock diseases and deaths on animal health and production. The poor fertility and poor livestock performance can be addressed through better management and crossbreeding with improved breeds.

Abbreviations

ADA: Agricultural development agents; CBPP: Contagious bovine pleuropneumonia; GIT: Gastro intestinal tract; HH: Household; LSD: Lumpy skin disease; OIE: Office International Des Epizootics; PPR: Pest petis des ruminants

Acknowledgements

The authors gratefully acknowledge for the financial fund and vehicle for transportation to Tigray Agricultural Research Institute (TARI) and Humera Agricultural Research Center (HuARC) making this study happen. We would also like to thank all the farmers interviewed, Agricultural Development Agents (ADA) and veterinarians for disease identification and diagnosis offered during the study period.

Funding

The study was funded by Tigray Agricultural Research Institute (TARI).

Authors' contributions

GMW, GGT, DGT, THA, HHK, SKW and BBG participated in the conception and design of the study, GMW collected data, GMW, GGT, DGT, THA, HHK, SKW, BBG, MBS and THA analyzed, interpreted the data. GMW drafted the initial manuscript. All authors read and approved the final manuscript, contributed the critical review and the content.

Competing interest

The authors declare that they have no competing interests.

Ethics approval and consent to participate

Ethical clearance was obtained from Institutional Review Board (IRB) of Aksum University, College of Agriculture, Shire Campus. The purpose of study was well explained to the study participants and informed consents were obtained through verbal consent form approved by institution ethical committee. Confidentiality was maintained at all levels of the study by avoiding identifiers such as any personal identifying characteristics; images, videos of study participants were kept anonymously. Participants' involvement in the study was on voluntary basis; participants who were unwilling to participate in the study and those who wish to quit their participation were informed to do so without any restriction.

Consent for publication

Since our data do not involve any personal identifying characteristics; images, videos, names and data kept anonymously of study participants; we believe that "Consent for publication" is not applicable.

Author details

[1]Department Animal Sciences, College of Agriculture, Aksum University, P.O .Box: 314, Shire Campus, Shire, Ethiopia. [2]School of Geology, College of Agriculture, Aksum University, Shire Campus, Shire, Ethiopia. [3]Department of Biomedical Science, Aksum University, Aksum, Ethiopia. [4]Department of Epidemiology & Biostatistics, School of Public Health, Aksum University, Aksum, Ethiopia. [5]Department of Reproductive Health, School of Public Health, Aksum University, Aksum, Ethiopia.

References

1. Pen M, Savage DSW, Lorn S, Seng M. Cattle feeding and management practices of small-holder farmers in Kampong Cham Province, Cambodia. IJERD. 2010;1(1):132–8.
2. Debele G, Guru M, Hundessa F, Duguma M. Assessment of farmers' management practices and factors affecting goats' production system in Adami Tulu Jido Kombolcha district of EastShawa zone, Ethiopia. Agric Biol J N Am. 2013;4(5):520–6.
3. Belay D, Getachew E, Azage T, Hegde B. Farmers' perceived livestock production constraints in Ginchi watershed area. Result of participatory rural appraisal Int J Livest Prod. 2013;4(8):128–34.
4. Shija DSN, Kusiluka LJM, Chenyambuga SW, Shayo D, Lekule FP. Animal health constraints in dairy goats kept under smallholder farming systems in Kongwa and Mvomero districts, Tanzania. J Vet Med Anim Health. 2014;6(11):268–79.
5. Anteneh A. Livestock and food production in Africa: challenge and opportunity for the national livestock and veterinary services. Revue Scientifique et Technique, Office International des Epizooties. 1989;8(3).
6. Centeral Statistics Agency. Agricultural sample survey;statistical agency Federal Democratic Republic of Ethiopia. Addis Ababa: Central Statistics Agency; 2011.
7. Kagira JM, Kanyari PWN. Questionnaire survey on urban and peri-urban livestock farming practices and disease control in Kisumu municipality, Kenya. J S Afr Vet Assoc. 2010;81(2):82–6.
8. Anteneh, A., Trends in sub-Saharan Africa's livestock industries*. Livestock Policy Unit, ILCA, P.O.Box 5689, Addis Ababa, Ethiopia, 1984.
9. Lawal-Adebowale OA. Dynamics of ruminant livestock Management in the Context of the Nigerian agricultural system livestock production, 2012.
10. Ashenafi FB. Livestock disease management and food safety brief. In: Feed the Future Innovation Lab for Livestock Systems; 2016.
11. Moabiemang G, Barbara NN, Demel T, Oluwatoyin DK. ETHNO-VETERINARY Practices amongst livestock farmers in ngamiland district, Botswana. Afr J Tradit Complement Altern Med. https://doi.org/10.4314/ajtcam.v10i3.16. 2013;10(3):490–502.
12. Getachew MW, Kefyalew AA, Berihun AD. Visceral leishmaniasis treatment outcome and its determinants in Northwest Ethiopia. Epidemiology and Health. 2017;39.
13. Duguma B, Tegegne A, Hegde B. Smallholder livestock production system in Dandi district, Oromia regional state, Central Ethiopia. Read and write. 2012;20:25–6.
14. Brigitte LM, Dieudonné KM, Wanjiku LC, Anja G, Michael P. Challenges and opportunities for smallholder livestock production in post-conflict south Kivu eastern DR Congo. Trop Anim Health Prod. 2012;44:1221–32.
15. Dereje F. Characterizing farming practices from three regions of Ethiopia on which enset (*Ensete ventricosum*) is widely profited as a multipurpose crop plant. Livest Res Rural Dev. 2009;21(12).
16. Gari G, Waret-szkuta A, Grosbois V, Jacquiet P, Roger F. Risk factors associated with observed clinical lumpy skin disease in Ethiopia. Epidemiol Infect. 2010;138(11):1657–66.
17. Pushpangadan P, Lijinu TP, Bincy AJ, Anzar S, Aswany T, Chitra MA, Harsha K, Sreedevi P, George V. Traditional Medicine in livestock management. J. Traditional and Folk Practices. 2016;04(1):43–9.
18. Yirga G, Mekonen T, Gebregergis B, Solomon B. Plants used in ethnoveterinary practices in MedebayZana District, northern Ethiopia. J Med Plants Res. 2012;6(3):433–8.
19. Nibret M, Basaznew B. Assessment of major animal production and health problems of livestock development in lay-Armacheho District, northwestern Ethiopia. American-Eurasian J Sci Res. 2012;7(3):136–41.
20. Lawal-Adebowale OA. Dynamics of Ruminant Livestock Management in the Context of the Nigerian Agricultural System. 2013. https://doi.org/10.5772/52923.
21. Brian P, Delia G. The impacts of livestock diseases and their control on growth and development processes that are pro-poor. Phil Trans R Soc B. 2009;364:2643–55.

19

Combined double chambered right ventricle, tricuspid valve dysplasia, ventricular septal defect, and subaortic stenosis in a dog

Iuliu Scurtu[1], Flaviu Tabaran[1*], Mircea Mircean[1], Gavril Giurgiu[1], Andras Nagy[1], Cornel Catoi[1] and Dan G. Ohad[2]

Abstract

Background: Double chambered right ventricle (DCRV) is a congenital heart anomaly where the right ventricle is divided into two chambers. We describe, for the first time, an unusual combination of DCRV combined with some other congenital heart defects.

Case presentation: A 1.2-year-old Golden Retriever was presented with lethargy, exercise intolerance and ascites. Physical examination revealed an irregularly irregular pulse and a grade V/VI, systolic, right cranial murmur. Electrocardiography revealed widened and splintered QRS complexes with a right bundle-branch block pattern. Radiography demonstrated right-sided cardiomegaly. Two-dimensional echocardiography identified a DCRV with tricuspid valve dysplasia. The patient died despite abdominocentesis and 4 days of oral pharmacotherapy, and necropsy revealed an anomalous fibromuscular structure that divided the right ventricle into two compartments. Another finding was tricuspid valve dysplasia with hypoplasia of the posterior and septal leaflets. The anterior leaflet was prominent, being part of the anomalous structure that divided the right ventricle. Necropsy also identified a perimembranous ventricular septal defect and mild subaortic stenosis. Histopathological examination of the fibromuscular band that separated the right ventricle identified longitudinally oriented layers of dense fibrous connective tissue and myocardial cells arranged in a plexiform pattern. The muscular component was well represented at the ventral area of the fibromuscular band, and was absent in the central zone. Superficially, the endocardium presented areas of nodular hyperplasia covering mainly the fibrous part of the abnormal structure. The nodules were sharply demarcated and were composed by loosely arranged connective tissue with myxoid appearance, covered by discrete hyperplastic endocardium.

Conclusions: Concomitant cardiac malformations involving DCRV, tricuspid valve dysplasia, perimembranous ventricular septal defect and mild subaortic stenosis have not been previously described in veterinary medicine, and are reported here for the first time. Moreover, this is the first report of a canine patient with tricuspid valve dysplasia (TVD) and DCRV where the anterior leaflet is part of an anomalous structure dividing the right ventricle (RV) into two separate compartments.

Keywords: Canine, Congenital heart disease, Echocardiography

* Correspondence: alexandru.tabaran@usamvcluj.ro
[1]Universitatea de Stiinte Agricole si Medicina Veterinara din Cluj-Napoca, Calea Manastur 3-5, 400372 Cluj-Napoca, Romania
Full list of author information is available at the end of the article

Background

A double chambered right ventricle (DCRV) is a rarely diagnosed congenital heart anomaly, where a fibromuscular band separates the right ventricle (RV) into two chambers [1, 2]. This condition has been described in dogs, human beings [3–5], cats [6], and alpacas [7]. The dog breeds most frequently affected by this anomaly are large, such as Golden Retriever [2, 8] and Boxer [9]. A case of DCRV was also reported in a Pug [10]. One study reported no sex predisposition [10] and another suggested that males were overrepresented [8]. There are two types of DCRV reported in human beings: a low (oblique) type [11] and a high (horizontal) type [5, 11]. In both types, an anomalous development of septoparietal trabeculation has been reported [11], but there is currently no consensus regarding the exact pathogenesis behind the obstructing muscle bundles [12].

In a veterinary study, DCRV represented 1.2% (14/1132) of identified congenital heart pathologies [13]. In human beings, DCRV evolves as an isolated anomaly in only exceptionally rare instances [3]. Similarly, in dogs, most frequently, DCRV can be associated with ventricular septal defect (VSD), atrial septal defect (ASD), tricuspid valve dysplasia (TVD), pulmonic stenosis (PS), subaortic stenosis (SAS) or patent ductus arteriosus (PDA) [2, 8, 10].

In human beings, a genetic predisposition has been postulated [14]. There were also cases reported with Down's syndrome and DCRV, and a possible relationship between these two conditions was proposed [15]. It was also suggested that there were multiple embryological and postnatal causes of DCRV, as cardiac morphogenesis is an extremely complex and interconnected process [5]. Another theory considered DCRV as an acquired cardiac defect of postnatal development, as the coexistence of discrete aortic stenosis might imply a genetic predisposition toward cellular proliferation [16].

In dogs, due to the lack of well-documented data, epidemiological and morphological features are not clearly understood [8]. The most frequently encountered presenting complaints include cough, exercise intolerance, cyanosis, and syncope [8]. A grade III-VI/VI systolic murmur is typically present, with the point of maximum intensity located over either the left or the right hemithorax [6, 8]. Forty four percent of humans with this condition are reportedly asymptomatic, while fatigue was present in 35%, exertional dyspnea in 17%, cyanosis in 12%, and palpitations in 10% of the cases [17].

Case presentation

A 1.2 year-old, 28 kg, male intact Golden Retriever, was referred to our Cardiology Service for ascites evaluation. History included lethargy, anorexia and exercise intolerance over the previous five days. Prior to the onset of these signs, the dog was viable and readily able to exercise.

Physical examination showed a severely dyspneic, depressed, dehydrated dog, with moist but pale mucous membranes and a body condition score of 3/9. Rectal temperature was 38.9 °C. The femoral arterial pulse was irregularly irregular and weak, and a right cranial precordial thrill was palpable. Heart auscultation identified a grade V/VI systolic murmur with the point of maximal intensity located ventrad to the right heart-base region. Jugular venous distention was also noted and ascites was confirmed. Respiratory sounds were normal over all lung lobes, while the respiratory rate was elevated at 60 rpm.

An electrocardiographic (ECG) rhythm strip identified atrial fibrillation (AF) with widened (80 milliseconds) and splintered QRS complexes, and a right bundle branch block (RBBB) pattern, with an average ventricular response rate of 190 beats/min (Fig. 1).

Radiographs revealed well-ventilated lung fields and severe, right-sided cardiomegaly. Vertebral heart score was severely increased at 13.3v (Fig. 2) (reference interval < 10 ± 0.5).

Two-dimensional echocardiography demonstrated a severely enlarged right atrium. There was evidence of congenital TVD: the tricuspid leaflets were malpositioned and displaced toward the right ventricular apex (Fig. 3a). A severe tricuspid insufficiency (TI) jet (Fig. 3d) with a 4.26 m/s peak flow velocity (compatible with a systolic pressure gradient of at least 72.6 mmHg across this valve) was recorded (Fig. 3c). The septal tricuspid leaflet was thickened and attached to very short chordae tendineae; the posterior tricuspid leaflet was also thickened. The right parasternal short axis view, at the level of the left ventricular papillary muscles, demonstrated systolic flattening of the interventricular septum (IVS), attributed to an elevated systolic right ventricular pressure (Fig. 4a). In that same view, an anomalous fibromuscular structure appeared to partially separate the right ventricular cavity into two compartments. A small, systolic, turbulent jet was identified between the two right-ventricular chambers (Fig. 4b).

Spectral Doppler interrogation of the abnormal jet was attempted but accurate velocity measurements could not be performed due to less–than–ideal angulation. However, based on the turbulent appearance of the color flow jet its velocity seemed subjectively high.

The left cardiac chambers and valves demonstrated normal structure and function, and only mild left ventricular (LV) hypertrophy was seen. The left ventricular free wall thickness in end diastole (LVFWd) was 9.9 mm (reference ranges 8.04–8.94 mm), and the interventricular septum thickness in end diastole (IVSd) was 12.08 mm (reference ranges 9.99–11.05) [18].

Pulmonary arterial flow had a normal profile and peak flow velocity. Aortic flow velocity was not accurately measured due to less-than-optimal beam-to-flow alignment.

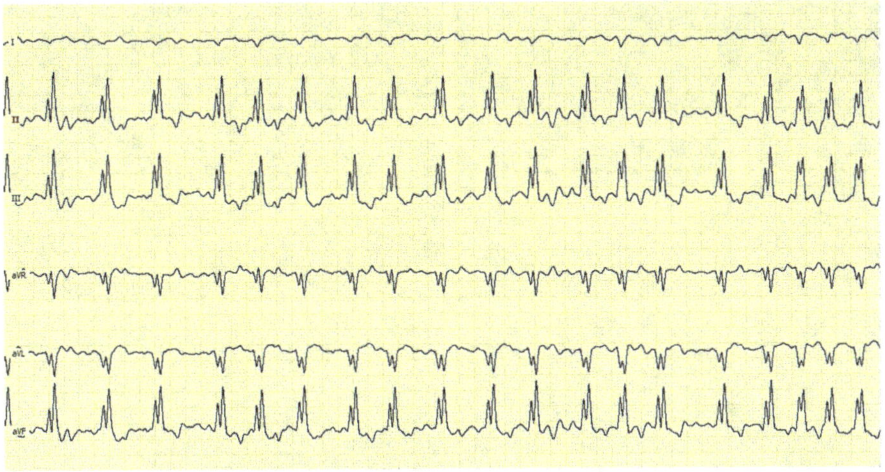

Fig. 1 A six-lead ECG strip from a 1.2-year-old male Golden Retriever demonstrating atrial fibrillation with widened (80 ms) and splintered QRS complexes, compatible with a RBBB pattern and mild right axis deviation of the ventricular depolarization mean electrical axis (1 cm/mV, 50 mm/s). Note that the QRS complex, while of small amplitude, is negative in Lead I

Serum biochemistry showed only mild liver enzyme elevation. Alanine transaminase (ALT) was 93 U/l (upper reference limit <40 U/l) and aspartate aminotransferase (AST) was 88 U/l (upper reference limit <40 U/l). Hematology was normal.

Five liters of a sero–sanguinotic fluid were removed from the abdominal cavity via abdominocentesis. The fluid contained a low protein (< 2.5 g/dL) concentration, containing only a few scattered cells, including mostly red blood cells, neutrophils, and desquamated mesothelial cells.

The dog unfortunately responded poorly to pimobendan (0.25 mg/kg q 12 h) and furosemide (2 mg/kg q 12 h), and went on to die suddenly four days later.

Necropsy revealed a severely enlarged right atrium (Fig. 5a). The septal and posterior leaflets of the tricuspid valve were both severely thickened. The septal leaflet was also adhered to the IVS (Fig. 5b). The tricuspid valve annulus was displaced ventrad and caudad, towards the right ventricular apex. The RV was partially divided into two separate compartments by a fibromuscular structure, which was more muscular near the RV apex and more fibrotic near the atrioventricular junction. The structure appeared to be part of the anterior tricuspid valve leaflet, without involving any of the papillary muscles. This impression was supported by the fact that the chordae tendineae of this specific leaflet were of normal length but their insertions were embedded inside the abnormal fibromuscular structure. This fibromuscular structure was attached to the RV apex, at an area rich with coarse septomarginal trabeculation. The two right ventricular compartments communicated only at the uppermost part of the abnormal fibromuscular structure (Fig. 5c, d). The diameters of the oval communicating ostium were 0.8 X 1.2 cm. One right ventricular compartment contained inflow tract components, while the other contained outflow components. A resistive perimembranous VSD measuring 4 mm in diameter was also

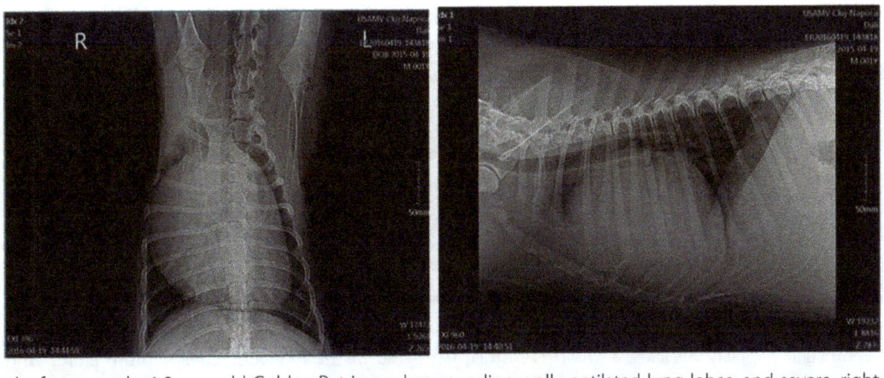

Fig. 2 Two radiographs from a male, 1.2-year-old Golden Retriever dog, revealing well-ventilated lung lobes, and severe, right-sided cardiomegaly (vertebral heart sum is 13.3v)

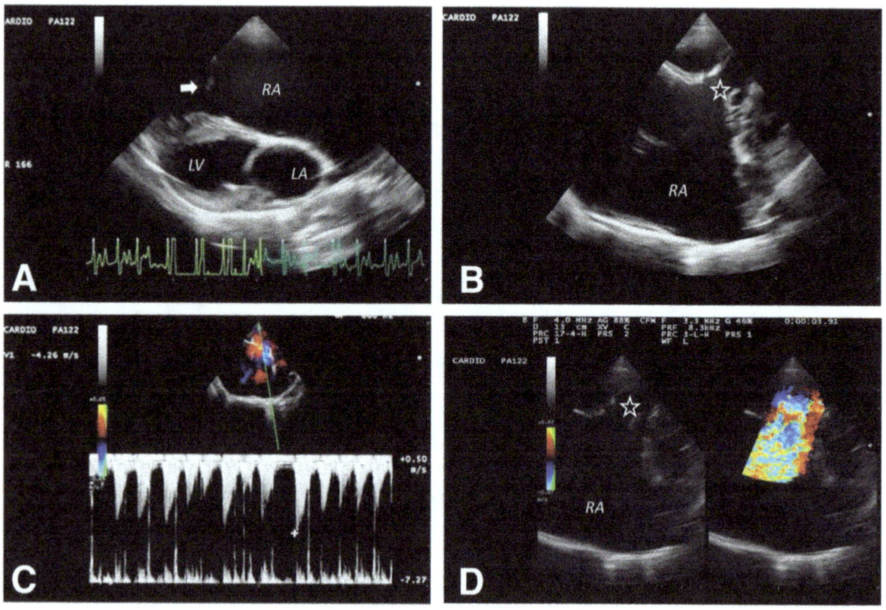

Fig. 3 Echocardiograms from a male, 1.2-year-old Golden Retriever dog with atrial fibrillation. **a** A systolic, right parasternal, long axis view demonstrating a severely enlarged right atrium with malpositioned (apically displaced) tricuspid valve leaflet insertions (arrow). **b** A modified left parasternal apical four-chamber view demonstrating incomplete coaptation of the tricuspid valve leaflets (asterisk). **c** A continuous wave Doppler signal from the left apical four-chamber view, demonstrating tricuspid insufficiency (TI) with a peak flow velocity of up to 4.26 m/s in many of the irregularly dispersed cardiac cycles. This velocity is compatible with a systolic pressure gradient of 72.6 mmHg between one of the right ventricular compartments and the right atrium. Note the "V-wave cut off" of the TI signal, suggestive of an elevated pressure in the receiving compartment. **d** A modified left parasternal apical four-chamber view depicting color Doppler evidence of severe TI; LA, left atrium; LV, left ventricle. RA, right atrium

detected on necropsy, below the aortic valve cusps. The VSD opened into the RV distal chamber. Beneath the aortic valve cusps, there was a small, proliferative, stenotic nodule, partially obstructing the left ventricular outflow tract (LVOT). A fibrotic ring encircled the LVOT as well, at a distance of 1.5 cm from the aortic valve cusps (Figs. 6 and 7). These two combined findings were compatible with mild SAS, which presumably had triggered systolic left ventricular (LV) pressure elevation, based on the mildly pre-mortem, echocardiographically increased LV wall thickness.

Histologically, the fibromuscular band that separates the right ventricle consists of longitudinal layers of dense fibrous connective tissue admixed with cardiomyocytes organized in a plexiform pattern (Fig. 7a, b). The muscular component was present mainly in the ventral area of the band, being largely absent in the central zone. Superficially, the endocardium presented areas of nodular hyperplasia covering mainly the fibrous tissue-rich part of the band (Fig. 7c). The nodules were sharply demarcated and composed of loose connective tissue with myxoid appearance covered by hyperplastic endocardium (Fig. 7d).

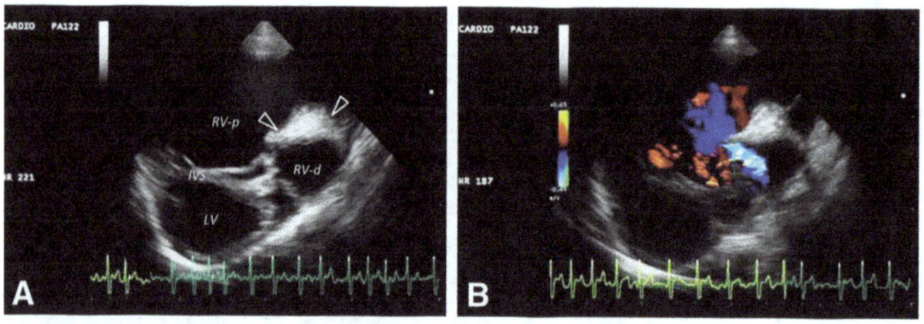

Fig. 4 Two-dimensional echocardiograms from the right parasternal short axis view of a male, 1.2-year-old Golden Retriever dog with atrial fibrillation at the level of the left ventricular papillary muscles. **a** There is systolic flattening of the interventricular septum along with a fibromuscular band (arrowhead) dividing the RV into two separate compartments. **b** Color flow Doppler imaging demonstrates a turbulent jet between the two right ventricular chambers. IVS, interventricular septum; RV–d, right ventricular distal chamber; RV–p, right ventricular–proximal chamber

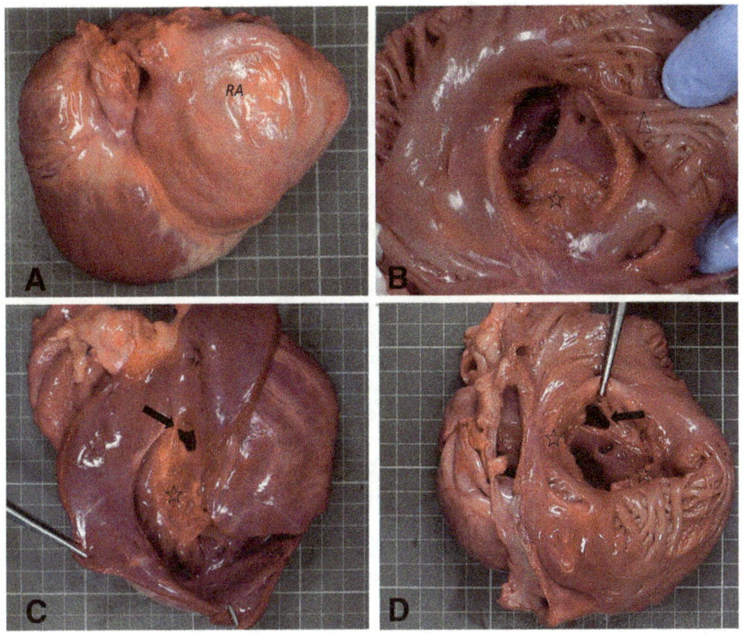

Fig. 5 Necropsy findings from a male, 1.2-year-old Golden Retriever dog. **a** The right lateral exterior aspect of the heart, demonstrating a severely enlarged right atrium. **b** The tricuspid valve apparatus seen from the opened right atrium, demonstrating a thickened septal leaflet (asterisk). An arrowhead shows pectinate muscles. **c** A large fibromuscular band (asterisk) seen from the distal RV chamber, divides the RV cavity and includes an oval ostium at its dorsal aspect, communicating between this and the other, proximal RV compartment (arrow). The ostium is seen from the compartment that contains the outflow tract structures. **d** The communicating ostium between the two RV compartments (arrow) seen from the RA, through the compartment that contains the inflow structures, including the tricuspid annulus and leaflets (asterisks). An arrowhead shows right atrial pectinate muscles. LA, left atrium; LV, left ventricle; RA, right atrium; RV–d, right ventricular distal chamber. Each small square represents 1 cm × 1 cm

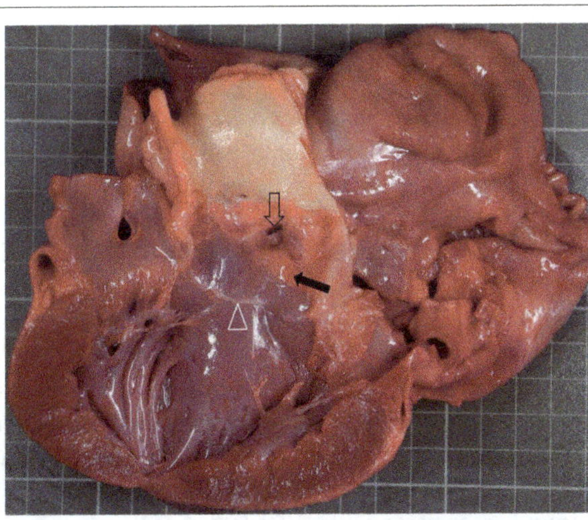

Fig. 6 Necropsy findings from a male, 1.2 year-old Golden Retriever dog, demonstrating the left ventricular outflow tract (LVOT) with a small, 4.0 mm wide, perimembranous VSD (transparent arrow) and a small sub-valvar stenotic nodule (black arrow). A fibrotic ring also encircles the LVOT (arrowhead). Mild concentric hypertrophy of the left ventricle (asterisks) is suspected. Ao, aorta; LA, left atrium; LV, left ventricle; RA, right atrium. Each small square represents 1 cm × 1 cm

Discussion and conclusions

To the best of the authors' knowledge, this is the first report of a patient with TVD and DCRV where the anterior tricuspid leaflet is part of an anomalous structure dividing the RV chamber in two compartments that communicated through a single ostium, situated in the dorsal part of the anomalous structure.

As there is no reason to expect that pulmonary hypertension was present, it is likely that one of the two RV compartments was highly pressurized in systole, which would explain both the high-velocity TI jet and the systolic interventricular IVS flattening towards the LV.

In the present case, VSD was restrictive and perimembranous, located just below the aortic valve cusps [19]. In both humans and dogs with DCRV, a concurrent VSD often opens into the more highly pressurized RV (proximal) chamber [11]. However, in the present case, the VSD actually opened into the more distal and lowly pressurized chamber.

The anatomical nature of the TVD in the present case can be thought of as reminiscent of the so-called Ebstein's anomaly in human beings [20]. In terms of intra-cavitary pressure, Ebstein's anomaly is characterized by "atrialization" of the dorsal aspect of the RV, due to a downward displacement of the tricuspid septal and lateral leaflet insertions, while the anterior leaflet seems

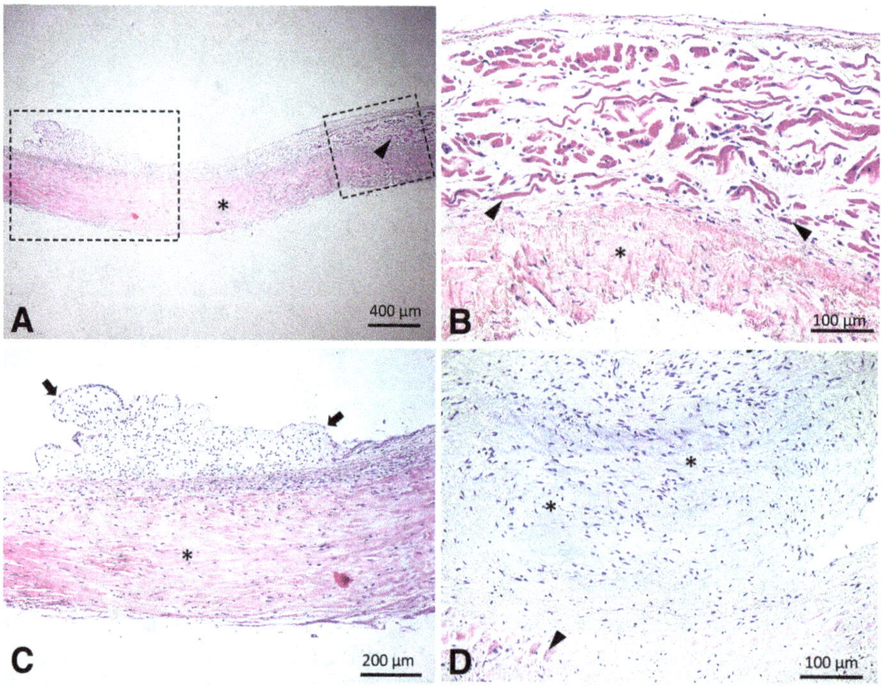

Fig. 7 Histopathological features of the fibromuscular band. **a** General view of the structure composed by dense, longitudinally oriented fibrous connective tissue (indicated by an asterisk) and myocardium (indicated by an arrowhead) located mostly at the ventral zone (close to the apex). The endocardium presents areas of nodular hyperplasia. **b** Detail of the area demarcated by the small rectangle in image 7A, presenting the plexiform pattern of the myocardium (indicated by the arrowheads) and the adjacent densely packed fibrous connective tissue (indicated by an asterisk). **c** Detail of the area demarcated by the large rectangle in image 7A. The fibromuscular band shows areas of hyperplasia, marked by sparsely cellular nodules of loose myxoid connective tissue covered by hyperplastic endocardium. **d** A myxoid nodule sharply demarcated from the surrounding myocardium (indicated by the arrowhead), composed of abundant, basophilic extracellular matrix and loosely arranged fibroblasts. H&E stain, ob. X 4 for image A, ×20 for images B and D, and ob.× 10 for image C

enlarged and appears to be "sail-like" [21]. An autosomal dominant mode of inheritance was proposed in Labrador Retrievers [21] and an autosomal recessive mode of inheritance was suggested in the Dogue de Bordeaux [22]. In the present case, the tricuspid valve septal and lateral leaflets were extremely thickened with restricted motion. The septo-anterior leaflet was prominent, being part of the fibromuscular band dividing the RV. The chordae tendineae of this leaflet were longer than normal, and were attached to the fibromuscular structure.

As the dog presented with clinical signs and physical examination findings of right-sided congestive heart failure (R-CHF), right atrial pressure was likely higher than 15 mmHg. This possibility is also subjectively supported by the "V-wave cutoff" appearance of the spectral Doppler TI-jet morphology (Fig. 3c). When added to the calculated 72.6 mmHg systolic pressure gradient across the tricuspid valve, this translates into an extremely elevated systolic pressure of at least 87.6 mmHg in the (proximal) highly pressurized RV compartment. In fact, the presence of AF suggests that the measured TI systolic pressure gradient was likely an underestimation of the true systolic pressure within this highly pressurized proximal RV compartment, which would suggest that the true systolic pressure within this compartment would have been much higher than 87.6 mmHg, while still in normal sinus rhythm. In addition, this patient's condition had been severe but also stable for a long enough period, to allow for the development of a severely enlarged right atrial diameter, which eventually contributed to the development of AF. This, in turn, must have exacerbated the hemodynamic compromise and ultimately hastened the onset and progression of R-CHF with not only ascites but also resultant clinical deterioration, to which the patient finally succumbed.

A fourth congenital anomaly observed in this case was a mild SAS, consisting of a fibrous band located 1.5 cm below the aortic valve cusps, and a proliferative nodule situated just below the VSD. In human beings, SAS is commonly associated with DCRV, [3, 4, 23].

To the best of the author's knowledge, this is the first veterinary case report of a combination of congenital TVD, DCRV, VSD and SAS, where a tricuspid valve leaflet is an integral anatomical component of the fibromuscular anomalous structure dividing the RV into two separate compartments.

Abbreviations

AF: Atrial fibrillation; ALT: Alanine transaminase; ASD: Atrial septal defect; AST: Aspartate aminotransferase; DCRV: Double chambered right ventricle; ECG: Electrocardiography; IVS: Interventricular septum; IVSd: Interventricular septum thickness in end diastole; LA: Left atrium; LV: Left ventricle; LVFWd: Left ventricular free wall thickness in end diastole; LVOT: Left ventricular outflow tract; PDA: Patent ductus arteriosus; PS: Pulmonic stenosis; RA: Right atrium; RBBB: Right bundle branch block; R-CHF: Right sided congestive right failure; RV: Right ventricle; RV–d: Right ventricular distal chamber; RV–p: Right ventricular proximal chamber; SAS: Subaortic stenosis; TI: Tricuspid insufficiency; TVD: Tricuspid valve dysplasia; VSD: Ventricular septal defect

Acknowledgements

Not applicable.

Funding

Not applicable.

Authors' contributions

IS and FT diagnosed the case and wrote the manuscript; OD analyzed ECG data, wrote and revised the manuscript; MM and GG revised the manuscript; CC and AN described the gross pathology and revised the manuscript. All the authors read and approved the final manuscript.

Consent for publication

The owner of the dog gave written informed consent to publish this case report and accompanying images.

Competing interests

The authors declare that they have no competing interests.

Author details

[1]Universitatea de Stiinte Agricole si Medicina Veterinara din Cluj-Napoca, Calea Manastur 3-5, 400372 Cluj-Napoca, Romania. [2]The Koret School of Veterinary Medicine, Robert H. Smith Faculty of Agriculture Food and Environment, Hebrew University of Jerusalem, P.O. Box 12, 76100 Rehovot, Israel.

References

1. Tanaka R, Shimizu M, Hirao H, Kobayashi M, Nagashima Y, Machilda N, Yamane Y. Surgical management of a double-chambered right ventricle and chylothorax in a Labrador retriever. J Small Anim Pract. 2006;47: 405–8.
2. Martin MJ, Orton CE, Boon JA, Mama KR, Gaynor JS, Bright JM. Surgical correction of double-chambered right ventricle in dogs. JAVMA. 2002;220(6): 770–4.
3. Hoffman P, Wocik AW, Rozanski J, Siudalska H, Jakubowska E, Wlodarska EK, Kowalski M. The role of echocardiography in diagnosing double chambered right ventricle in adults. Heart. 2004;90:789–3.
4. Park IJ, Kim YH, Lee K, Park HK, Park BC. Isolated double chambered right ventricle presenting in adulthood. Inter J Cardio. 2007;121:e25–7.
5. Loukas M, Housman B, Blaak C, Kralovic S, Tubbs RS, Anderson HA. Double-chambered right ventricle: a review. Cardiovasc Path. 2013;22:417–3.
6. Koffas H, Fuentes VL, Boswood A, Connolly DJ, Brockman DJ, Bonagura JD, Meurs KM, Koplitz S, Baumwart R. Double chambered right ventricle in 9 cats. J Vet Inter Med. 2007;21:76–80.
7. Poser H, Pria AD, De Benedictis GM, Stelletta C, Berlanda M, Guglielmini C. Ventricular septal defect and double chambered right ventricle in an alpaca. J of Vet Card. 2014;17(1):71–6.
8. Fukushima R, Tanaka R, Suzuki S, Hamabe R, Machida N, Nakao S, Saida Y, Takashima K, Matsumoto H, Koyama H, Hirose H, Yamane Y. Epidemiological and morphological studies of double-chambered right ventricle in dogs. J Vet Med Sci. 2011;73(10):1287–3.
9. Willard MD, Eyster GE. Double-chambered right ventricle in two dogs. J Am Vet Med Assoc. 1981;178(5):486–8.
10. Koie H, Kurotobi EN, Sasaki T. Double-chambered right ventricle in a dog. J of vet. Med Sci. 2000;62:651–3.
11. Alva C, Ho SY, Lincoln CR, Rigby ML, Wright A, Anderson RH. The nature of obstructive muscular bundles in double chambered right ventricle. J Thor. Cardiovasc Surg. 1999;117:1180–9.
12. Kahr PC, Gonzalez RA, Kempny A, Orwat S, Uebing A, Dimopoulos K, Swan L, Baumgartner H, Gatzoulis MA, Diller PG. Long term natural history and postoperative outcome of double chambered right ventricle – experience from two tertiary adult congenital heart centers and review of the literature. Intern J Cardio. 2014;174(3):662–8.
13. Oliveira P, Domenech O, Silva J, Vannini S, Bussadori R, Bussadori C. Retrospective review of congenital heart disease in 976 dogs. J Vet Int Med. 2011;25:477–3.
14. Moustafa S, Patton DJ, Alvarez N, Al Shanawani M, AlDossari K, Connelly MS, Prieur T, Mookadem F. Double chambered right ventricle septal defect in adult: case series and review of the literature. J Cardiovas. Ultrasound. 2015; 23(1):48–51.
15. Eltohami EA, Hajar HA, Folger GM Jr. Double-chambered right ventricle and Down's syndrome: a proposed new association. Angiology. 1994;45:119–23.
16. Oliver JA, Garrido A, Gonzalez A, Benito F, Mateos M, Aroca A, Sanz E. Rapid progression of midventricluar obstruction in adults with double – chambered right ventricle. J Thorac Cardiovasc Surg. 2003;126:711–7.
17. Cil E, Saraclar M, Ozkutlu S, Ozme S, Bilgic A, Ozer S. Double-chambered right ventricle: experience with 52 cases. Int J Cardiol. 1995;50(1):19–29.
18. Boon JA, Apendix 2. Canine M–Mode Reference Ranges. In: Veterinary Echocardiography. 2nd ed. Willey – Blackwell; 2011. p. 538.
19. Bomassi E, Misbach C, Tissier R, Gouni V, Sechi ET, Petit AM, Desmyter A, Damoiseaux C, Pouchelon JL, Chetboul V. Signalment, clinical features, echocardiographic findings, and outcome of dogs and cats with ventricular septal defects: 109 cases (192 – 2013). JAVMA. 2015;247(2):166–75.
20. Andelfinger G, Wright KN, Lee H, Siemens L, Benson D. Canine tricuspid valve malformation, a model of human Ebstein anomaly, maps to dog chromosome 9. J Med Genet. 2003;40:320–4.
21. Restivo A, Cameron AH, Anderson RH, Allwork SP. Divided right ventricle: a review of its anatomical varieties. Pediatr Cardiol. 1984;5:197–204.
22. Ohad DG, Avrahami A, Waner T, David L. The occurrence and suspected mode of inheritance of congenital subaortic stenosis and tricuspid valve dysplasia in Dogue de Bordeaux dogs. The vet. Journal. 2013;197:351–7.
23. Penkoske PA, Duncan N, Collins RL. Surgical repair of double chambered right ventricle with or without ventriculotomy. J Thor Cardiovasc Sur. 1987; 93:385–93.

20

A randomized, double-blind, prospective, placebo-controlled study of the efficacy of a diet supplemented with curcuminoids extract, hydrolyzed collagen and green tea extract in owner's dogs with osteoarthritis

Fanny Comblain[1], Nicolas Barthélémy[2], Michael Lefèbvre[2], Cédric Schwartz[3], Isabelle Lesponne[4], Samuel Serisier[4], Alexandre Feugier[4], Marc Balligand[2] and Yves Henrotin[1,5*]

Abstract

Background: We have previously demonstrated that a mixture of Curcuminoids extract, hydrolyzed COllagen and green Tea extract (CCOT) inhibited inflammatory and catabolic mediator's synthesis by bovine and human chondrocytes. A randomly allocated, double-blind, prospective, placebo-controlled study was performed to evaluate the efficacy of a diet containing this CCOT mixture on dogs with naturally occurring osteoarthritis (OA). Therefore, 42 owner's dogs with OA were randomly assigned to receive for 3 months an experimental diet (control) or the same diet supplemented with CCOT.

Results: Ground reaction forces did not show statistical differences between groups. After 3 months of feeding, there was a significant reduction of pain at manipulation in the CCOT group, but not in the control group. The evolution for pain at manipulation depended on the diet. The three other parameters evaluated by veterinary subjective assessment (lameness, pain at palpation and joint mobility) did not show statistical differences. Concerning owner subjective assessment, pain severity score worsened in the control group but remained stable in CCOT group. The evolution for pain severity depended on the diet. No statistical difference was found for pain interference, except for the ability to rise to standing from lying down, which was significantly improved in the CCOT compared to the control group. Serum OA biomarkers did not show statistical differences.

Conclusions: Objective variables measured, such as ground reaction forces and OA biomarkers, did not show statistical differences. However, indicators of pain appeared reduced in dogs receiving CCOT mixture for 3 months. The difference of evolution between groups suggests that a greater number of dogs may be necessary to reach a stronger effect on other parameters.

Keywords: Osteoarthritis, Dog, Diet, Curcumin, Hydrolyzed collagen, Green tea polyphenols

* Correspondence: yhenrotin@ulg.ac.be
[1]Bone and Cartilage Research Unit, Arthropôle Liège, University of Liège, Liège, Belgium
[5]Physical Therapy & Rehabilitation Department, Princess Paola Hospital, Vivalia, Marche-en-Famenne, Belgium
Full list of author information is available at the end of the article

Background

Osteoarthritis (OA) is a chronic, painful, degenerative and inflammatory condition that affects the synovial joints. It is highly prevalent in dogs [1, 2] with 20% of the canine population over one year old affected [3, 4]. This musculoskeletal disease is related to chronic pain, lameness, loss of joint function and mobility, functional disability and reduced quality of life [5]. The management of OA in dogs is a lifetime commitment, involving a multimodal approach. The main recommendation is to control symptoms by reducing pain, improving mobility and hence quality of life; whilst protecting joints from OA [6].

To decrease pain and inflammation associated with OA, non-steroidal anti-inflammatory drugs (NSAIDs) are commonly prescribed [5]. Indeed, in clinical practice, many dogs suffering from OA are long term treated with NSAIDs such as carprofen [6]. NSAIDs act mostly by inhibiting cyclo-oxygenase and thus reducing the concentration of pro-inflammatory prostaglandins. Unfortunately, the use of NSAIDs may be associated with adverse effects, especially gastrointestinal tract ulcerations [7, 8]. Corticosteroid injection in dogs is usually reserved for severe end stage OA and for cases that have become refractory to other treatments [5]. Beside pain relief, preventing cartilage degradation is an important objective for treatment. This requires the long term use of safe therapies, while the absence of any cure reinforces the importance of prevention [9]. Such prevention and alternative solutions could come from nutrition or from dietary supplements. Indeed, these latter present the advantage of having few or no known side effects.

In a preliminary in vitro study [10], we have demonstrated that a mixture of curcuminoids extract, hydrolyzed collagen and green tea extract (CCOT) inhibited inflammatory and catabolic mediator's synthesis by bovine and human chondrocytes. These findings suggest a scientific rationale for the evaluation of these natural ingredients in a clinical trial. Curcumin is the major component of turmeric, a yellow spice derived from the rhizomes of the plant *Curcuma longa*. Evidence has been published for its potency to target multiple inflammatory diseases [11]. The main characteristic of hydrolyzed collagen is its amino acid composition, which is identical to collagen, thus providing high levels of glycine and proline, two amino acids essential for the stability and regeneration of cartilage [12, 13]. Green tea contains polyphenolic fractions called catechins and, among them, epigallocatechin-3-gallate, which exhibits antioxidant, anti-tumoral and anti-mutagenic activities [14].

This randomly allocated, double-blind, prospective, placebo-controlled clinical trial aimed to evaluate the effects of a diet containing CCOT mixture on client owned dogs with OA using objective variables such as force plate analysis and serum OA biomarkers (Coll2–1 and Coll2–1 NO_2) as well as subjective variables such as orthopedic evaluation and owner assessment [15].

Methods

Dogs

Dogs with OA were recruited among the patients of the Veterinary Hospital of the University of Liege, or through advertisements in pet stores, veterinarians' dog magazines, daily papers, websites with animal news, grooming salons and pet associations. The (potential) participants were informed about the purpose and design of the trial.

Inclusion criteria were the presence of clinical (such as lameness) and radiographic (such as the presence of osteophytes, subchondral bone sclerosis) signs of OA on at least one limb, to be older than 18 months and weigh over 10 kg with a body condition score lower than 8 (on a 9-point scale) [16], without evidence of systemic disease identified by history and results of physical examination, serum biochemical analysis and urinalysis.

Non-inclusion criteria were as follows: signs of lumbosacral disease or neurologic deficit, acute traumatic injuries (including OA acute crises), treatment with NSAIDs, corticosteroids or antimicrobials within 14 days before enrolment, surgery on any joint within 6 months before enrolment, aggressive behavior, and pregnancy or likelihood of becoming pregnant during the study. For ethical reasons, analgesics (tramadol, 2–5 mg/kg, 2–3 times a day) were allowed, except within 48 h before the evaluation.

Dogs were excluded from the study for the following reasons: development of an adverse reaction, injury or illness that required treatment or surgical intervention, excessive pain or other complications as determined by the investigator, lack of owner compliance with study restrictions, and death of the dog because of natural causes or owner-elected euthanasia.

Study diets

The 2 study diets were an experimental diet (control) or the same diet supplemented with CCOT mixture (CCOT) (Table 1). Both dry dog food products had similar nutritional and energy content (3515 kcal/kg) and similar visual aspect. Energy requirements for dogs were based on the equation published by the National Research Council in 2006: 95 kcal/kg$^{0.75}$ body weight [17, 18]. Both diets were supplied by the manufacturer in identical neutral bags but differentiated by their code names. The diet with the CCOT mixture contained 0.43 g curcuma extract per 1000 kcal, 4.27 g hydrolyzed collagen per 1000 kcal and 0.85 g green tea extract per 1000 kcal. Curcuma extract (Indena, Paris, France) contained between 18 and 22% of curcuminoids and was associated with a phosphatidylcholine complex to

Table 1 Composition of both study diets

	Unit	Control	CCOT
Moisture	%	12,2	12,1
Protein	%	20,5	20,5
Fat	%	11,7	11,7
Ash	%	6,0	5,9
Crude fiber	%	4,0	4,0
Total dietary fiber	%	9,0	9,0
Nitrogen free extract	%	40,2	39,9
Glycine	%	0,7	1,0
Hydroxyproline	%	0,002	0,2
Proline	%	1,1	1,2
Curcuminoids extract	%	0	0,15
Hydrolyzed collagen	%	0	1,5
Green tea polyphenols	%	0	0,3

increase its bioavailability [19]. Peptides constituting hydrolyzed collagen (Gelita, Eberbach, Germany) were composed of 30 amino acids peptides. Glycine and proline represented more than 35% of total amino acids content. Green tea extract (Naturex, Avignon, France) contained 25% polyphenols, which represented 12.5% catechins representing more than 9.3% epigallocatechin-3-gallate.

Study protocol

The study was designed as a 3-month double-blind, randomly allocated, prospective, placebo-controlled clinical trial, adhering to the CONSORT guidelines [20]. All owners received a detailed written description of the protocol and provided written informed consent before the inclusion of their dog in the study. The protocol was approved by the Institutional Animal Care and Use Ethics Committee of the University of Liège (reference 12–1330) and by the Royal Canine Ethics Committee. They adhere to a high standard of veterinary care. Investigators collected blood samples at the first screening visit for serum biochemistry which validated dog eligibility for the study. Eligible dogs were randomly assigned (using Microsoft Office Excel 2013) to receive either the control diet or the CCOT supplemented diet. A statistician generated the random allocation sequence. Block size was 10. Allocation ratio was 1:1. The allocation sequence was not concealed but neither pet owners, neither veterinarians nor investigators had knowledge of the diet to which dogs were assigned. A veterinarian enrolled dogs. Upon enrollment in the study, pet owners were instructed to feed their dogs on a transition diet (same composition as control but kibble of a different shape) over 14 days. In this way, all eligible dogs received the same diet (without any potential active compound included within the diet) before starting the study. Feeding guidelines were provided to owners with the intent for dogs to maintain a constant body weight and condition as well as to be fed according to their usual feeding regimen (free choice or meal). An investigator assigned dogs to interventions. Dogs were weighed each month.

Adverse events

During the study, all adverse events were reported to the investigator, who noted the event characteristics including severity, occurrence and suspected association with the food.

Objective measurement: force plate analysis

Ground reaction forces were measured with kinetic analysis using biomechanical force platforms (Kistler, Winterthur, Switzerland) at the Laboratory of Human Motion Analysis at the University of Liège. At study start (T0 = inclusion +14 days of transition diet), the limb most affected by lameness, as shown by peak vertical force (PVF) gait analysis and orthopedic examination, and with radiographic OA lesions was defined as "the most affected limb" and followed throughout the study. Dogs were acclimated to the force plate before data collection. Data for the right and left sides were collected from separate passes across the plate. The limb most affected by lameness, as shown by PVF gait analysis and orthopedic examination, and with radiographic OA lesions was considered as the most affected limb and its contralateral limb was considered as less affected limb (compared to its contralateral most affected limb). Ground reaction forces were recorded at T0 and after 3 months of diet (T3). The owner trotted dogs across the force plate, and an investigator observed and filmed each pass to confirm foot strikes and gait. A test was considered valid when only one limb landed on the force plate at a time, while the dog was trotted across it at a velocity of 1.8 to 2.2 m/s and acceleration-deceleration variation of ±0.5 m/s^2. The dog's forward velocity was measured with a 3D sensor (Charnwood Dynamics, Rothley, United Kingdom) placed on the back of the dog. Five valid tests were obtained for each limb.

PVF, braking and propulsive peak forces, vertical impulse, braking and propulsive impulses, and loading and unloading rates were measured and analyzed using the software CODAmotion (V6.78.1) (Charnwood Dynamics). All parameters were normalized by body weight (BW) (Newton) and expressed in % of BW. Data from five valid tests of each most affected and less affected limb were averaged as previously described [21]. PVF has been defined as the primary outcome of our study. Based on this outcome, we determined the positive and negative responder's rates for control and COT groups [22]. We used the minimal detectable change, at the 95%

level (MDC95), which reflected a real change. A change of at least 3.6% BW in PVF measurement, when expressed relatively to baseline values, at the 95% level, needed to occur to be confident [22].

Subjective measurement: orthopedic evaluation

At inclusion visit and T3, dogs were examined by a veterinarian specialized in orthopedic surgery. Two orthopedists participated in the study. One orthopedist evaluated 24 dogs, and another 18 dogs. The same veterinarian performed a dog's assessment at T0 and at T3. Lameness (1 to 5), pain at manipulation (0 to 10), pain at palpation (1 to 5) and joint mobility (1 to 5) were evaluated as previously described [23, 24]. The scoring system is described in Table 2. Pain at manipulation was evaluated on a scale from 0 to 10, 0 corresponding to no pain, and 10 corresponding to extreme pain [24]. Pain upon limb manipulation was evaluated by animals' vocalization or other observations of pain during the extension and flexion of all four limbs for a period of several minutes.

Subjective measurement: owner assessment

Owners evaluated their dog's condition at T0 and T3 by completing a validated Canine Brief Pain Inventory (CBPI), a questionnaire assessing pain severity (PS) and pain interference (PI) [15]. The questionnaire was translated in French. The same owner evaluated his/her dog at T0 and T3. The 4 PS questions (worst pain in the last 7 days, least pain in the last 7 days, average pain in the last 7 days and pain right now) were scored on a numeric scale from 0 (no pain) to 10 (extreme pain). The scores of each question were averaged to generate the global PS score. Each criterion was considered with the same weighing. The 6 PI questions (i.e., how much the pain interfered with the dog's typical function: general activity, enjoyment of life, ability to rise to standing from lying down, ability to walk, ability to run and ability to climb up) were scored on a numeric scale from 0 (does not interfere) to 10 (completely interferes). The scores of each question were averaged to generate the global PI score. Each criterion was considered with the same weighing.

Table 2 Clinical scoring system for assessing dogs with osteoarthritis

Criterion	Grade	Clinical evaluation
Lameness	1	Walk normally
	2	Slightly lame when walking
	3	Moderately lame when walking
	4	Severely lame when walking
	5	Reluctant to rise and will not walk more than five paces
Pain at palpation	1	None
	2	Mild signs; dog turns head in recognition
	3	Moderate signs; dog pulls limb away
	4	Severe signs; dog vocalizes or becomes aggressive
	5	Dog will not allow palpation
Joint mobility	1	Full range of motion
	2	Mild limitation (10 ~ 20%) in range of motion; no crepitus
	3	Mild limitation (10 ~ 20%) in range of motion; crepitus
	4	Moderate limitation (20 ~ 50%) in range of motion; ± crepitus
	5	Severe limitation (>50%) in range of motion; ± crepitus

Objective measurement: OA biomarkers

Blood samples were collected each month (T0, after 1 month of diet (T1), after 2 months of diet (T2) and T3) and OA biomarkers (Coll2–1 and Coll2–1 NO2) were quantified by competitive immunoassays (Artialis SA, Liège, Belgium). All Coll2–1 and Coll2–1NO2 tests have been performed by Artialis in collaboration with Bone and Cartilage Research Unit.

These assays are competitive immunoassays utilizing a synthetic peptide pre-coated onto the ELISA plate for the quantification of the corresponding antigen in samples. A binding competition between the immobilized peptide and the peptide contained in the standards or samples takes place upon addition of the antibodies. After removal of the unbound peptide, a peroxidase-conjugated goat anti-rabbit antibody is added into each well to detect and quantify the level of competitive binding. After washing of the unbound detection antibody, the antibody-antigen complex is detected by a chromogenic reaction with 3, 3′, 5, 5′-tetramethylbenzidine (TMB). The reaction is stopped by adding acid to give a colorimetric endpoint that is subsequently determined spectrophotometrically.

Coll2–1 was quantified in dog sera by competitive ELISA in triplicate with polyclonal rabbit antisera (ab-Coll2–1; Artialis) using buffers specifically developed to measure these fragments in dog serum (confidential composition). A 6-fold dilution of samples has been applied. Intraassay coefficient of variation (CV) was 3.6% and interassay CV was 9.8%.

Coll2–1-NO2 was quantified in dog sera by competitive ELISA according to the methodology cited above, in triplicate, with polyclonal rabbit antisera (D37; Artialis) using buffers specifically developed to measure these fragments in dog serum (confidential composition). A 2-fold dilution of samples has been applied. Intraassay CV was 5.8% and interassay CV was 4.7%.

Statistical analysis

The number of dogs needed, on a statistical point of view, was calculated from a previous study evaluating the effect of an extract of turmeric in OA dogs on PVF [9]. Using the related effect size, this study was powered at 80% with an alpha risk at 5%. A two-tailed test was performed. Including a 10–20% margin for fallout during the study, the optimal initial number of dogs was determined between 46 and 50.

There was no change to trial outcomes after the trial commenced. PVF was calculated in terms of PVF evolution as Δ T3-T0. PVF was assessed with a mixed model including diet, limb effect (most/less affected), and interaction between diet and limb effect as fixed effects. As given that BW influenced PVF, BW was entered as covariate in PVF statistical analysis. Lameness, pain at manipulation, pain at palpation and joint mobility were also assessed using a mixed model including time, diet, and the related interaction between time and diet as the main effects. Dog was defined as a random term in mixed models. PS and PI were assessed using generalized linear model. Diet, defined as the main effect, was investigated on Δ T3-T0. Generalized linear model or mixed model were analyzed using SAS 9.3. According to data features and residuals distribution of each model, the outcomes were previously rank transformed or not. Homoscedasticity was checked on residuals with a white test at a level of 1%. All data were expressed as mean ± standard deviation. The analysis was two-sided. A *p*-value ≤0.05 was considered as statistically significant.

Results

Dogs

One hundred and fifty five dog owners responded to the advertising. After a phone interview to get additional information, 115 owners were invited with their dog to the first screening visit. Of those 115 screened dogs, 48 were found eligible for the study and were randomly assigned to receive CCOT ($n = 23$) or control ($n = 25$) diet for 3 months. Two dogs in the CCOT and 4 in the control groups were excluded from the study for the following reasons: development of an illness that required treatment (such as NSAIDs) or surgical intervention (3 control dogs), appearance of neurologic deficit (1 CCOT dog), lack of owner compliance with study restrictions (1 control dog), and death of the dog because of owner-elected euthanasia due to deterioration of general condition of the dog (1 CCOT dog). Consequently, 42 dogs completed the study, including 21 from the CCOT group and 21 from the control group (Fig. 1). Only dogs that completed the study were included in the analysis (per-protocol population). Two dogs in the control group needed rescue analgesia during the study: one for 8 days and one for 7 days. The periods of recruitment and follow-up lasted for more than two years (from February 2013 to April 2015). The trial ended because between 46 and 50 dogs were enrolled in the study.

There were no significant differences concerning population characteristics between control and CCOT groups at T0 and T3 (Table 3). In the control group, the following breeds were represented: mixed breed ($n = 6$),

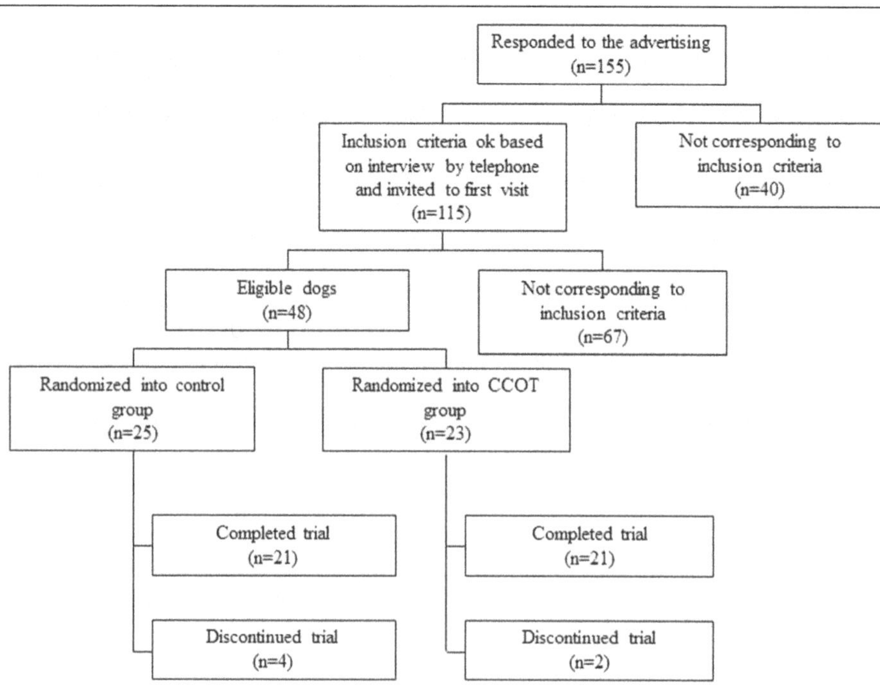

Fig. 1 Flow diagram through study

Table 3 Characteristics of dogs which completed the study

Characteristics	Control	CCOT	*p*-value
Total number of subjects	21	21	NA
Male/female	8/13	10/11	NA
Castrated male/sterilized female/intact	2/9/10	6/7/8	NA
Age at T0 (years)	7.50 ± 2.85	7.56 ± 3.07	0.952
Body weight at T0 (kg)	34.91 ± 11.66	36.43 ± 12.63	0.563
Body weight at T3 (kg)	35.17 ± 11.60	36.13 ± 12.95	0.717
Peak vertical force at T0 (% BW)	69.65 ± 19.86	61.81 ± 11.56	0.618
Pain at manipulation at T0	3.65 ± 2.50	4.19 ± 2.40	0.988
Pain severity at T0	2.46 ± 2.08	2.67 ± 1.82	0.680
Pain interference at T0	3.44 ± 2.71	3.26 ± 2.47	0.898
Most affected joint at T0			
Carpus	1	0	NA
Elbow	5	2	NA
Stifle	2	6	NA
Hip	13	13	NA

Data were expressed as distributions (number of dogs) for categorical characteristics and as mean ± SD for continuous characteristics
T0 study start, *T3* after 3 months of diet, study end, *NA* not applicable, *BW* body weight

German Shepherd Dogs ($n = 5$), Bernese Mountain Dogs ($n = 2$), Border Collies ($n = 2$), and 1 each of Australian Shepherd, Bordeaux Mastiff, Braque d'Auvergne, German Shorthaired Pointer, Golden Retriever, Rottweiler. In the CCOT group, the following breeds were represented: Golden Retrievers ($n = 5$), Border Collies ($n = 2$), Cockers ($n = 2$), German Shepherd Dogs ($n = 2$), Labradors ($n = 2$), Newfoundland ($n = 2$) and 1 each of Airedale Terrier, Bernese Mountain Dog, German Mastiff, mixed breed, Pitbull-type dog, Saint-Bernard.

Tolerance

The CCOT diet was well tolerated. There was no significant change in dogs' body weight nor evidence of side effects over the duration of the study. Three dogs in CCOT group and 2 dogs in control group had mild diarrhea but it was minor and transient.

Objective measurement: force plate analysis

We recruited only few dogs affected by front and hind limbs OA, and those dogs were « clinically » lame only on one leg (usually the front limb). We did not recruit any dogs with lameness on both front and hind limbs.

PVF values for the most severely affected limb were not significantly different between control and CCOT groups at T0 ($p = 0.618$) and T3 ($p = 0.953$). There was no significant PVF change with time in control group (T0: 69.65 ± 4.33% BW; T3: 69.63 ± 3.18% BW; $p = 0.999$) and in CCOT group (T0: 61.81 ± 2.52% BW; T3: 67.44 ± 3.32% BW; $p = 0.283$). The PVF change (Δ T3-T0) was not different between groups ($p = 0.319$) (Fig. 2).

Different levels of change in PVF measurement were observed in dogs. The positive responder's rate was greater in CCOT group (47.6%) than in control group (42.9%). Moreover, the negative responder's rate was greater in control group (23.8%) than in CCOT group (14.3%). Indeed, among the 21 dogs in CCOT group, 13 (61.9%) had clinically meaningful changes, which were positive in 10 (47.6%) or negative in 3 (14.3%) dogs. Among the 21 dogs in control group, 14 (66.7%) had clinically meaningful changes, which were positive in 9 (42.9%) or negative in 5 (23.8%) dogs (Fig. 3).

There were no significant differences between groups for the vertical impulse, the braking and propulsive peak forces, the braking and propulsive impulses and the loading and unloading rates changes between T0 and T3 (data not shown).

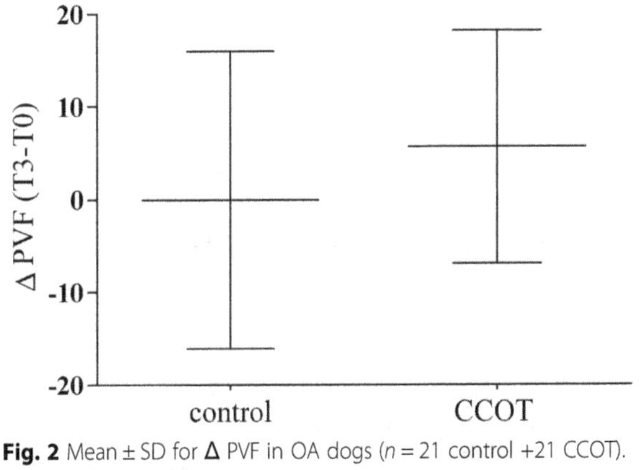

Fig. 2 Mean ± SD for Δ PVF in OA dogs ($n = 21$ control +21 CCOT). PVF = peak vertical force

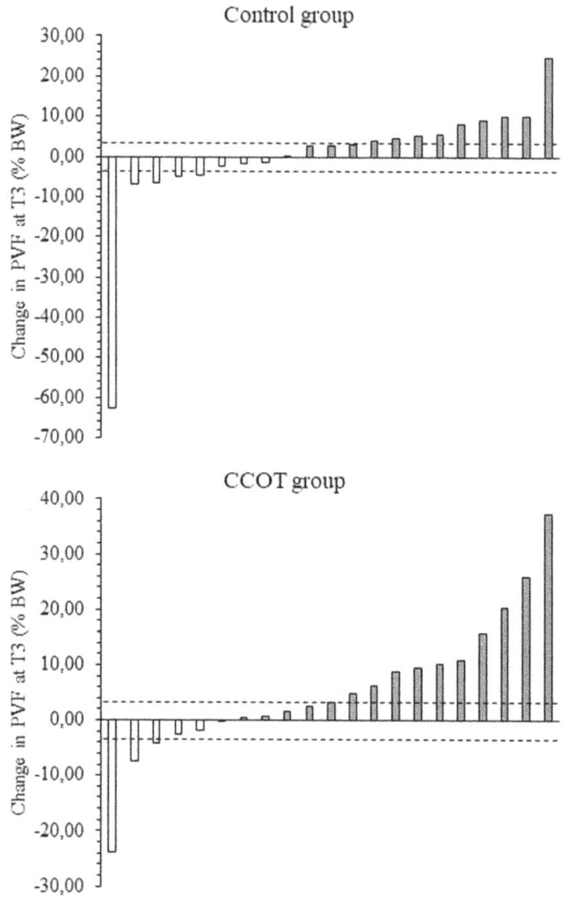

Fig. 3 Individual changes in PVF measured at T3 in OA dogs. Changes were the difference between T3 and T0. Dashed lines represent the minimal detectable change, when expressed relatively to baseline values, at the 95% level. T0 = study start; T3 = study end

Subjective measurement: veterinary evaluation

Pain at manipulation was significantly decreased in the CCOT group (T0: 4.19 ± 0.52; T3: 2.86 ± 0.51; $p = 0.037$) but not in the control group (T0: 3.65 ± 0.56; T3: 3.7 ± 0.4, $p = 0.999$). Furthermore, the evolution for pain at manipulation depended on the diet ($p = 0.036$) (Fig. 4). There was no significant difference between groups for lameness, pain at palpation and joint mobility at T0 and T3 (Table 4).

Subjective measurement: owner assessment

Regarding owner's assessment, PS did not change in the control (T0: 2.46 ± 0.45; T3: 3.58 ± 0.51; $p = 0.071$) or the CCOT group (T0: 2.67 ± 0.4; T3: 2.42 ± 0.38: $p = 0.35$). The PS change (ΔT3-T0) was significantly different between CCOT and control groups ($p = 0.009$) (Fig. 5a). There was no significant difference for PI change between CCOT (T0: 3.26 ± 0.54; T3: 2.96 ± 0.45; $p = 0.101$) and control groups (T0: 3.44 ± 0.59; T3: 3.86 ± 0.66; $p = 0.633$) ($p = 0.063$) (Fig. 5b). However, when each question of the PI score was analyzed separately, PI change

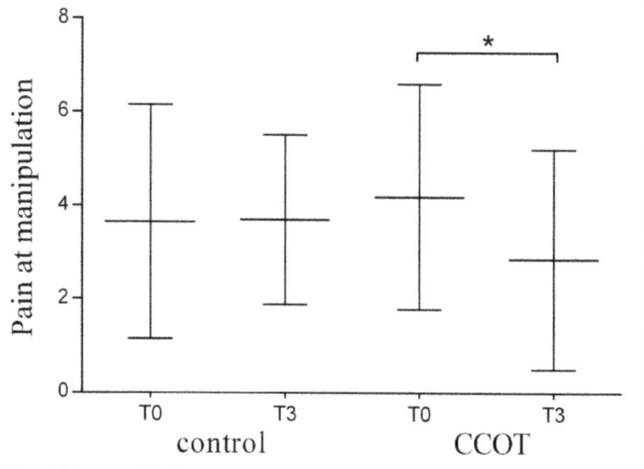

Fig. 4 Mean ± SD for pain at manipulation at T0 and T3 in OA dogs ($n = 21$ control +21 CCOT). T0 = study start; T3 = study end; *$p < 0.05$

(Δ T3-T0) on the ability to rise to standing from lying down was significantly improved in CCOT group compared to control group ($p = 0.029$).

Objective measurement: OA biomarkers

Coll2–1 and Coll2–1 NO_2 serum concentrations were not significantly different between control and CCOT groups at T0 and T3. No significant changes over time in Coll2–1 and Coll2–1 NO_2 serum concentrations were observed in both groups.

Discussion

The results of this study suggest that there is some benefit in feeding symptomatic OA dogs with a diet containing the CCOT mixture, even if the primary outcome (PVF, objective variable) was not improved.

Interestingly, our study showed that the veterinary subjective assessment pain at manipulation was decreased by more than 30% by CCOT diet. These data are consistent with that of a study evaluating the effects of curcuma extract in owner's dogs [9]. Another study

Table 4 Mean ± SD for lameness, pain at palpation and joint mobility of the most severely affected limb in OA dogs

	T0	T3	Time*diet *p*-value
Lameness			
Control ($n = 21$)	1.8 ± 0.77	1.95 ± 1.05	0.244
CCOT ($n = 21$)	2.19 ± 0.87	1.86 ± 0.96	
Pain at palpation			
Control ($n = 21$)	2.45 ± 0.94	2.55 ± 0.94	0.195
CCOT ($n = 21$)	2.62 ± 0.92	2.1 ± 0.94	
Joint mobility			
Control ($n = 21$)	2.3 ± 1.08	2.75 ± 1.25	0.815
CCOT ($n = 21$)	2.71 ± 1.42	2.7 ± 1.22	

T0 study start, *T3* after 3 months of diet

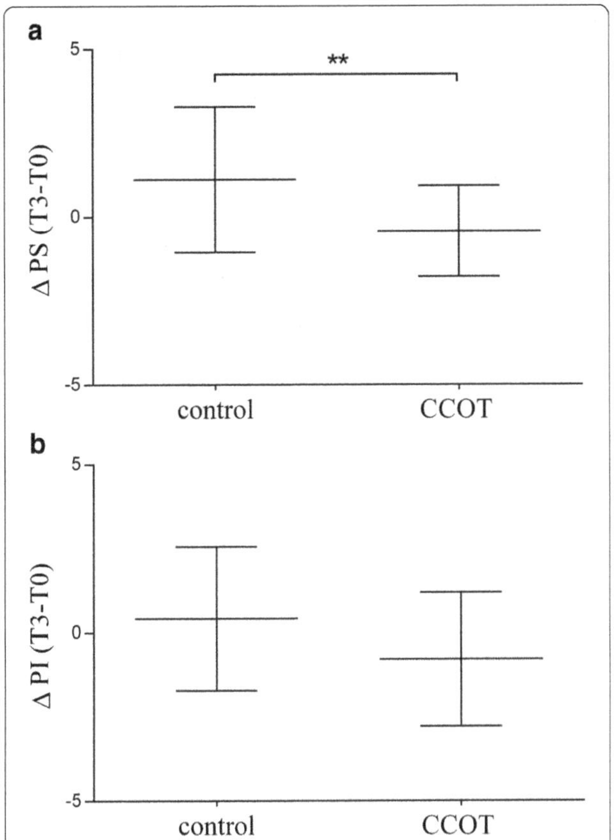

Fig. 5 Mean ± SD for **Δ** PS (**a**) and **Δ** PI (**b**) in OA dogs ($n = 21$ control +21 CCOT). PS = pain severity; PI = pain interference; $**p < 0.01$

evaluating the effect of undenatured type II collagen also demonstrated a decrease in pain upon limb manipulation [25]. Pain improvement was not associated with lameness improvement. Indeed, constraints and movement amplitudes are different. This may also be explained by the fact that manipulation investigates pain coming from the peri-articular tissue while lameness could be partially generated by pain triggered by subchondral bone loading.

Assessments by owners are subjective measures but, when such measures are used, a composite score is more effective than individual scores [26]. In the present study, we used the validated CBPI which includes two composite scores: PS and PI [15]. Regarding owner's assessment, the evolution for PS, as assessed by ΔT3-T0, was significantly different between CCOT and control groups, with the CCOT group staying stable and the control group worsening. In contrast, no significant difference was observed for PI between CCOT and control groups. This suggests that CCOT could affect pain but not limb function. Nevertheless, when questions corresponding to PI were analyzed separately, we found that change (ΔT3-T0) in the ability to rise to standing from lying down was significantly improved in the CCOT compared to the control group. This is consistent with a study showing that fish oil induced a significant improvement on the ability to rise from a resting position, to play and to walk in OA dogs [27]. It has been shown that the CBPI was not correlated with changes in force plate data [21]. Pain mechanism during the weight bearing is different. Moreover, owners considered that showing improvements in quality of life (performing activities of daily living) is much more important than demonstrating enhancements in force plate data and increased or decreased use of a single limb at a walk or trot [21]. Gait analysis has the limitation of only evaluating an animal at one specific time point, outside of its normal environment. On the contrary, CBPI quantifies the owners' assessment of clinically relevant chronic pain–related behaviors with the dog in its routine environment over an extended period of time as well as how their dog is doing "right now" [21].

However, PVF is often recognized as the most appropriate measure for assessing the effects of therapeutic modalities in OA dogs and is frequently used in clinical trials [26, 28, 29]. PVF was increased by a diet supplemented with fish oil omega-3 fatty acids [26, 30], with type II collagen [24] and with green lipped mussel [31] but not by an extract of curcuma [9]. PVF presents some weaknesses, however. It is less reliable when used in owner's dogs. The fact that data for the most and less affected limbs were mostly collected from separate runs could also bring a bias. Minimal body weight of included dogs was 10 kg. It may have been better to start with higher body weight of dogs (e.g. 20 kg). Historically the weight limitation was related to the ability for the force plate to record a single stride (the size of the plate was too big to have only one leg striking the plate at the same time). Indeed, a small dog will have a faster joint angular velocity than a big dog. That is why we compared the difference between T0 and T3 on the same dog, at the same velocity. We were based on a study in which minimal body weight was 11.4 kg [26]. Additionally, the gait analysis data combined thoracic and pelvic limbs. This was problematic because PVF for the front limb is higher than PVF for the hind limb. There was a higher number of front limb OA dogs in control group ($n = 6$) than in COT group ($n = 2$). Therefore PVF was calculated as Δ T3-T0 but this heterogeneity may add a bias to our study.

Moreover, PVF decrease has been demonstrated to be more important in dogs affected by stifle OA than by hip OA [32]. So we can speculate that the low ratio of stifle OA in our population explains in part the absence of effects of CCOT on PVF. Indeed in our study, 19% of dogs had stifle OA while 62% had hip OA. Our population was heterogeneous in terms of OA location. Some dogs also had indirect signs of OA (such as a decreased range of motion or discrete discomfort on manipulation) in multiple limbs. An improvement in one limb could hidden pain in others limbs. This is a limitation of this study. However heterogeneous groups of dogs mimics the real clinical situation in veterinary medicine. One could consider this heterogeneity as a strength of our study.

The owner was the leash-driver for kinetics gait analysis. This is good for lowering stress associated with the manipulation for the dog. But this could be another source of inter-individuals variability, which may be controlled by the same manipulator for each dog. Before the beginning of the study, we compared kinetic analysis when dogs were guided by their owners or by the manipulator. We concluded that dogs were less troubled when they were guided by their owners. It was the same owner who guided his/her dog at T0 and at T3. Indeed, the dog response to a foreign manipulator is another inter-individual variability. Anyway, all the trials were recorded at the same velocity, acceleration (with the dog not turning its head). Dogs were also guided by their owners in other similar studies [30, 33].

Because mean changes often obscure the individual change, we presented individual changes in PVF for both control and CCOT groups. We also calculated positive and negative responder's rates. The positive responder's rate was greater in CCOT group (47.6%) than in control group (42.9%) whereas the negative responder's rate was greater in control group (23.8%) than in CCOT group (14.3%). Reporting the percentages of dogs which met the MDC_{95} requirements provided additional insightful interpretations other than considering only the overall mean change scores [22]. The MDC_{95} that reflected a real change in PVF measurement has been established in a recent study [22]. The MDC_{95} was found at 2% BW, indicating that any change in PVF for OA dog would be considered as measure noise below 2% BW, and a clinically significant change over 2% BW. However, when expressed relatively to baseline values, the MDC_{95} was found to be 3.6% BW [22]. As given that the change in PVF was measured between T0 (baseline) and T3, we choose this limit (3.6%) to calculate responder's rates in our study.

Chronic pain is complex to measure. Even if the force plate is considered as one of the most appropriate measure of outcome as it is the most objective, so far, it is unknown if it is the most sensitive (pertinent) for chronic OA.

To our knowledge, this is the first time that serum OA biomarkers were measured to assess the effects of a diet supplemented with CCOT mixture in OA dogs. Collagen degradation is one of the main features of cartilage breakdown during OA. Coll2–1 and Coll2–1 NO_2 serum concentrations were correlated with the macroscopic and histological changes in dogs with OA induced by transection of the anterior cruciate ligament [34]. We failed to observe an effect of CCOT on Coll2–1 and Coll2–1 NO_2 serum levels. This may be explained by the higher heterogeneity of biomarker values in our population than in a model of surgically induced OA dogs.

No age effect was observed (data not shown) on the outcomes of interest but the study was not designed for this purpose.

Our study presented some limitations such as its short duration and the number of dogs included. Even though the number of dogs needed was statistically calculated a priori based on the PVF data, the lack of information to fully represent targeted population variability (i.e. breed effect, gender effect...) might have underestimated required sample size. Additionally, higher numbers are required for subjective veterinary and owner assessments compared to gait analysis. A larger number of dogs and a reduced inter-individual variability could increase the benefit of the CCOT diet and subsequently reinforce the likelihood of measurable improvements of PVF and OA biomarkers serum concentrations. Moreover, the fact that the bags were clearly marked with codes that differentiated the groups and that the randomization sequence was not concealed could add bias to the study.

Conclusions

Objective variables measured, such as ground reaction forces and OA biomarkers, did not show statistical differences. Regarding the objective outcome PVF, the positive responder's rate was greater in CCOT group than in control group whereas the negative responder's rate was greater in control group than in CCOT group, albeit not statistically tested. The study reveals that dogs receiving diet supplemented with CCOT mixture for 3 months showed less pain at manipulation. The three other parameters evaluated by veterinary subjective assessment (lameness, pain at palpation and joint mobility) did not show statistical differences. Regarding the subjective owner assessment, the evolution of PS showed significant difference between CCOT and control groups. No statistical difference was found for PI, except for the ability to rise to standing from lying down, which was significantly improved in the CCOT compared to the control group. These results suggest that, even if the CCOT diet does not seem to improve lameness (on kinetics and clinical rating) in our studied OA dogs, it could present some benefits on chronic pain and its impact on activities of daily living in OA dogs.

Abbreviations

BW: body weight; CBPI: Canine Brief Pain Inventory; CCOT: a mixture of curcuminoids extract, hydrolyzed collagen and green tea extract; CV: coefficient of variation; NSAIDs: non-steroidal anti-inflammatory drugs; OA: osteoarthritis; PI: Pain Interference; PS: Pain Severity; PVF: peak vertical force; T0: at study start; T3: after 3 months of diet; TMB: 3, 3', 5, 5'-tetramethylbenzidine

Acknowledgements
The authors are grateful to Royal Canin SAS who funded the present research. The authors thank Artialis SA for performing Coll2-1 and Coll2-1NO_2 tests. The authors are grateful to Anne-Françoise Donneau for her help in calculating the number of dogs needed. The authors would like to thank all the dogs' owners who accepted to seriously participate in this study.

Funding
The research leading to these results was supported by a grant of Royal Canin SAS. Royal Canin SAS has given final approval of the version to be published.

Authors' contributions
FC, NB, CS, IL, SS, MB and YH conceived and designed the study. FC, NB, ML, CS and MB acquired the data. FC, NB, CS, IL, AF, MB and YH analyzed the data. AF made the statistical analyzes. All authors revised the article critically for important intellectual content. All authors have given final approval of the version to be published. All authors agreed to be accountable for all aspects of the work.

Consent for publication
Not applicable.

Competing interests
FC receives her PhD fellow from Royal Canin SAS. IL and SS are employed by Royal Canin. YH receives honoraria from Artialis, Bepharbel, Bioiberica, Danone, Expanscience, Galapagos, Ibsa, Merck, Pierre Fabre, KiOmed Pharma and Tilman. YH is the founder and President of Artialis SA, a biomarker manufacturer and KiOmed Pharma, two spin-off companies of the University of Liege. FC, SS and YH are inventors for patent WO/2014/184246.

Author details
[1]Bone and Cartilage Research Unit, Arthropôle Liège, University of Liège, Liège, Belgium. [2]Department of Clinical Sciences, Faculty of Veterinary Medicine, University of Liège, Liège, Belgium. [3]Laboratory of Human Motion Analysis, University of Liège, Liège, Belgium. [4]Royal Canin Research Center, Aimargues, France. [5]Physical Therapy & Rehabilitation Department, Princess Paola Hospital, Vivalia, Marche-en-Famenne, Belgium.

References

1. Paster ER, LaFond E, Biery DN, Iriye A, Gregor TP, Shofer FS, Smith GK. Estimates of prevalence of hip dysplasia in golden retrievers and Rottweilers and the influence of bias on published prevalence figures. J Am Vet Med Assoc. 2005;226(3):387–92.
2. Smith GK, Paster ER, Powers MY, Lawler DF, Biery DN, Shofer FS, McKelvie PJ, Kealy RD. Lifelong diet restriction and radiographic evidence of osteoarthritis of the hip joint in dogs. J Am Vet Med Assoc. 2006;229(5):690–3.
3. Moreau M, Rialland P, Pelletier JP, Martel-Pelletier J, Lajeunesse D, Boileau C, Caron J, Frank D, Lussier B, del Castillo JR, et al. Tiludronate treatment improves structural changes and symptoms of osteoarthritis in the canine anterior cruciate ligament model. Arthritis Res Ther. 2011;13(3):R98.
4. Johnston SA. Osteoarthritis. Joint anatomy, physiology, and pathobiology. Vet Clin North Am Small Anim Pract. 1997;27(4):699–723.
5. Henrotin Y, Sanchez C, Balligand M. Pharmaceutical and nutraceutical management of canine osteoarthritis: present and future perspectives. Vet J. 2005;170(1):113–23.
6. Aragon CL, Hofmeister EH, Budsberg SC. Systematic review of clinical trials of treatments for osteoarthritis in dogs. J Am Vet Med Assoc. 2007;230(4):514–21.
7. Moreau M, Dupuis J, Bonneau NH, Desnoyers M. Clinical evaluation of a nutraceutical, carprofen and meloxicam for the treatment of dogs with osteoarthritis. Vet Rec. 2003;152(11):323–9.
8. Forsyth SF, Guilford WG, Haslett SJ, Godfrey J. Endoscopy of the gastroduodenal mucosa after carprofen, meloxicam and ketoprofen administration in dogs. J Small Anim Pract. 1998;39(9):421–4.
9. Innes JF, Fuller CJ, Grover ER, Kelly AL, Burn JF. Randomised, double-blind, placebo-controlled parallel group study of P54FP for the treatment of dogs with osteoarthritis. Vet Rec. 2003;152(15):457–60.
10. Comblain F, Sanchez C, Lesponne I, Balligand M, Serisier S, Henrotin Y. Curcuminoids extract, hydrolyzed collagen and green tea extract Synergically inhibit inflammatory and catabolic Mediator's synthesis by normal bovine and osteoarthritic human chondrocytes in monolayer. PLoS One. 2015;10(3):e0121654.
11. Henrotin Y, Priem F, Mobasheri A. Curcumin: a new paradigm and therapeutic opportunity for the treatment of osteoarthritis: curcumin for osteoarthritis management. Spring. 2013;2(1):56.
12. Walrand S, Chiotelli E, Noirt F, Mwewa S, Lassel T. Consumption of a functional fermented milk containing collagen hydrolysate improves the concentration of collagen-specific amino acids in plasma. J Agric Food Chem. 2008;56(17):7790–5.
13. Ohara H, Iida H, Ito K, Takeuchi Y, Nomura Y. Effects of pro-Hyp, a collagen hydrolysate-derived peptide, on hyaluronic acid synthesis using in vitro cultured synovium cells and oral ingestion of collagen hydrolysates in a guinea pig model of osteoarthritis. Biosci Biotechnol Biochem. 2010;74(10):2096–9.
14. Henrotin Y, Lambert C, Couchourel D, Ripoll C, Chiotelli E. Nutraceuticals: do they represent a new era in the management of osteoarthritis? - a narrative review from the lessons taken with five products. Osteoarthr Cartil. 2011;19(1):1–21.
15. Brown DC, Boston RC, Coyne JC, Farrar JT. Ability of the canine brief pain inventory to detect response to treatment in dogs with osteoarthritis. J Am Vet Med Assoc. 2008;233(8):1278–83.
16. Laflamme DP. Development and validation of a body condition score system for dogs. Canine Practice July/August. 1997;22:10–5.
17. NRC: Nutrient requirements of dogs and cats. Washington DC: National Academic Press. In: *Energy*. edn. Edited by Council NR; 2006: 22–48.
18. Bermingham EN, Thomas DG, Cave NJ, Morris PJ, Butterwick RF, German AJ. Energy requirements of adult dogs: a meta-analysis. PLoS One. 2014;9(10):e109681.
19. Chaurasia S, Patel RR, Chaubey P, Kumar N, Khan G, Mishra B. Lipopolysaccharide based oral nanocarriers for the improvement of bioavailability and anticancer efficacy of curcumin. Carbohydr Polym. 2015;130:9–17.
20. Schulz KF, Altman DG, Moher D. Group C: CONSORT 2010 statement: updated guidelines for reporting parallel group randomised trials. BMC Med. 2010;8:18.
21. Brown DC, Boston RC, Farrar JT. Comparison of force plate gait analysis and owner assessment of pain using the canine brief pain inventory in dogs with osteoarthritis. J Vet Intern Med. 2013;27(1):22–30.
22. Moreau M, Pelletier JP, Lussier B, d'Anjou MA, Blond L, Pelletier JM, del Castillo JR, Troncy E. A posteriori comparison of natural and surgical destabilization models of canine osteoarthritis. Biomed Res Int. 2013;2013:180453.
23. Nganvongpanit K, Pothacharoen P, Suwankong N, Ong-Chai S, Kongtawelert P. The effect of doxycycline on canine hip osteoarthritis: design of a 6-months clinical trial. J Vet Sci. 2009;10(3):239–47.
24. Gupta RC, Canerdy TD, Lindley J, Konemann M, Minniear J, Carroll BA, Hendrick C, Goad JT, Rohde K, Doss R, et al. Comparative therapeutic efficacy and safety of type-II collagen (UC-II), glucosamine and chondroitin in arthritic dogs: pain evaluation by ground force plate. J Anim Physiol Anim Nutr. 2012;96(5):770–7.
25. Peal A, D'Altilio M, Simms C, Alvey M, Gupta RC, Goad JT, Canerdy TD, Bagchi M, Bagchi D. Therapeutic efficacy and safety of undenatured type-II collagen (UC-II) alone or in combination with (–)-hydroxycitric acid and chromemate in arthritic dogs. J Vet Pharmacol Ther. 2007;30(3):275–8.
26. Roush JK, Cross AR, Renberg WC, Dodd CE, Sixby KA, Fritsch DA, Allen TA, Jewell DE, Richardson DC, Leventhal PS, et al. Evaluation of the effects of dietary supplementation with fish oil omega-3 fatty acids on weight bearing in dogs with osteoarthritis. J Am Vet Med Assoc. 2010;236(1):67–73.
27. Roush JK, Dodd CE, Fritsch DA, Allen TA, Jewell DE, Schoenherr WD, Richardson DC, Leventhal PS, Hahn KA. Multicenter veterinary practice assessment of the effects of omega-3 fatty acids on osteoarthritis in dogs. J Am Vet Med Assoc. 2010;236(1):59–66.

28. Gillette RL, Angle TC. Recent developments in canine locomotor analysis: a review. Vet J. 2008;178(2):165–76.
29. Rialland P, Bichot S, Moreau M, Guillot M, Lussier B, Gauvin D, Martel-Pelletier J, Pelletier JP, Troncy E. Clinical validity of outcome pain measures in naturally occurring canine osteoarthritis. BMC Vet Res. 2012;8:162.
30. Hielm-Bjorkman A, Roine J, Elo K, Lappalainen A, Junnila J, Laitinen-Vapaavuori O. An un-commissioned randomized, placebo-controlled double-blind study to test the effect of deep sea fish oil as a pain reliever for dogs suffering from canine OA. BMC Vet Res. 2012;8:157.
31. Rialland P, Bichot S, Lussier B, Moreau M, Beaudry F, del Castillo JR, Gauvin D, Troncy E. Effect of a diet enriched with green-lipped mussel on pain behavior and functioning in dogs with clinical osteoarthritis. Can J Vet Res. 2013;77(1):66–74.
32. Madore E, Huneault L, Moreau M, Dupuis J. Comparison of trot kinetics between dogs with stifle or hip arthrosis. Vet Comp Orthop Traumatol. 2007;20(2):102–7.
33. Hielm-Bjorkman A, Tulamo RM, Salonen H, Raekallio M. Evaluating complementary therapies for canine osteoarthritis part I: green-lipped mussel (Perna canaliculus). Evid Based Complement Alternat Med. 2009;6(3): 365–73.
34. Henrotin Y, Martel-Pelletier J, Msika P, Guillou GB, Deberg M. Usefulness of specific OA biomarkers, Coll2-1 and Coll2-1NO2, in the anterior cruciate ligament OA canine model. Osteoarthr Cartil. 2012;20(7):787–90.

Stunning of common carp: Results from a field and a laboratory study

Karina Retter[1], Karl-Heinz Esser[2], Matthias Lüpke[3], John Hellmann[1,4], Dieter Steinhagen[1*] and Verena Jung-Schroers[1]

Abstract

Background: Common carp *Cyprinus carpio* is an important food fish in Central Europe, which in some regions is consumed as part of local tradition. The majority of carp are sold by small retailers and not processed in commercial processing plants. The overall objective of this study was to monitor how animal welfare is safeguarded during the stunning and slaughtering of carp for retail sale. For this, the stunning and slaughtering process was monitored on 12 carp farms. Four welfare-related parameters were assessed: (i) stunning success, (ii) injuries related to the applied stunning method, (iii) time between stunning and slaughter, and (iv) visible responses of carp during slaughtering. In addition, indicators of physiological stress were measured. In order to analyse whether the absence of behavioural indicators of consciousness after electrical stunning was correlated with unconsciousness a complementary laboratory study was performed. Here, carp were exposed to electrical current densities between 0.09 and 0.41 A/dm^2. The presence of behavioural responses and visually-evoked responses (VER) in the electro-encephalogram in response to light flashes as indicators for an absence of consciousness was recorded.

Results: The carp farms applied manual percussive (18%) or electrical (23%) stunning methods, while the majority of farms used a combination of electrical stunning immediately followed by manual percussive stunning (59%). In the latter condition, 92.6% of stunned carp displayed no behavioural indicators of consciousness and significantly fewer injuries related to mishits compared to sole percussive stunning. In the laboratory study, behavioural indicators of consciousness recovered in carp between 1 and 9 min following removal of the electrical current. However, VER could be recorded already at 30 ± 8 s post stunning. This indicates a fast recovery of carp from electrical stunning when exposed to current densities in the range of those generated by commercially available stunning instruments for fish.

Conclusions: Under field conditions, percussion (applied manually) and electrical stunning might be poor inducers of unconsciousness before slaughter, while a combination was most effective. In order to undertake improvements in electrical stunning, further investigations into the current density, required for inducing prolonged insensibility in carp during electrical stunning, are needed.

Keywords: Carp, Stunning procedures, Animal welfare, Electrical stunning, Visually-evoked responses

Background

The demand for consuming fish is steadily increasing not only because of a growing global population, but also due to consumers preferring fish as a healthy food [1]. The consumers expect high quality fish meat, which is produced with minimal environmental impact, safeguarding animal welfare [2, 3]. Even though farmed fish are often not addressed as animals to care for, but as crops to harvest [4] and the moral status of fish is unresolved, finfish being vertebrates enjoy in Europe the same legal protection as farm animals. Finfish are, for instance, included in the EU Council Regulation (EC 1099/2009) [5] on the protection of animals at the time of killing. This regulation determines that "animals shall be spared any avoidable pain, distress or suffering during their killing ..." (Article 3.1EC No. 1099/2009) [5]. According to this regulation, farm "animals shall only be killed after stunning" and "the loss of consciousness and sensibility shall be maintained until the death of the animal" (Article 4, EC No. 1099/2009) [5]. For farmed fish, the European Food

* Correspondence: dieter.steinhagen@tiho-hannover.de
[1]Fish Disease Research Unit, Institute for Parasitology, University of Veterinary Medicine, Bünteweg 17, D-30559 Hannover, Germany
Full list of author information is available at the end of the article

Safety Authority (EFSA) issued a scientific opinion on welfare aspects of the principal methods for stunning and killing in 2004 [6] and concluded that "many fish killing processes are designed for commercial efficiency rather than welfare priorities." Hence, "many existing commercial killing methods expose fish to substantial suffering over a prolonged period of time" [6]. This report [6] further highlighted that because of large differences in "ecological adaptations and evolutionary developments" between farmed fish species, appropriate methods for stunning and killing must be developed and optimised for each species under consideration [6, 7].

One of the major freshwater fish species farmed in mainland Europe is the common carp (*Cyprinus carpio* L., 1758). Common carp is mainly raised in shallow ponds in monoculture or in polyculture with fish from different cyprinid species, which occupy slightly different ecological niches in the pond system [8]. The common carp is regarded as a domesticated species [9] which is well adapted to the husbandry systems it is reared in [10]. In some regions in Central Europe, the consumption of carp during the "carp season", which lasts from autumn to spring, is part of the local tradition. In these regions, the majority of carp are sold as whole fish on farms, by small retailers, in supermarkets or in restaurants. The majority of fish are killed on demand, only a small proportion of the production is processed in commercial plants [7]. In accordance with EFSA [7], percussion and/ or whole-body electrical stunning in water, followed by evisceration are the main methods used in European carp aquaculture for stunning and killing carp. Percussive stunning is performed for each fish singly with a sharp blow (or some blows) on the head of the carp with a wooden or plastic club ("priest") [11]. In a risk assessment [7], a mishit or a hit with insufficient force, which does not render fish unconscious, resulting in the fish being further processed while still conscious are considered major hazards associated with percussive stunning. An alternative to percussive stunning could be electrical stunning of fish by passing an electrical current through the fish immersed in tank water by submerged electrodes, or by applying the electrical current to the head of the fish outside the water [11]. Hazards related to electrical stunning include the application of currents and voltages, which are insufficient for rendering fish unresponsive to external stimuli (considered as unconscious) instantaneously [7]. This also would result in continuing with the processing of fish despite it still being responsive to external stimuli, i.e., conscious. In a study on the efficiency of electrical stunning, Lambooij et al. [11] observed that carp exposed to an overall current density of 0.14 A/dm^2 for 1 s were stunned immediately. Hence, it was concluded that applying electrical current at this density would result in an effective stunning of carp at marketable size (approx. 1–1.5 kg body weight [11]).

To ensure whether the applied stunning method induces a loss of consciousness, it is necessary to recognise whether the fish is in a stage of insensibility. Consciousness can be assessed by electro-encephalogram (EEG) recordings; in particular, responses to stimuli such as visual evoked-responses (VER) or somato-sensory evoked responses [12]. Such sensory-evoked responses indicate that the brain can support the processing of an external sensory stimulus. If an external stimulus can be processed it can be assumed that the brain is capable of supporting consciousness [12]. Possible brainstem/ behavioural indicators of consciousness like the control of body posture, regular operculum movements or eye roll reflex can be used in some fish species in which the behavioural indicators correlate with neural activity [13]. In carp, the presence of these behavioural/ brain stem responses may be used as evidence for consciousness. Nevertheless, it is questioned whether their absence reliably indicates a loss of sensory perception [7]. EEG recordings, however, are only suitable in laboratory settings and cannot be applied on farms. Therefore, adequate training of operators in recognising behavioural indicators of consciousness for safeguarding humane killing of carp is essential [14].

For the German carp aquaculture, no data are available how animal welfare is safeguarded at the time of stunning and killing of farmed carp. Percussion and whole-body electrical stunning in water are prescribed to be applied to farmed carp as stunning methods by the German Regulations for Animal Welfare during Slaughter (Tierschutz-Schlachtverordnung, TierSchlV [15]). In the current pilot study, we analysed for the first time how the stunning and killing process of carp are implemented on carp farms with regard to the applied stunning method, the stunning success and the occurrence of major hazards. In previous laboratory experiments, we analysed whether the absence of behavioural indicators of consciousness correlated with a loss of neural activity.

Methods

Laboratory study

A laboratory study was conducted to evaluate whether commercially available stunning instruments generate electrical parameters necessary for a successful electrical stunning of carp. A further aim was to analyse whether a loss of behavioural/ brain stem indicators of consciousness, such as control of body posture, operculum movements and eye roll reflex correlate with a loss of VER as evidence of unconsciousness.

Fish and husbandry

Common carp (*Cyprinus carpio L.*; $n = 56$) with size ranging from 28.3 to 37.4 (32.5 ± 2.43) cm and weighing 0.613 to 1.548 (1.085 ± 0.230) kg were collected from a carp farm and kept in groups of two to three individuals in 400 l tanks filled with tap water at ambient temperature for about one week in the laboratory facilities of the Fish Disease Research Unit, University of Veterinary Medicine Hannover, Germany. All animal experiments were performed under approval of the Lower Saxony State Office for Consumer Protection and Food Safety, Germany (LAVES, Oldenburg, Germany) (reference number 09/1714) regarding internationally accepted veterinary standards and federal guidelines.

Position of electrodes

For the monitoring of VER, EEG electrodes had to be positioned intracranially over the *cerebellum* and *tectum opticum*. The recording electrode was situated on the right hemisphere of the *tectum opticum*, the electrodes over the *cerebellum* and the left hemisphere of the *tectum opticum* were used as grounding electrodes and to suppress current artefacts [16, 17]. To determine the exact positioning on the skull of these electrodes, in total, 24 carp specimens were euthanised using buffered MS222 (Pharmaq, UK) at a concentration of 0.5 g/l. Subsequently, these carp were either deep frozen and cut longitudinally intol cm slices or dissected to determine the positions of the *tectum opticum* and *cerebellum* in relation to external features of the head and the variation in these measurements among individuals.

Implantation of the electrodes and recording of visual-evoked responses (VER) of the brain

Prior to implanting the electrodes, the carp were anaesthetized using buffered MS222 at a concentration of 0.15 g/l. For maintenance of narcosis a dosage of 0.075–0.100 g/l buffered MS222 was applied to the gills of the carp in a closed water circuit system. For positioning of the electrodes, the exact locations of *cerebellum* and *tectum opticum* were determined using the measurements from the previously dissected carp. The electrodes were fixed to the skull by means of a bonding agent used in dentistry (GULMA comfort bond, Kulzer, Germany). Briefly, above the positioning locations, the skin was removed from the skull until the cranial bone was dorsally exposed in an area of about 2 × 2 cm. The bone was subsequently treated with 20% phosphoric acid (GLUMA Etch 20-Gel) and with the bonding agent GLUMAComfort Bond (Chemicals from Heraeus Kulzer, Germany), which was polymerised by the light of a polymerization lamp (LITEMA, Germany) in order to prepare the skull area for firm attachment of the electrodes and the filling composite (see below). Then, three holes, each 1.5 mm in diameter were drilled into the cranial bone above the *cerebellum* and the two hemispheres of the *tectum opticum*. EEG electrodes (0.4 mm silver plated copper wire (Conrad, Germany) fixed in a 0.9 × 40 mm cannula (Braun, Germany), which was shortened to 1.5 cm and connected to a shielded copper wire (Conrad, Germany), were inserted through the holes and advanced for approximately 1 to 1.5 cm. Thereafter, the electrodes were fixed by a mix of the bonding agent (GLUMA Comfort Bond) and a filling composite (CHARISMA, Heraeus Kulzer, Germany), which then was polymerised using the polymerisation lamp.

To amplify recorded signals, recording and reference electrodes were connected to a differential amplifier (Differential-Amplifier WPI DAM 50; band-pass filter10 Hz to 3 kHz, 1000-fold amplification, World Precision Instrument, USA). To further eliminate irrelevant interfering signals a downstream bandpass filter (Ithaco 4213 Electronic Filter, Ithaco, USA), was set to the same frequency range. Amplified and filtered signal cycles of 116 ms duration were averaged (512 signals) using a digital oscilloscope (Hitachi Digital VC 7504, Hitachi Europe, Germany) in order to reduce background noise as far as possible and to increase the amplitude of the neural signal. Light stimuli were generated by means of a stroboscope (eurolite Action Strobe 300, Conrad, Germany), which was triggered by a pulse generator (HSE Stimulator P, Harvard Apparatus, UK) to generate light pulses of 1.5 ms. The trigger signal was displayed as a rectangular pulse on the second channel of the oscilloscope for temporal correlation of the VER with the light stimulus. During presentation of light stimuli and recording the room was kept dark.

Whole body electrical stunning

All carp subjected to electrical stunning were individually equipped with EEG electrodes and placed in a U-shaped adjustable PVC grid or a fenestrated aquarium with plastic grids on the sides and internal adjustable separators in order to restrain possible movements of the carp. Then the carp were placed individually in a polyethylene tank equipped with plate electrodes for applying electrical stunning. In all stunning experiments, the conductivity of water was adjusted to 600 µS/cm and the temperature was kept in the range of the water in the holding tank (16.1–22.7 °C). Two different systems were used for applying the current: In one system, stainless-steel plate-electrodes, each having an area of 22 dm^2, were placed at a distance of 31 to 34 cm at the top and the bottom (t/b) of a polyethylene tank with a volume of 117 l and a viewing window at the front side. In this tank, carp were fixed with the fenestrated aquarium. In the second system, stainless-steel plate-electrodes, each 9.45 dm^2, were placed at a distance of 22.0–22.2 cm laterally from the carp in a plastic tank with a volume of 26.7 l. In this tank, the carp were restrained in the flexible U-shaped plastic grid, which was closed at the top and fixed at the upper margin of the tank in order to allow the carp to keep an upright body position.

Prior to applying electrical stunning, carp were monitored for any signs of consciousness, such as maintenance of an upright body posture and regular operculum movements. Then, EEG recordings were taken with and without light stimuli to confirm the correct position of the EEG electrodes and whether recorded signals were indeed visually-evoked responses of the carp's brain (Fig. 1).

Next, the EEG-measuring devices were disconnected from the experimental carp and the plate electrodes were connected to a power supply delivering either a voltage of 50 V (sinusoidal a. c.; constructed by the technical service of LAVES, in order to mimic stunning devices present on carp farms) or 150 V (KT No.8.99, Karl Schermer, Hannover, Germany, modified by the aforementioned technical service for an application on aquaculture farms). Applied voltages and currents were measured with a multimeter (Voltcraft® VC 170, Digital Multimeter, Conrad Electronic, Switzerland) and achieved current densities were calculated by using the following formula:

$$\text{Current density}\left[\frac{\text{A}}{\text{dm}^2}\right] = \text{conductivity of water}\left[\frac{\text{S}}{\text{dm}}\right] * \frac{\text{voltage [V]}}{\text{distance of plate electrodes [dm]}}$$

$$\text{Amperage [A]} = \text{current density}\left[\frac{\text{A}}{\text{dm}^2}\right] * \text{area of aplate electrode}\left[\text{dm}^2\right]$$

An electrical alternating voltage of 50 V and 50 Hz was applied for 5 min (time recommended by the aforementioned technical service) with electrodes placed in lateral positions as well as above and below the fish (bottom/ top position). An electrical alternating voltage of 150 V and 50 Hz was applied in experiments with the same electrode positions for 1 min (time set by the instrument). After stunning, the connection to the EEG-measuring devices was immediately re-installed and EEG responses of carp to light flashes were recorded. Hereby, first VER were registered by30 ± 8 s post stunning. The recordings were then continued until 30 min post stunning. The presence or absence of the behavioural indicators vestibulo-ocular reflex – (VOR), operculum movement– (OM) and righting behaviour – (RB) was recorded for up to 55 min post stun. Furthermore, changes in skin colour were registered after applying the electrical current. All carp were euthanised with buffered MS222 (500 mg/l) after the end of the experiment.

Field study

To monitor the stunning process of carp under field conditions and to evaluate the stunning success of the different methods used, on 12 carp farms located in the German regions of Bavaria, Saxony and Lower Saxony the processes of stunning and slaughtering were analysed during routine marketing operations. On some of the farms, different methods for stunning and slaughtering were used. Therefore, a total of 17 stunning and killing processes were analysed. For each process, the applied stunning method and, in case of electrical stunning, relevant parameters such as electrical current density, conductivity of the water and application time of the electric current were registered. During and directly after the electrical current flow, behavioural responses were noted and after applying the electrical current, the percentage of carp showing behavioural characteristics of consciousness or reflexes was documented. If percussive stunning was used as a stunning method, it was applied to each carp in turn with two quick blows to the skull using a wooden or plastic club. For percussive stunning, the percentage of carp experiencing mishits (the stroke hitting the skull but not in the brain region) and which displayed behavioural indicators of consciousness after the blow was recorded. For both stunning methods, it was noted whether a stunning procedure was re-applied to insufficiently stunned carp. Finally, the time span between stunning and slaughtering of the carp by exsanguination and/or evisceration was noted.

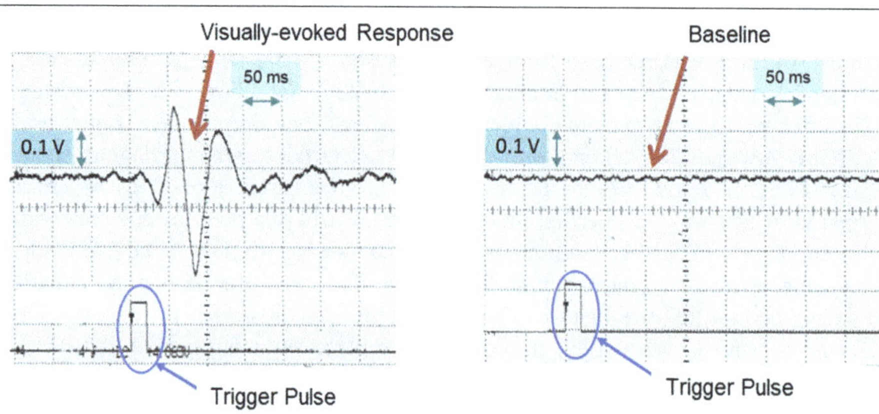

Fig. 1 Averaged visually- evoked response (VER, $n = 512$ signals) in the electro- encephalogram of carp. Left panel: Neuronal responses were triggered by light flashes. The onset of the light flash corresponds to the onset of the trigger pulse. Right panel: Averaged control condition without light stimulus

Furthermore, on each farm, directly after stunning blood samples were collected from the caudal vein of six to ten carp individuals in syringes with lithium-heparinised beads (Sarstedt, Germany) to prevent blood clotting. From the blood samples, the haematocrit was determined immediately using a haematocrit centrifuge. In addition, a part of the blood sample was centrifuged at 600 x *g* at 4 °C for 15 min, the supernatant plasma was collected and transported on ice to the laboratory. There it was frozen at – 80 °C and kept until use for chemical analysis. Blood cortisol levels were measured by solid phase enzyme-linked immunosorbent assay (ELISA, RE52611, IBL International, Germany). Calcium, glucose, lactate, magnesium, potassium, sodium, and total protein, were analysed with an automated blood analyser (ABX Penta 400, Horiba, Kyoto, Japan) as possible stress indicators. The carp were also examined for the occurrence of injuries caused by the stunning procedure.

Statistical analysis

For statistical analysis the computer program SigmaPlot (Systat Software GmbH, Germany) was used. Normality was tested with a *Shapiro Wilk Test* and homoscedasticity by computing a Spearman's rank correlation between the absolute values of the residuals and the observed value of the independent variable at $p < 0.05$. When variances were considered equal and the data were distributed normally, an ANOVA, followed by Tukey's post-hoc test was used to detect statistical differences between groups. When the test for normality failed, the Kruskal Wallis ANOVA on ranks test, followed by Dunn's post hoc test, were used for data analysis. Differences between groups were considered as significant at $p < 0.05$.

Results

Laboratory study

In order to analyse whether electrical parameters generated by commercially available stunning instruments may induce a loss of behavioural indicators of consciousness and whether this was correlated with an unresponsiveness to external stimuli, carp were subjected to electrical stunning parameters from commercially available stunning units under laboratory conditions and VER were recorded thereafter. The applied electrical parameters, the current density and attained field strengths are listed in Table 1.

When the electrical current was applied, carp were motionless, the body muscles were contracted and breathing movements suspended. Immediately after the electrical current was switched off, all carp showed no behavioural indicators of consciousness and weakened muscle contraction. Between 50 s and 10 min after stunning, OM reappeared in 28 out of the 32 stunned specimens. OM reappeared in carp stunned for 5 min at 0.09 A/dm^2 after 2.3–9.0 min (25–50 percentile: 3–8 min, median 6.0 min), and at 0.14 A/dm^2, 5.0–10.0 min (25–50 percentile: 6–8 min, median 6.8 min) post stunning. In carp stunned for 1 min at 0.28 A/dm^2 OM reappeared after 0.8–3.5 (25–50 percentile: 1.0–2.1 min, median 1.6 min) min and at 0.41 A/dm^2 between 1.0 and 7.0 min (25–50 percentile: 1.5–2.6 min, median 2.0 min, see Table 2). The reappearance of OM was followed by a reoccurrence of the VOR as an additional sign of recovery in 28 out of the 32 stunned specimens between 1 and 25 min (see Table 4) and 19 out of 27 individuals tried to right themselves between 4 and 55 min post stunning. Only four of the 32 stunned carp showed no signs of recovery.

Table 1 Electrical stunning of carp: achieved electrical parameters

Voltage, position of the plate electrodes, stunning duration	Current density [A/dm^2]	Electric field strength [V/dm]
50 V, t/b, 5 min	0.09 ± 0.003	15.5 ± 0.39
50 V, lateral, 5 min	0.14 ± 0.00	22.7 ± 0.07
150 V, t/b, 1 min	0.28 ± 0.005	46.9 ± 0.73
150 V, lateral, 1 min	0.41 ± 0.00	68.2 ± 0.00

Conductivity of water: 600 µS/cm; given are mean ± standard deviation
t/b: plate electrodes positioned at top and bottom; lateral: plate electrodes positioned laterally of stunned carp

Visually-evoked responses

Before applying the electrical current all carp specimens responded to light flashes by generating a visually-evoked response in the EEG. About 30 s after stunning (i.e., the time needed for reconnecting the electrodes to the recording system) a VER could be observed in 31 of the 32 carp specimens. Only from one carp, which was stunned at 0.14 A/dm^2 for 5 min, could no VER be recorded after applying the current flow. From all carp, VER were obtained before behavioural characteristics, indicating that a recovery could be observed.

Field study

In the 17 analysed stunning processes, the carp were stunned by percussion in a total of three processes, by electrical-stunning in four processes, and by an initial electrical stunning followed by percussion in ten processes. In ten processes, the carp were electrically stunned in a water bath, in three processes a dry electrical-stunning method was used, and once a combination of dry and water-bath stunning was applied. For electrical-stunning in a water-bath, plate-electrodes were used in six cases, grid electrodes in three cases and bar electrodes in one case. The farmers used commercially available or self-modified stunning devices.

After percussive and electrical stunning, 69.2 and 71.9% of the carp, respectively displayed no behavioural indicators of consciousness (Table 3). When electrical

Table 2 Temporal recurrence of behavioural characteristics in carp after exposure to electrical current

		Current density and stunning duration			
		0.09 A/dm^2	0.14 A/dm^2	0.28 A/dm^2	0.41 A/dm^2
		5 min	5 min	1 min	1 min
VER before	n/total	8/8	8/8	8/8	8/8
VER after	n/total	8/8	7/8	8/8	8/8
Survival	n/total	8/8	4/8	8/8	8/8
OM	n/total	8/8	4/8	8/8	8/8
	min-max (min)	2.25–9	5–10	0.83–3.5	1–7
	median (min)	6	6.75	1.6	2
VOR	n/total	8/8	4/8	8/8	8/8
	min-max (min)	6.5–18	8–25	1–10	4–18
	median (min)	8.75	16.25	3.3	11
RB	n/total	4/4	2/8	7/7	6/8
	min-max (min)	15–25	17–25	4–19.5	14–55
	median (min)	19.5	21	6	27

VER visually evoked responses, *OM* operculum movements, *VOR* vestibulo-ocular reflex, *RB* righting behaviour

stunning followed by percussion was used, 92.6% of the carp did not show any behavioural indicators of conciousness.

After percussive stunning, three out of 13 carp (23.1%) showed injuries in paramedian positions of their heads, resulting from mishits. After electrical stunning, four out of 32 fish (12.5%) received external injuries, for instance, during dry electrical stunning, resulting from contact with the electrodes (Table 3).

An overview of the stunning success, the percentage of carp displaying no behavioural indicators of consciousness post stunning, the percentage of carp receiving injuries from the stunning process, of those showing behavioural indicators of consciousness at the time of slaughter, and the time until exsanguination are presented in Table 3.

During wet electrical stunning, stunning tanks were filled with water at an electrical conductivity between 337 and 1200 μS. The stunning devices generated an electrical voltage between 29 and 54 V, which resulted in an electrical current density of between 0.023 and 0.146 A/dm^2. When considering water conductivity, especially when the conductivity was very low (< 400μS) or very high (> 1000 μS), the percentage of successfully stunned carp was low (50.0%). An overview of water conductivity and electrical parameters achieved during stunning are presented in Table 3.

Most of the carp were killed within 0.5 and 3.0 min after stunning, mainly by evisceration (ten cases), by gill cuts, or destruction of the heart (seven cases).

In order to monitor stress associated with the stunning and killing methods applied on the farms, physiological parameters, including cortisol, glucose, lactate and sodium levels of blood plasma were measured and compared between the applied stunning methods. Mean plasma concentrations of the divalent ions calcium and magnesium ranged between 2.2 and 2.9 mmol l^{-1} (Ca^{2+}) and 1.1 and 1.6 mmol l^{-1}(Mg^{2+}) and did not differ between carp after percussive or electrical stunning. Significant differences between the stunning methods were observed in cortisol, glucose, haematocrit and sodium measurements (Table 4). Mean cortisol measurements ranged between 62.1 and 337.7 ng mL^{-1}and were significantly elevated on farms in which carp were stunned by percussion compared to farms, which used electrical stunning or electrical stunning followed by percussion. Likewise, glucose measurements varied to a large extent, with mean farm levels ranging between 2.7 and 16.6 mmol l^{-1} (Table 4). Plasma glucose levels were significantly lower in carp subjected to electrical stunning compared to carp stunned by percussion, or by electrical stunning followed by percussion (Table 4). Mean plasma sodium levels varied between 115.2 and 151.5 mmol $l^{-1}$with significantly lower values after electrical stunning compared to percussion, or electrical stunning followed by percussion. Haematocrit values ranged between 25.5 and 41.8% and were significantly lower in carp subjected to percussive stunning compared to electrical stunning, or electrical stunning followed by percussion. Mean lactate levels per farm ranged between 1.0 and 41.8 mmol l^{-1}, but did not differ in carp after percussion or electrical stunning (Table 4). A direct correlation between insufficient stunning and high cortisol and glucose levels or decreased sodium and haematocrit measurements (data not shown) could not be detected.

Discussion

The welfare of carp during stunning and slaughtering was considered by EFSA [7] and it was noticed that fewer than 10% of carp for human consumption were processed in commercial processing plants. Instead,

Table 3 Stunning and killing of carp: Overview of applied stunning methods, electrical parameters, stunning success and time

		Electrical parameters				Stunning success	Injuries/ mis-hits	Time until exsanguination	Behavioural signs at time of slaughtering
Stunning procedure no.	Number of fish N total: 113	Water conductivity [µS/cm; MIN-MAX]	Voltage [V; MIN-MAX]	Electrical current densities [A/dm^2; MIN-MAX]	Stunning time (min)	[%; (n/ total number of fish)]	[%; (n/ total number of fish)]	[minutes; minimum - maximum]	[%; (n/total number of fish)]
Stunning by percussion									
1	5	n.a.	n.a.	n.a.	n.a.	80.0 (4/5)	20.0 (1/5)	0.5–2	60.0 (3/5)
2	2	n.a	n.a	n.a	n.a	100.0 (2/2)	100.0 (2/2)	30	0.0 (0/2)
3	6	n.a	n.a	n.a	n.a	50.0 (3/6)	0.0 (0/6)	0.5–1	50.0 (3/6)
Summary Percussion	13	n.a	n.a	n.a	n.a	69.2 (9/13)	23.1 (3/13)	0.5–30	46.2 (6/13)
Electrical stunning									
4	10	453	47	0.0213	6	90.0 (9/10)	0.0 (0/10)	2	90.0 (1/10)
5	6	337	36	0.0267	2	50.0 (3/6)	50.0 (3/6)	2.5	50.0 (3/6)
6	10	n.a. (Dry stunning)	n.a.	n.a	1	80.0 (8/10)	10.0 (1/10)	1	20.0 (2/10)
7	6	398	36	0.0276	1	50.0 (3/6)	0.0 (0/6)	0.5	50.0 (3/6)
Summary Electrical stunning	32	337–1179	36–47	0.0213–0.0276	1–6	71.9 (23/32)	12.5 (4/32)	0.5–2.5	28.1 (9/32)
Electrical stunning followed by percussion									
8	6	1200	33	0.0759	2	50.0 (3/6)	0.0 (0/6)	0.5–2	66.0 (4/6)
9	10	441	54	0.0238	5	100.0 (10/ 10)	20.0 (2/10)	30	0.0 (0/10)
10	10	526	39	0.0409	0.5	100.0 (10/ 10)	20.0 (2/10)	1–3	0.0 (0/10)
11	2	/ (Dry stunning)	/	/	1.5–2	100.0 (2/2)	50.0 (1/2)	1–3	0.0 (0/2)
12	10	587	38	0.0441	0.5	90.0 (9/10)	0.0 (0/10)	0.5–2	10.0 (1/10)
13	6	939	33	0.0808	1	100.0 (6/6)	0.0 (0/6)	0.5–1	16.7 (1/6)
14	6	939	33	0.0808	1	100.0 (6/6)	0.0 (0/6)	2–5	16.7 (1/6)
15	6	939	33	0.0808	1	100.0 (6/6)	0.0 (0/6)	0.5–1	0.0 (0/6)
16	6	822	29	0.1464	2	100.0 (6/6)	0.0 (0/6)	0.5–1	0.0 (0/6)
17	6	/ (Dry stunning)	/	/	1.75	83.3 (5/6)	0.0 (0/6)	2–5	16.7 (1/6)
Summary Electrical stunning followed by percussion	68	441–959	29–54	0.0238–0.1464	0.5–5	92.6 (63/68)	7.4 (5/68)	0.5–30	11.8(8/68)

most carp were processed in supermarkets, by small retailers or on fish farms. Substantive data on the stunning and killing methods used were not available, but in a questionnaire to EU member states percussion and electrical stunning were reported as being most commonly used [7]. Applying percussive or electrical stunning is also stipulated by the German Regulations for Animal Welfare and Slaughter. Therefore, only these methods or a combination of these two were applied on carp farms visited in the present study. The exact procedures for applying these methods, in particular, parameters for electrical stunning are not stipulated and therefore, the practical application of stunning and killing varied on almost every farm.

Every applied stunning method should render carp unresponsive to external stimuli (considered as unconscious) in order to ensure humane killing [7], and the presence of behavioural responses like operculum movements, eye roll

Table 4 Clinical chemical parameters in blood of carp after different stunning methods

Stunning procedure	N [number of fish]	Calcium [mmol/l][c]	Cortisol [ng/mL][c]	Glucose [mmol/l]	Hematocrit [%]	Lactate [mmol/l]	Magnesium [mmol/l]	Potassium [mmol/l]	Sodium [mmol/l]	Total protein [g/l]
Percussive stunning										
1	5	2.5 ± 0.12	246.9 ± 142.25	7.3 ± 2.48	28.5 ± 5.54	4.8 ± 2.58	1.1 ± 0.21	2.5 ± 0.38	133.0 ± 4.38	27.1 ± 1.94
2	2	2.2 ± 0.38	276.5 ± 7.78	16.6 ± 9.26	25.5 ± 3.53	8.7 ± 1.33	1.5 ± 0.21	2.0 ± 1.10	151.5 ± 13.44	50.5 ± 4.95
3	6	2.4 ± 0.10	193.7 ± 54.18	2.7 ± 1.00	26.8 ± 2.92	5.7 ± 1.93	1.3 ± 0.11	2.5 ± 0.12	136.8 ± 3.37	21.5 ± 4.32
Summary Percussion	13	2.4 ± 0.18[a]	228.3 ± 99.94[a]	6.7 ± 5.63[b]	27.4 ± 4.16[a]	5.8 ± 2.44[a]	1.2 ± 0.21[a]	2.5 ± 0.43[a]	137.3 ± 8.08[b]	28.1 ± 10.40[a]
Electrical stunning										
4	10	2.9 ± 0.20	119.6 ± 82.48	2.6 ± 0.78	38.7 ± 8.88	8.9 ± 2.38	1.3 ± 0.27	1.8 ± 0.40	129.6 ± 8.54	29.4 ± 4.88
5	6	2.3 ± 0.30	91.4 ± 32.94	3.9 ± 0.74	31.9 ± 4.34	1.2 ± 0.42	1.3 ± 0.17	2.7 ± 0.46	136.4 ± 17.32	28.9 ± 6.82
6	10	2.3 ± 0.21	62.1 ± 44.71	3.2 ± 2.10	32.5 ± 3.81	3.5 ± 2.36	1.1 ± 0.18	2.1 ± 0.25	117.2 ± 8.77	24.2 ± 6.23
7	6	2.5 ± 0.16	217.8 ± 35.18	3.4 ± 0.90	33.2 ± 3.19	10.2 ± 2.35	1.4 ± 0–18	5.1 ± 0.93	134.2 ± 0.02	24.0 ± 3.85
Summary Electrical stunning	32	2.5 ± 0.32[a]	114.0 ± 76.54[b]	3.2 ± 1.37[a]	34.4 ± 6.32[b]	5.9 ± 4.12[a]	1.2 ± 0.25[a]	2.7 ± 1.28[a]	128.112.68[a]	26.7 ± 5.94[a]
Electrical stunning followed by percussion										
8	6	2.5 ± 0.15	253.0 ± 72.35	6.0 ± 3.02	35.5 ± 4.28	4.1 ± 2.47	1.1 ± 0.16	3.3 ± 0.32	144.8 ± 8.32	35.0 ± 10.29
9	10	2,6 ± 0.19	263.047.89	5.1 ± 1.10	35.3 ± 4.57	9.0 ± 2.00	1.6 ± 0.24	1.9 ± 0.54	147.0 ± 15.91	28.1 ± 5.30
10	10	2,5 ± 0.33	89.7 ± 29.33	3.7 ± 0.96	31.9 ± 5.25	1.7 ± 1.30	1.2 ± 0.27	5.5 ± 8.82	138.1 ± 12.13	23.7 ± 8.15
11	2	2.4 ± 0.03	62.9 ± 22.45	3.9 ± 1.34	29.5 ± 7.78	1.1 ± 0.26	1.3 ± 0.04	2.7 ± 0.24	143.0 ± 4.24	20.5 ± 2.12
12	10	2.2 ± 0.32	71.6 ± 16.23	2.2 ± 0.35	25.6 ± 2.55	1.0 ± 0.43	1.2 ± 0.08	2.6 ± 0.44	131.3 ± 8.89	23.3 ± 2.50
13	6	2.7 ± 0.20	66.6 ± 59.36	4.3 ± 1.81	37.9 ± 6.24	3.8 ± 1.22	1.4 ± 0.12	2.8 ± 0.62	133.8 ± 2.56	24.2 ± 3.43
14	6	2.6 ± 0.10	81.7 ± 43.78	4.2 ± 0.74	40.2 ± 6.11	6.9 ± 1.67	1.5 ± 0.16	2.8 ± 0.61	133.0 ± 6.84	26.7 ± 2.88
15	6	2.8 ± 0.49	337.7 ± 104.13	6.3 ± 2.23	41.8 ± 9.22	2.8 ± 1.09	1.2 ± 0.14	3.6 ± 0.37	115.5 ± 10.82	34.0 ± 4.15
16	6	2.5 ± 0.07	112.2 ± 36.02	4.4 ± 0.37	38.3 ± 6.32	3.5 ± 0.65	1.4 ± 0.09	3.2 ± 0.54	135.8 ± 2.14	28.3 ± 3.83
17	6	2,2 ± 0.18	135.7 ± 47.36	3.7 ± 1.77	35.3 ± 7.34	3.9 ± 1.05	1.1 ± 0.14	2.6 ± 0.16	117.7 ± 9.71	19.8 ± 3.97
Summary Electrical stunning followed by percussion	68	2.5 ± 0.31[a]	151.32 ± 105.96[b]	4.2 ± 1.83[b]	34.7 ± 7.26[b]	3.9 ± 3.00[a]	1.3 ± 0.23[a]	3.1 ± 3.43[b]	134.3 ± 13.66[b]	26.5 ± 6.86[a]

Mean ± standard deviation

Statistical evaluation was performed on measurements from individual fish in order analyse whether stunning success in individual fish had an impact on clinical chemical parameters of the blood

[a] measurements of this parameter are not significantly different between farms

[b] measurements of this parameter are significantly different between farms

[c] Data distributed normally, statistical evaluation by ANOVA followed by Tukey's post hoc test. Other parameter: Data distributed not normally, statistical evaluation by ANOVA on ranks followed by Dunn's post hoc test. Data for a clinical chemical parameter sharing the same superscript letter are not significantly different (total $n = 113$)

or flight reaction upon touching can be used as evidence of consciousness [16].

Electrical stunning is considered as humane because a fish becomes insensible immediately after exposure to an electrical field provided that sufficient current is administered [11]. Rainbow trout remain motionless and apparently insensible for several seconds even after a 1-s exposure to an electrical field of sufficient field strength. This suggests that the onset of insensibility may occur within less than 1 s [18]. The persistence of insensibility after removal of the electrical field increased with increasing exposure duration [13, 18, 19]. However, the exposure to an electrical field of insufficient field strength can cause paralysis without loss of consciousness. In this state, the fish shows no reflexes or behavioural characteristics, but the perception is not totally disrupted [6, 20–22]. Eels subjected to electrical stunning at a voltage of 50 V for a prolonged period of time turned upside down and stopped breathing for a limited period of time when the electrical current was switched off. This was followed by sluggish behaviour [23]. This observation suggests that in this case applying the electrical current resulted in a phase of exhaustion during which the eels seemed to be unconscious and insensible to external stimuli but were not stunned immediately. Hence, this treatment was considered to be painful for the eels [23]. The study on electrical stunning in eels [23] indicated that the absence of behavioural traits and signs of recovery might not be sufficient for an assessment of insensibility in fish. Instead, EEG recordings, in particular the observation of evoked responses, should be applied [6, 20, 22, 23]. This, however, is only applicable under laboratory conditions. Therefore, in the present study, laboratory experiments were performed to confirm whether the absence of behavioural responses of carp would correlate with unresponsiveness to external stimuli, which then could be considered as unconsciousness. Carp were exposed to an electric field generated by commercially available stunning devices and VER of the brain and signs of recovery were recorded after removing the electric field. With a stunning device operating at 50 V, current densities of 0.09 and 0.14 A/dm^2 were achieved and with a device operating at 150 V current densities of 0.28 und 0.41 A/dm^2 were achieved, both at a water conductivity of 600 μS/cm. In all cases, prolonged stunning induced a loss of righting behaviour, OM and VOR, but VERs were present in all carp at the time of recording, i.e., at about 30 s after removing the electric field. In a previous study, epileptiform insults could be recorded in EEGs of carp immediately after electrical stunning with a current density of 0.14 or 0.73 A/dm^2 [11]. In this state, carp were considered to be unconscious and insensible [22, 24, 25]. After applying 0.14 A/dm^2 for 1 s, epileptiform insults could be recorded for 34 ± 10 s. Carp recovered and started responding to painful stimuli 30 s to 10 min after the application [11]. The presence of epileptiform insults in the EEG of carp after stunning suggests that at 0.14 A/dm^2 a stage of insensibility could be induced. In our experiments, EEG electrodes had to be disconnected during exposure of carp to the electric field and were reconnected immediately after the electrical current was switched off. Therefore, the recording of brain activity could only be started about 30 s after stunning. At this time, VER to light stimuli could already be recorded from carp exposed to current densities of 0.14 to 0.41 A/dm^2. In rainbow trout, the duration of insensibility could be extended by increasing the current magnitude or the duration of exposure [13, 18]. In our experiments, the reoccurrence of behavioural indicators of consciousness was influenced by the duration of exposure, but not the recovery of VER. Our findings could be interpreted as follows: Namely, that insensibility, if at all, was induced for a short period of time and the carp recovered at some point within 30 s. The temporary absence of behavioural indicators of consciousness might then have resulted from exhaustion due to a prolonged duration of stunning. Hence, on farms, recognition of unconsciousness is extremely difficult in carp since the absence of the behavioural traits operculum movement or eye roll reflex do not necessarily indicate a loss of consciousness as result of an effective stunning. Nevertheless, if these behavioural traits can be observed in carp after a stunning operation, these carp have certainly not been stunned.

On several farms, where carp were stunned either by percussion or by electrical stunning alone, these behavioural traits were still observed in some individuals after the stunning procedure or even during slaughter, which represents a compromised welfare for the fish. In a risk assessment of stunning methods, EFSA [7] listed mishits at the wrong place or with too little force and subsequent processing of fish still during consciousness as possible hazards during percussive stunning. This could be substantiated by our observations on farms (present study), where about 23% of the carp showed signs of hits at a wrong place on the head and were processed while showing behavioural signs. For electrical stunning, exposure to insufficient current and subsequent processing still during consciousness, were estimated as serious hazards by EFSA experts [7] and could also be confirmed during our field study. In contrast, in the majority of carp stunned by a combination of electrical stunning followed by percussion, behavioural indicators of consciousness were not observed. Nevertheless, in an overall assessment of this method, a relatively high proportion of carp, that of 7.4%, still displayed operculum movements, which have to be interpreted as signs of consciousness. However, in seven out of the ten stunning and killing processes in which this stunning method was applied, behavioural indicators of consciousness were absent in all carp. This underlines the importance of an adequate training of operators in performing the stunning and recognising behavioural indicators of consciousness in order to safeguard humane slaughter of carp.

Plasma electrolytes, cortisol and glucose levels were monitored as possible indicators for stress during the stunning and killing process. In particular, measurements of cortisol, glucose and sodium levels varied to a great extent between individuals processed with a particular stunning and killing procedure. When the different procedures were considered, cortisol levels were higher in carp stunned by percussion, while glucose and sodium levels were lower in carp stunned by electrical stunning. Normal cortisol levels in carp are between 5 and 15 ng/ml [26].

Elevated cortisol and glucose levels were found in carp after a stress event [27]. Therefore, the data presented here might indicate that stunning by percussion could be more stressful for carp. However, the wide variations in these measurements between the assessed individual processes underlines the importance of the pre-slaughter process on animal welfare in addition to the stunning method. The handling of carp before stunning differed greatly on the investigated farms, and most likely, the differences in cortisol, glucose or sodium levels were influenced by hazards related to the pre-slaughter process in addition to the stunning method. This view could be supported by our observation that the increase in cortisol levels was not correlated to lower stunning success on farms.

The technical devices used for electrical stunning on the farms differed widely in design and generated electrical parameters. Most farmers used commercially available stunning devices, which were specified for "stunning of fish". During stunning of carp in a water bath, the achieved current densities varied between 0.016 and 0.146 A/dm^2. In several of the settings the current densities were lower than 0.1 A/dm^2, a current density which was recommended for successful stunning of rainbow trout [13, 17]. At lower current densities, operculum movements recovered in rainbow trout between 30 and 50 s post stunning [18]. On several farms, the interval between stunning and slaughter was longer than 30–50 s, which also could explain why in some carp individuals signs of consciousness could be observed at the time of slaughtering. On the majority of farms, recovery of carp before slaughter was prevented by a combination of electrical stunning and percussion. In addition, on these farms, recovered carp were re-stunned by percussion, which might indicate a high staff awareness of good professional practice in the stunning and slaughtering process.

Conclusion

Our laboratory study showed that after electrical stunning with devices operating at 50 V, carp are unconscious for only a very short period of time (max. 30 s), if at all. Any operculum movement of a carp therefore has to be rated as a sign of perceptiveness. Our field observations indicate that under farm conditions, both percussive and electrical stunning of carp require careful attention. Farmers have to be aware of behavioural signs of consciousness and to re-stun carp by percussion as soon as indicators such as regular operculum movements or the vestibulo-ocular reflex are visible after a stunning method has been applied. As many farmers were aware of this difficulty, an initial electrical stunning and a subsequent re-stunning of carp by percussion were implemented into the work flow on several of the visited farms. With this procedure, the farmers could ensure that carp were not showing behavioural traits of consciousness at the time of slaughter. As even carp showing no signs of behavioural traits might be perceptive shortly after stunning, slaughtering of carp should be performed immediately afterwards.

Conditions for electrical stunning need to be optimised. In particular, investigations into the current density, which is required for inducing insensibility and determining how the period of insensibility could be increased to more than a few seconds, are needed.

Acknowledgements
The stunning devices used during the laboratory study were made available by Dr. D. Kleingeld at LAVES, Lower Saxony. We thank F. Sherwood-Brock for language proofreading.

Funding
The field study was financially supported by the German Federal Ministry of Food and Agriculture (BMEL) through the Federal Office for Agriculture and Food (BLE).

Authors' contributions
VJS and JH planned, conducted and evaluated the field study. DS, KHE and ML planned the laboratory study, KR conducted and evaluated the laboratory study under the supervision of KHE and DS. VJS and DS drafted the manuscript, KR and DS wrote the manuscript. All authors contributed to writing and editing the manuscript and approved the final version.

Consent for publication
Not applicable.

Competing interests
The authors declare that they have no competing interests.

Author details
[1]Fish Disease Research Unit, Institute for Parasitology, University of Veterinary Medicine, Bünteweg 17, D-30559 Hannover, Germany. [2]Institute of Zoology, University of Veterinary Medicine, Bünteweg 17, D-30559 Hannover, Germany. [3]Institute for General Radiology and Medical Physics, University of Veterinary Medicine, Bünteweg 17, D-30559 Hannover, Germany. [4]Landesamt für Natur, Umwelt und Verbraucherschutz Nordrhein-Westfalen (LANUV), Fisheries Ecology, Heinsberger Straße 53, D-57399 Kirchhundem, Albaum, Germany.

References

1. Food and Agricultural Organisation, FAO. The State of World Fisheries and Aquaculture 2010. Rome: Food and agricultural organisation; 2010.
2. Aarest B, Beckmann S, Bigne E, Beveridge M, Bjørndal T, Bunting J, McDonagh P, Mariojouls C, Muir J, Prothero A, Reisch L, Smith A, Tveteras R, Young J. The European consumers' understanding and perception of the organic food regime: the case of aquculture. Br Food J. 2004;106:93–105.
3. Feucht Y, Zander K. Of earth ponds, flow-through and closed recirculation systems – German consumers' understanding of sustainable aquaculture and its communication. Aquaculture. 2015;438:151–8.
4. Lund V, Mejdell CM, Röcklinsberg H, Anthony R, Håstein T. Expanding the moral circle: farmed fish as objects of moral concern. Dis Aquat Org. 2007;75:109–18.
5. Council Regulation (EC) no 1099/2009 of 24 September 2009 on the protection of animals at the time of killing. Off J Eur Union 2009;L 303/1. https://eur-lex.europa.eu/legal-content/EN/TXT/?uri=celex:32009R1099. Accessed July 2017.
6. EFSA. Welfare aspects of the main systems of stunning and killing the main commercial species of animals. EFSA J. 2004;45:1–29.

7. EFSA. Species-specific welfare aspects of the main systems of stunning and killing of farmed carp. EFSA J. 2009;1013:1–37.
8. FAO. Cyprinus carpio. In: Cultured Aquatic Species Information Program, Food and Agriculture Organisation of the United Nations, Fisheries and Aquaculture Department. 2016, Available at: http://www.fao.org/fishery/culturedspecies/Cyprinus_carpio/en. Accessed July 2017.
9. Balon EK. About the oldest domesticates among fishes. J Fish Biol. 2004;65(Suppl A):1–27.
10. EFSA. Animal welfare aspects on husbandry systems for farmed fish: carp. Scientific opinion of the panel on animal health and welfare. EFSA-Journal. 2008;843:1–28.
11. Lambooij E, Pilarczyk M, Bialowas H, Van den Boogaart JGM, Van de Vis JW. Electrical and percussive stunning of the common carp (Cyprinus carpio L.): neurological and behavioural assessment. AgricultEngin. 2007;37:171–9.
12. Van de Vis H, Kestin S, Robb D, Oehlenschlager J, Lambooij B, Munkner W, Kuhlmann H, Kloosterboer K, Tejada M, Huidobro A, Ottera H, Roth B, Sorensen NK, Akse L, Byrne H, Nesvadba P. Is humane slaughter of fish possible for industry? Aquac Res. 2003;34:211–20.
13. Robb DHF, Roth B. Brain activity of Atlantic salmon (Salmo salar) following electrical stunning using various field strengths and pulse durations. Aquaculture. 2003;216:363–9.
14. Ashley PJ. Fish welfare: current issues in aquaculture. Appl AnimBehavSci. 2007;104:199–235.
15. Tierschutzschlachtverordnung, TierSchlV. Verordnung zum Schutz von Tieren im Zusammenhang mit der Schlachtung oder Tötung zur Durchführung der Verordnung (EG) Nr. 1099/2009 des Rates (German regulation for anmal welfare during slaughter). 2012;BGBl 1 S 2982 (in German).
16. Kestin SC, van de Vis JW, Robb DH. Protocol for assessing brain function in fish and the effectiveness of methods used to stun and kill them. Vet Rec. 2002;150:302–7.
17. Reimers U. Untersuchungen zur Elektrobetäubung von Regenbogenforellen (Oncorhynchus mykiss).Dr. med. vet.-Dissertation.2008;Tierärztliche Hochschule Hannover (in German), available at: http://elib.tiho-hannover.de/dissertations/reimersu_ss08.pdf . Accessed 30 May 2017.
18. Lines JA, Robb DH, Kestin SC, Crook SC, Benson T. Electric stunning: a humane slaughter method for trout. Aquacult Engin. 2003;28:141–54.
19. Lambooij E, Pieterse C, Potgieter CM, Snyman JD, Nortje GL. Some neural and behavioural aspects of electrical and mechanical stunning in ostriches. Meat Sci. 1999;52:339–45.
20. Robb DHF. KestinSC.Methods used to kill fish: field observations and literature reviewed. Anim Welf. 2002;11:269–82.
21. Poli BM, Parisi G, Scappini F, Zampacavallo G. Fish welfare and quality as affected by pre-slaughter and slaughter management. Aquacult Int. 2005;13:29–49.
22. Lambooij E, Grimsbo E, Van de Vis JW, Reimert HGM, Nortvedt R, Roth B. Percussion and electrical stunning of Atlantic salmon (Salmo salar) after dewatering and subsequent effect on brain and heart activities. Aquaculture. 2010;300:107–12.
23. Lambooij E, van den Vis JW, Kuhlmann H, Münkner W, Oehlenschläger J, Kloosterboer RJ, Pieterse C. A feasible method for humane slaughter of eel (Anguilla anguilla L.): electrical stunning in fresh water prior to gutting. Aquac Res. 2002;33:643–52.
24. Lopes da Silva FH. The assessment of unconsciousness: general principles and practical aspects. In: Eikelenboom G, editor. Stunning of animals for slaughter. The Hague: Martinus Nijhoff Publisher; 1983. p. 3–12.
25. Roth B, Imsland A, Moeller D, Slinde E. Effect of electric field strength and current duration on stunning and injuries in market-sized Atlantic salmon held in seawater. N Am J Aquacult. 2003;65:8–13.
26. Goos B, Consten D. Stress adaptation, cortisol and pubertal development in the common carp, Cyprinus carpio. Mol Cell Endocrin. 2002;197:105–16.
27. Cowan M, Azpeleta C, Lopez-Olmeda JF. Rhythms in the endocrine system of fish: a review. J Comp Physiol B. 2017;187:1057–89.

22

Diffusion-weighted imaging of the brains of dogs with idiopathic epilepsy

Antje Hartmann[1*], Steffen Sager[2], Klaus Failing[3], Marion Sparenberg[3] and Martin J. Schmidt[2]

Abstract

Background: Idiopathic epilepsy is one of the most common neurological disorders in dogs. Unfortunately, up to 30% of dogs with idiopathic epilepsy show no improvement under antiepileptic drug treatment. Diffusion-weighted imaging is used in human medicine to identify epileptogenic foci in the brain to allow for more invasive treatments such as deep brain stimulation or surgical removal.

The aim of this study was to ass the feasibility of interictal diffusion-weighted MRI in dogs and to evaluate the distribution of diffusion in the brains of dogs with idiopathic epilepsy (IE) and to compare these values to previously published values from healthy beagle dogs.

Client-owned dogs with the final diagnosis of IE were included in this study. MRI examination was carried out using a 1.0Tesla superconductive magnet. Diffusion-weighted images using a single shot echo planar imaging sequence (SSh-EPI) with a b value of $b = 0$ s/mm^2 and $b = 800$ s/mm^2 were acquired in a dorsal and transverse plane with diffusion gradients in all three planes (x-, y- and z-plane). An ADC (apparent diffusion coefficient) map of the isometric image of each acquired slice was generated.

Regions of interest (ROIs) were manually drawn around the caudate nucleus, the thalamus, the piriform lobe including the amygdala, the hippocampus, the semioval center and the temporal cerebral cortex by one of the authors. ROI drawings were repeated 5 times at different time points to assess intra-obersver variability. A multi-way mixed-model analysis of variance (ANOVA) and two-way ANOVA were used during statistical analysis. A p value of $p < 0.05$ was considered significant.

Results: Dogs with IE showed a significantly increased ADC in the amygdala within the piriform lobe and in the semioval center ($p < 0.05$) compared with the healthy control group.

Conclusion: Changes in the piriform lobe in cases of epilepsy are reported infrequently in human and veterinary medicine. Similar to our results, ADC changes in the interictal phase usually include an increase in ADC due to cell loss and increased intercellular spaces. Diffusion MRI might be a promising technique for the examination of canine epileptic patients lacking other gross neuromorphological abnormalities.

Keywords: Magnetic resonance imaging, Canine, MRI, Apparent diffusion coefficient, ADC, Seizure

Background

Idiopathic epilepsy (IE) is considered the most common neurological disorder in dogs, with a reported incidence of 0.5–5% [1–4]. IE is characterized by the presence of recurrent seizures without any underlying clinical disorder causing the seizures; thus, a genetic basis is presumed [1, 5, 6]. Dogs usually exhibit a normal neurological examination in the interictal phase. The diagnosis of IE is based on the exclusion of other diseases [1, 7–9]. The onset of the disease in dogs is usually between 1 and 6 years, but an onset between 6 months and 10 years is possible [1, 8, 9]. Lifelong medication with antiepileptic drugs is necessary, however, treatment failure can occur in up to 30% of dogs [1, 10]. These unresponsive dogs become an increasingly critical issue, and innovative diagnostic and therapeutic strategies will be needed in the future.

Analogous to human patients [11], the concept of an epileptogenic zone has been proposed for dogs as a functional area of the cortex initiating and propagating

* Correspondence: drantjehartmann@gmail.com
[1]Department of Clinical Veterinary Medicine, Vetsuisse Faculty, University of Bern, Länggassstraße 128, 3012 Bern, Switzerland
Full list of author information is available at the end of the article

seizures that cannot be defined by anatomical imaging [12]. Surgical resection or isolation of the brain area that triggers the seizures, e.g., partial or total temporal lobe resection or subpial transection, represent more invasive treatment options in human patients with refractory epilepsy. Such procedures can lead to seizure reduction [13–20]. For temporal lobe epilepsy (TLE) in particular, early surgery for patients with mesial TLE is superior to medical therapy [21]. Epilepsy surgery has also begun to attract veterinary attention [22]. However, surgical techniques require presurgical mapping of the cortex and the exact localization of the epileptogenic zone. In dogs with no gross neuromorphologic abnormality diffusion-weighted imaging might be employed to help visualize patho-physiological processes in the brain parenchyma [23, 24]. Diffusion-weighted imaging (DWI) has been used to detect the epileptogenic zone in human epileptic patients and in animal models of epilepsy [12, 25, 26].

DWI measures the degree of thermal motion of a substance based on Brownian motion within the imaged tissue. In the brain, the movement of water molecules in three compartments contributes to the measured degree of diffusion: intravascular perfusion, extracellular diffusion and intracellular diffusion. Thus, the measured degree of diffusion not only includes diffusion-based motion but also perfusion. In addition, a variety of factors influence the motion of water molecules in tissues. To acknowledge this variation, the term apparent diffusion coefficient (ADC) is used [27–29].

Reduction in diffusion in human patients with temporal lobe epilepsy is described during the ictus and postictally [30], whereas increased diffusion has been described in cases of presumed hippocampal sclerosis [31]. An experimental study of dogs showed an initial decrease (3–6 h) in diffusion after kainic acid-induced complex partial status epilepticus, which was followed by an increase in diffusion after 12 and 24 h and a normalization after 48 h. The authors suggested that diffusion-weighted imaging can be useful to detect the epileptogenic focus or assess potential epileptic brain damage in dogs [25].

The aim of our study was to assess the feasibility of interictal DWI to detect areas with altered diffusion in comparison to healthy control dogs and to analyze the distribution of diffusion in the brain of dogs with idiopathic epilepsy (IE).

Methods

Study design

The study was conducted prospectively. All investigations were performed in strict compliance with the restrictions of the German Animal Protection Law. All dogs were client-owned and lived with their owners. The owners of the dogs gave permission for their animals to be used in this study. Approval from the Committee on the Ethics of Animal Experiments of the Justus-Liebig-University and the local Hessian government was not required as all examinations were performed for diagnostic reasons at the owner's request. All owners were informed that the data of their dogs might be used for this study, which they agreed upon. The MRI protocol was similar to a previous study that was approved by the Committee on the Ethics of Animal Experiments of the Justus-Liebig-University Giessen and local Hessian government (reference number: V54-19c2015(1)GI18/17 Nr. 78/2011) [32].

Study population and MRI examination

During the study period (January 2013 to January 2014), 89 dogs were presented to the neurology unit of the Justus-Liebig-University of Giessen because of seizures. Only dogs with a final diagnosis of IE were included in this study. IE was defined following the proposal of the international veterinary epilepsy task force [9] as recurrent, generalized, tonic-clonic seizures with autonomic clinical signs (salivation, urination) and an impaired state of consciousness during the previous 4 weeks. Dogs showing a single seizure, partial seizures or complex partial seizures were not included. The classification of seizures was performed by video analysis.

Dogs must have been between 1 and 3 years old when the first seizures occurred. The general and neurological examination carried out by a board certified neurologist needed to be normal interictally. Laboratory results (complete blood count, serum chemistry profile and serum ammonia, pre- and postprandial serum bile acids), standard MRI and the CSF analysis needed to be unremarkable. Dogs with a history of dystocia during birth, head trauma and dogs that received antiepileptic drug treatment were excluded from the study.

The anesthetic protocol and MRI system were identical to the settings published for normal dogs using a using a 1.0 Tesla[1] superconductive system and a SENSitivity Encoding (SENSE) coil[2] [32]. The following sequences were acquired: dorsal, sagittal and transverse T2-weighted images (TE: 85 ms; TR: 4000 ms), transverse T2-weighted FLAIR images (TE: 97.5 ms; TR: 3962 ms; TI: 2000 ms), transverse T2*-weighted gradient echo images (TE: 21 ms; TR: 454 ms), transverse T1-weighted images (TE: 15 ms TR: 593 ms) and dorsal 3D T1-weighted gradient echo images (TE: 6.9 ms; TR: 25 ms). T1-weighted images were acquired pre- and post-contrast medium administration. Diffusion-weighted images using a single shot echo planar imaging sequence (SSh-EPI) with a b value of $b = 0\ s/mm^2$ and $b = 800\ s/mm^2$ were acquired in a dorsal and transverse plane with diffusion gradients in all three planes (x-, y- and z-plane) before contrast medium administration identical to the published protocol in normal dogs [32]. The slice orientation was parallel to the base of the skull for dorsal images and perpendicular to it for transverse images. Slices were oriented such that one slice crossed the thickest part of the caudate nucleus.

Further image processing was identical to the published processing in normal dogs. Isometric images including the diffusion effects from all three image planes were automatically generated. Using the integrated software, an ADC (apparent diffusion coefficient) map of each acquired slice was generated [32].

A drawing of the region of interest (ROI) was performed in accordance with a previously published study in healthy dogs. ROIs were manually drawn around the caudate nucleus, the thalamus, the piriform lobe including the amygdala, the hippocampus, the semioval center and the temporal cerebral cortex [32] (Fig. 1). Subjective visibility of the structure on the respective image determined whether a transverse or a dorsal image was used to draw the region of interest (ROI). Most structures were only visible on one slice. If a region was visible on more than one slice, the slice that showed the largest extent of the region was used. Images of the other sequences were available as anatomical references at time of ROI placement. The ROIs were drawn as large as possible while avoiding the inclusion of other structures. The ROI drawings were repeated 5 times at different time points. The integrated software calculated the ADC in $\mu m^2/s$ (= $10^{-6} mm^2/s$) [32]. All ROI drawings were performed by the second author of this study. Time gap between the individual measurements was 3–4 weeks.

Statistical analysis was performed using the software BMDP/Dynamic, Release 8.1 [32, 33]. A two-way analysis of variance (ANOVA) with repeated measures was used to evaluate the effect in diseased versus healthy dogs by comparing the results of this study to values

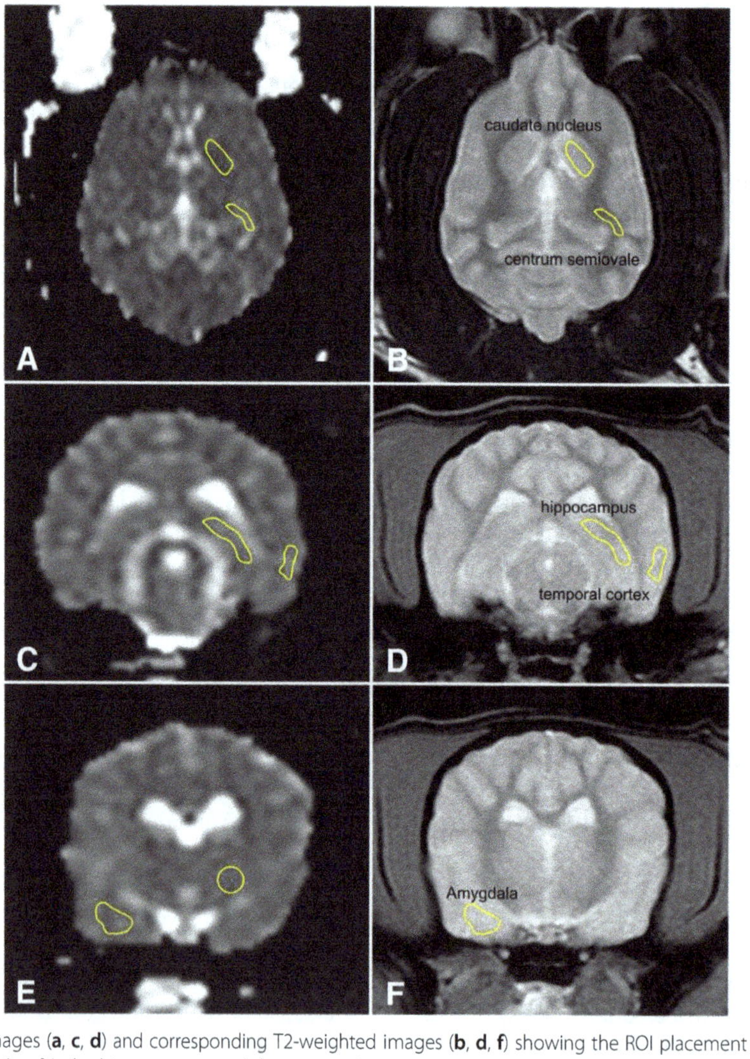

Fig. 1 Diffusion weighted images (**a**, **c**, **d**) and corresponding T2-weighted images (**b**, **d**, **f**) showing the ROI placement around the caudate nucleus and semioval center (**a** + **b**), the hippocampus and the temporal cerebral cortex (**c** + **d**), the amygdala in the piriform lobe and the thalamus (**e** + **f**)

obtained earlier in healthy beagle dogs (program BMDP2V; ANOVA and covariance with repeated measures). The results from the previous study in healthy beagle dogs are already published [32]. The level of significance was $p < 0.05$ for all tests.

For consistency with our first study about brain diffusion in healthy dogs and for being able to better compare possible differences intra-observer variability, the effect of the brain side (right versus left), as well as assessing differences between the different anatomic regions were assessed in addition. The intra-observer variability was evaluated by calculating the mean variation by a multi-way mixed-model analysis of variance with a random observer effect (program BMDP8V). The related coefficient of variation [%] was calculated by dividing this standard deviation by the grand mean multiplied by 100. A two-way analysis of variance (ANOVA) with repeated measures was used to examine the effect of anatomical region and side (left versus right) (program BMDP2V; ANOVA and covariance with repeated measures). A multi-way mixed model analysis of variance (program BMDP8V) was used to determine the region-specific standard deviation with respect to repeated measurements and to perform a region-specific side (left versus right) comparison.

Results

Seventeen dogs met the inclusion criteria. The mean age of the dogs was 3.09 ± 2.35 years. The mean body weight 29.23 ± 8.28 kg (Table 1).

The caudate nucleus had an ADC of 871.47 ± 179.67 $\mu m^2/s$ (mean ± standard deviation (SD)). The ADC of the thalamus was 811.51 ± 175.96 $\mu m^2/s$. The piriform lobe including the amygdala had an ADC of 963.80 ± 174.69 $\mu m^2/s$. The hippocampus had an ADC of 1015.03 ± 231.79 $\mu m^2/s$. The ADC of the semioval center was 790.98 ± 229.63 $\mu m^2/s$. The temporal cerebral cortex had an ADC of 875.65 ± 225.48 $\mu m^2/s$.

Significant differences were found comparing the data from this study to previously published data in normal dogs for the piriform lobe including the amygdala ($p = 0.02$) and the semioval center ($p < 0.01$). Diffusion was increased in the piriform lobe and the semioval centre in diseased dogs compared to normal dogs.

The caudate nucleus and the piriform lobe showed significant differences between the right and left side. With higher values for the left sided structures. However, not all regions showed higher values in the left side. Table 2 gives an overview of the ADC values, including minima, maxima and range for the right and left cerebral hemisphere individually.

The intra-observer variability was slightly higher as for normal dogs (intra-observer variability in normal dogs in general 2% [32]). With an average variation of 2.8% with the greatest degree of variation occurring in the semioval center and the least degree of variation in the piriform lobe.

Discussion

Diffusion changes in epilepsy are well documented in human medicine [34–36] and have also been described in an experimental study of kainic acid-induced complex partial status epilepticus in dogs [25]. In general, a

Table 1 Characteristics of included dogs

Breed	Age in years	Weight in kilograms	Sex	Time between last seizure and MRI in days
Australian Shepherd	8	28	mn	1
Giant Schnauzer	2	35	m	1
Airedale terrier	3	29	mn	1
Border Collie	1	21	m	1
Landseer	2	47.1	w	8
Mixed breed	1	14.2	w	2
Labrador retriever	9	35	mn	1
Entlebucher Mountain Dog	4	38.5	m	2
French bulldog	2	15	mn	2
Labrador retriever	2	26.5	m	4
Mixed breed	1	31.9	w	2
Wirehaired Pointer	4	25	w	9
Mixed breed	2	33	mn	1
Border collie	4	21.7	m	1
Golden retriever	3	32	m	2
Labrador retriever	1	33	w	2
Golden retriever	4	31	m	3

Table 2 ADC values given in μm²/s of the different brain regions listed by side for diseased and healthy dogs

Region	Seite	Mean ADC [μm²/s]		SD ADC [μm²/s]		Min ADC [μm²/s]		Max ADC [μm²/s]	
		diseased	normal	diseased	normal	diseased	normal	diseased	normal
Caudate nucleus	Right	836.44[a]	843.3	172.26	94.3	761.08	751.7	982.58	1089.5
	Left	906.5[a]	962.4	187.08	103.2	827.13	864.4	1140.69	1125.0
Thalamus	Right	819.8	792.2	167.14	31.0	767.29	741.7	893.92	833.2
	Left	803.22	823.4	184.78	30.1	706.33	794.9	868.62	874.8
Piriform lobe[c] (incl. Amygdala)	Right	958.96[b]	895.0	184.23	50.6	856.72	806.0	1086.76	962.5
	Left	968.64[b]	935.9	165.15	37.7	869.62	898.0	1049.03	1008.3
Hippocampus	Right	1027.93	1052.9	230.04	109.7	882.39	902.4	1230.62	1236.3
	Left	1002.14	1035.7	233.54	109.0	880.96	919.5	1138.59	1270.8
Semioval centerΔ	Right	786.36	717.6	241.4	73.8	641.39	597.0	894.95	808.9
	Left	795.59	725.2	217.85	83.0	666.33	609.5	893.94	851.8
Cerebral cortex	Right	866.16	820.2	236.35	71.5	763.57	738.5	975.18	960.6
	Left	885.14	857.1	214.61	63.4	761.81	809.0	1055.38	962.6

Significant differences between the right and left cerebral hemisphere were found for the caudate nucleus ($p < 0.0001$) and the piriform lobe including the amygdala ($p < 0.01$). Significant differences between normal and diseased dogs were found for the piriform lobe including the amygdala and for the seminoval centre. Normal values are from the publication about normal dogs [32]

ADC apparent diffusion coefficient, *Max* maximum ADC, *Min* minimum ADC, *SD* standard deviation; [a] highly significant difference between right and left hemisphere <0.0001; [b]significant difference between right and left hemisphere $p < 0.01$; [c]significant difference between normal and diseased dogs $p = 0.02$; Δ significant difference between normal and diseased dogs $p < 0.01$

transient reduction in diffusion with low ADC values is described. Changes are considered to be the result of cytotoxic or intramyelinic edema [25, 30, 31, 36]. A significant difference was found in the diffusion between normal and idiopathic epileptic dogs in the piriform lobe including the amygdala and the semioval center, with significantly higher ADC values in affected dogs.

The diagnosis of idiopathic epilepsy was made by the exclusion of other diseases based on a normal general and neurological examination and normal blood work, as well as by standard MRI and cerebrospinal fluid analysis. Dogs with a history of dystocia during birth, or head trauma or dogs that had previously received AED where excluded to avoid any effect on our results. The dogs examined were between 1 year and 9 years old. The usual age at which dogs present with idiopathic epilepsy ranges from 1 to 6 years; however, an onset between 6 months and 10 years is possible [1, 8, 9]. In older dogs, cryptogenic epilepsy must be considered as a differential diagnosis for dogs showing epileptic seizures without any other abnormalities. Differentiation between idiopathic and cryptogenic epilepsy is difficult. A focal onset of seizures is considered a sign for the presence of an intracranial lesion, and thus for a cryptogenic epilepsy if no lesion is visible [7, 8, 37, 38]. Dogs in which a focal onset of seizures was described by the owner or was visible on the videotapes were not included in the study population. Additionally, only dogs in which the onset of the disease was between 1 and 3 years were included, making cryptogenic epilepsy unlikely.

In humans, an increase in the mean diffusivity in various brain regions, including white and gray matter, has been described with aging. These changes are thought to be due to Wallerian degeneration leading to gray matter loss and fiber alterations [39, 40]. Studies examining the effect of age on diffusion in the canine brain are lacking. Standard MRIs revealed changes in canine brain morphology similar to findings described for the human aging brain [41, 42]. A histopathological study examining the brains of young (1–5 years) and aged (8–18 years) dogs found changes identical to changes described in the aging human brain [43]. Therefore, it seems reasonable to assume similar changes in brain diffusion in dogs as described for humans.

However, exclusion of the two dogs exceeding the 6 year threshold (96 and 108 months, respectively) did not alter the results of our study, and therefore we decided to keep them in the study population.

As discussed previously for normal patients, the MRI system, vendor, magnetic field strength, coil and b-value can lead to variations in the ADC [32]. However, the settings for this study were identical to the described settings in healthy dogs. Thus, variations due to technical differences in the study design can be excluded as a cause of the differences in the ADC.

Overall a significant increase in diffusion as expressed by a higher ADC in the piriform lobe including the amygdala of diseased dogs (963.80 ± 174.69 μm²/s) compared with healthy dogs (915.44 ± 159.84 μm²/s) was found. Changes due to seizures are usually transient, but experimental data suggest that ADC changes may persist for days [30, 44, 45]. Changes in the piriform lobe and amygdala, which is located within the piriform lobe and is included in the ROI in this region, are only occasionally described in cases of epilepsy. Necrosis of the hippocampus and piriform lobe was described in a series of cats with epileptic seizures identified on post mortem histopathology. Unfortunately, no information about the time interval between the last seizure event and necropsy is provided in this study [46]. An experimental study in rats describes a decrease in the ADC 12 h after seizure induction [47]. After kainic acid-induced complex partial status epilepticus in dogs, an initial decrease in ADC, 3 and 6 h after seizure induction, with normalization after 48 h has been described in the hippocampus and amygdala. Unfortunately, it is unclear if the examinations in this study were performed during the ictus or after the seizures stopped [25]. Decreased diffusion during status epilepticus in various brain regions, including the piriform cortex and amygdala, has also been described by others in experimental studies using rats [48, 49]. Reduction in diffusion in human patients during the ictus and postictally is considered the result of a shift in water from the extracellular to the intracellular compartment, leading to cell swelling, thus reducing diffusion [30, 34, 35, 45, 50].

Interictal normalization of diffusion occurs in most cases [30, 34, 35, 45, 50]. However, some studies have described ADC changes in the hippocampus interictally with an increased ADC on the ictogenic side in human patients. The authors concluded that these changes were due to a loss of structural organization and an expansion of the extracellular space. We can only speculate about the reason for the increase in ADC in the piriform lobe including the amygdala; however, it seems reasonable to assume similar mechanisms as described for the hippocampus, with loss of structural organization and an expansion of the extracellular space.

We also encountered differences in diffusion in the hippocampus, with lower values in diseased dogs (1015.03 ± 231.79 $\mu m^2/s$) compared with healthy dogs (1044.29 ± 165.21 $\mu m^2/s$). However, these differences were not significant.

We can only speculate regarding possible causes of the increased ADC in the semioval center (diseased: 790.98 ± 229.63 $\mu m^2/s$; healthy: 721.39 ± 126.28 $\mu m^2/s$). An increase in the ADC in the subcortical white matter was described in 2/8 human patients, whereas the remaining 6/8 showed a decreased ADC. The reduced ADC was assumed to be the result of a vasogenic edema due to focally increased perfusion and vascular permeability. The authors of that study did not provide an explanation for the increased ADC they found in two patients [51]. Similar to the hippocampus, the semioval center is a small region and its borders could not always be clearly identified; thus, the inclusion of adjacent cerebral cortex might have occurred. The increased ADC values might therefore be due to an increased ADC of the cortex, rather than being related to an increased ADC of the semioval center. A relatively large standard deviation supports this theory. Although not significant, the ADC in the cerebral cortex in diseased dogs (875.65 ± 225.48 $\mu m^2/s$) was higher than in healthy dogs (843.15 ± 98.24 $\mu m^2/s$). The increased ADC of the cerebral cortex is possibly related to what is known as a functional deficit zone in human medicine. The functional deficit zone is defined as an area of the cortex that is functionally abnormal in the interictal period. Proposed mechanisms include a direct destructive effect of the epileptogenic zone on the deficit zone or a functionally mediated process such as abnormal neuronal transmission. However, the exact mechanism is not yet fully understood [52].

Otherwise, the recorded values were similar to those reported in healthy dogs [32]. Lower values were found for the thalamus (811.51 ± 175.96 $\mu m^2/s$), reflecting its white and gray matter composition, and higher values were found for the caudate nucleus (871.47 ± 179.67 $\mu m^2/s$), representing a gray matter structure.

Similar to healthy dogs, we found a significant difference between the right and left cerebral hemisphere in the ADC for the caudate nucleus and the piriform lobe including the amygdala. However, we did not encounter any tendency of a consistently higher diffusion value in one cerebral hemisphere in contrast to healthy dogs [32]. This finding might be due to differences in sex distribution in our study population of 12 males and 5 females in contrast to only 2 males and 8 females in the study of healthy dogs, leading to obfuscation of related differences.

The limitations of this study include the small study population, such that type 2 error cannot be excluded. Applying less strict inclusion criteria might have allowed for a larger study population. However, unacceptable bias would have occurred if the difference in case numbers between the study population (diseased dogs) and the control group of healthy dogs were larger. Another limitation is the heterogeneity of the study population with respect to age, breed and sex in comparison to the homogenous control group consisting only of Beagle dogs of similar age and body weight. In addition we cannot prove if changes are consequence or cause of epilepsy in this dogs.

Conclusion

In summary, we found a significant increase in the ADC in the piriform lobe including the amygdala and the semioval center in dogs with IE compared with healthy dogs. One possible explanation for the increased ADC in the piriform lobe including the amygdala might be the loss of structural organization and an expansion of the extracellular space. The increased ADC in the semioval center might be related to the inclusion of part of the cerebral cortex in the ROI and a functional deficit zone. Despite the fact, that the encountered differences should be interpreted with caution interictal DWI seems to be a promising technique for the examination of canine epileptic patients lacking other gross neuromorphological abnormalities.

Endnotes

[1]Philips Intera Gyroscan, Philips Healthcare, Hamburg, Germany

[2]SENSE-flex M coil, Philips Healthcare, Hamburg, Germany

Abbreviations

ADC: Apparent diffusion coefficient; ANOVA: Analysis of variance; DWI: Diffusion weighted MRI; IE: Idiopathic epilepsy; kg: Kilogram; Max: Maximum; Min: Minimum; MRI: Magnetic resonance imaging; ROI: Region of interest; S: Second; SD : Standard deviation; μm2: Micrometer squared

Acknowledgments

The technical assistance of Ella Wenz is gratefully acknowledged. The work was performed at the Department of Veterinary Clinical Sciences, Clinic for Small Animals, Justus-Liebig-University Giessen, Germany.

Funding

No funding was received for this study.

Authors' contributions

AH, SS and MJS contributed to the development and writing of the paper. AH and SS performed the MRI examination and the measurements in all dogs. KF and MS performed the statistical analysis. All authors read and critically revised and approved the final manuscript.

Consent for publication

Not applicable.

Competing interests

The authors declare that they have no competing interests.

Author details

[1]Department of Clinical Veterinary Medicine, Vetsuisse Faculty, University of Bern, Länggassstraße 128, 3012 Bern, Switzerland. [2]Department of Veterinary Clinical Sciences, Small Animal Clinic, Justus-Liebig-University Giessen, Frankfurter Straße 108, 35392 Giessen, Germany. [3]Unit for Biomathematics and Data Processing Faculty of Veterinary Medicine Justus Liebig-University, Frankfurter Straße 95, 35392 Giessen, Germany.

References

1. Thomas WB. Idiopathic epilepsy in dogs and cats. Vet Clin North Am Small Anim Pract. 2010;40:161–79.
2. Löscher W. Animal models of intractable epilepsy. Prog Neurobiol. 1997;53:239–58.
3. Bellumori TP, Famula TR, Bannasch DL, Belanger JM, Oberbauer AM. Prevalence of inherited disorders among mixed-breed and purebred dogs: 27,254 cases (1995-2010). J Am Vet Med Assoc. 2013;242:1549–55.
4. Kearsley-Fleet L, O'Neill DG, Volk HA, Church DB, Brodbelt DC. Prevalence and risk factors for canine epilepsy of unknown origin in the UK. Vet Rec. 2013;172:338.
5. Potschka H, Fischer A, Löscher W, Patterson N, Bhatti S, Berendt M, De Risio L, Farquhar R, Long S, Mandigers P, Matiasek K, Muñana K, Pakozdy A, Penderis J, Platt S, Podell M, Rusbridge C, Stein V, Tipold A, Volk HA. International veterinary epilepsy task force consensus proposal: outcome of therapeutic interventions in canine and feline epilepsy. BMC Vet Res. 2015;11:177.
6. Hülsmeyer V-I, Fischer A, Mandigers PJJ, DeRisio L, Berendt M, Rusbridge C, Bhatti SFM, Pakozdy A, Patterson EE, Platt S, Packer RMA, Volk HA. International veterinary epilepsy task Force's current understanding of idiopathic epilepsy of genetic or suspected genetic origin in purebred dogs. BMC Vet Res. 2015;11:175.
7. Podell M, Fenner W, Powers J. Seizure classification in dogs from a nonreferral-based population. J Am Vet Med Assoc. 1995;216:1721–8.
8. Chandler K. Canine epilepsy : what can we learn from human seizure disorders ? Vet J. 2006;172:207–17.
9. De Risio L. International veterinary epilepsy task force consensus proposal: diagnostic approach to epilepsy in dogs. BMC Vet Res. 2015;11:148.
10. Buckmaster PS, Smith MO, Buckmaster CL, LeCouteur RA, Dudek FE. Absence of temporal lobe epilepsy pathology in dogs with medically intractable epilepsy. J Vet Intern Med. 2002;16:95–9.
11. Lüders HO, Najm I, Nair D, Widdess-Walsh P, Bingman W. The epileptogenic zone: general principles. Epileptic Disord. 2006;8(Suppl2):S1–9.
12. Hasegawa D. Pathophysiological and presurgical analysis of epilepsy in dogs and cats. Vet J. 2016;215:64–74.
13. Loddenkemper T, Pan A, Neme S, Baker KB, Rezai AR, Dinner DS, Montgomery EB Jr, Luders HO. Deep brain stimulation in epilepsy. JClinNeurophysiol. 2001;18:514–32.
14. Andrade DM, Zumsteg D, Hamani C, Hodaie M, Sarkissian S, Lozano AM, Wennberg RA. Long-term follow-up of patients with thalamic deep brain stimulation for epilepsy. Neurology. 2006;66:1571–3.
15. Boon P, Vonck K, De Herdt V, Van Dycke A, Goethals M, Goossens L, Van Zandijcke M, De Smedt T, Dewaele I, Achten R, Wadman W, Dewaele F, Caemaert J, Van Roost D. Deep brain stimulation in patients with refractory temporal lobe epilepsy. Epilepsia. 2007;48:1551–60.
16. Fregni F, Pascual-Leone A. Technology insight: noninvasive brain stimulation in neurology-perspectives on the therapeutic potential of rTMS and tDCS. Nat Clin Pract Neurol. 2007;3:383–93.
17. RH W, Bruening R, Noachtar S, Arnold S, Berchtenbreiter C, Bartenstein P, Drzezga A, Tatsch K, Reiser M. MR measurement of regional relative cerebral blood volume in epilepsy. J Magn Reson Imaging. 1999;9:435–40.
18. Pendse N, Wissmeyer M, Altrichter S, Vargas M, Delavelle J, Viallon M, Federspiel A, Seeck M, Schaller K, Lövblad KO. Interictal arterial spin-labeling MRI perfusion in intractable epilepsy. J Neuroradiol. 2010;37:60–3.
19. Wolf RL, Alsop DC, Levy-Reis I, Meyer PT, Maldjian JA, Gonzalez-Atavales J, French JA, Alavi A, Detre JA. Detection of mesial temporal lobe hypoperfusion in patients with temporal lobe epilepsy by use of arterial spin labeled perfusion MR imaging. Am J Neuroradiol. 2001;22:1334–41.
20. Spencer SS, Schramm J, Wyler A, O'Connor M, Orbach D, Krauss G, Sperling M, Devinsky O, Elger C, Lesser R, Mulligan L, Westerveld M. Multiple subpial transection for intractable partial epilepsy: an international meta-analysis. Epilepsia. 2002;43:141–5.
21. Engel J, McDermott M, Wiebe S, Langfitt JT, Stern JM, Dewar S. Early surgical therapy for drug- resistant temporal lobe epilepsy. J Am Vet Med Assoc. 2012;307(09):922–30.
22. Martle V, Van Ham L, Raedt R, Vonck K, Boon P, Bhatti S. Non-pharmacological treatment options for refractory epilepsy: an overview of human treatment modalities and their potential utility in dogs. Vet J. 2014;199:332–9.
23. Weishaupt D, Köchli VD, Marincek B. Wie Funktioniert MRI?: Eine Einführung in Physik Und Funktionsweise Der Magnetresonanzbildgebung. 6th ed. Heidelberg: Springer; 2009.
24. Westbrook C, Rot CK, Talbot J. MRI in practice. 4th ed. Chichester: Wiley-Blackwell; 2011.
25. Hasegawa D, Orima H, Fujita M, Nakamura S. Diffusion-weighted imaging in kainic acid-induced complex partial status epilepticus in dogs. Brain Res. 2003;983:115–27.
26. Yogarajah M, Duncan JS. Diffusion-based magnetic resonance imaging and tractography in epilepsy. Epilepsia. 2008;49:189–200.

27. Clark CA, Barker GJ, Tofts PS. An in vivo evaluation of the effects of local magnetic susceptibility-induced gradients on water diffusion measurements in human brain. J Magn Reson. 1999;141:52–61.
28. Niendorf T. Methodische Grundlagen moderner Magnet-Resonanz-Bildgebungsverfahren und ihre Anwendung in der Neurologie. Klin Neurophysiol. 2000;31:2–17.
29. Neil JJ. Diffusion imaging concepts for clinicians. J Magn Reson Imaging. 2008;27:1–7.
30. Diehl B, Najm I, Ruggieri P, Tkach J, Mohamed A, Morris H, Wyllie E, Fisher E, Duda J, Lieber M, Bingaman W, HO L. Postictal diffusion-weighted imaging for the localization of focal epileptic areas in temporal lobe epilepsy. Epilepsia. 2001;42:21–8.
31. Wieshmann UC, Clark CA, Symms MR, Barker GJ, Birnie KD, Shorvon SD. Water diffusion in the human hippocampus in epilepsy. Magn Reson Imaging. 1999;17:29–36.
32. Hartmann A, Söffler C, Failing K, Schaubmar A, Kramer M, Schmidt MJ. Diffusion-weighted magnetic resonance imaging of the normal canine brain. Vet Radiol Ultrasound. 2014;55:592–8.
33. Dixon W. BMDP statistical software manual, volume 1 and 2. Berkeley, Los Angeles, London: University of California Press; 1993.
34. Wieshmann UC, Symms MR, Bartlett PA, Shorvon SD, Clark CA, Barker GJ. Diffusion weighted MRI demonstrates abnormal pyramidal tract in hemiparesis. J Neurosurg Psychiatry. 1999;66:797–8.
35. Szabo K, Poepel A, Pohlmann-Eden B, Hirsch J, Back T, Sedlaczek O, Hennerici M, Gass A. Diffusion-weighted and perfusion MRI demonstrates parenchymal changes in complex partial status epilepticus. Brain. 2005; 128(Pt 6):1369–76.
36. Oster J, Doherty C, Grant PE, Simon M, Cole AJ. Diffusion-weighted imaging abnormalities in the Splenium after seizures. Epilepsia. 2003;44:852–854.
37. Berendt M, Gram L. Epilepsy and seizure classification in 63 dogs: a reappraisal of veterinary epilepsy terminology. J Vet Intern Med. 1999;13:14–20.
38. Jaggy A, Bernardini M. Idiopathic epilepsy in 125 dogs: a long-term study. Clinical and electroencephalographic findings. J Small Anim Pract. 1998;39:23–9.
39. Hsu J, Leemans A, Bai C, Lee C, Tsai Y, Chiu H, Chen W. Gender differences and age-related white matter changes of the human brain : a diffusion tensor imaging study. NeuroImage. 2008;39:566–77.
40. Pfefferbaum A, Adalsteinsson E, Rohlfing T, Sullivan EV. Diffusion tensor imaging of deep gray matter brain structures : effects of age and iron concentration. Neurobiol Aging. 2010;31:482–93.
41. Su M, Tapp PD, Vu L, Chen Y, Chu Y. A longitudinal study of brain morphometrics using serial magnetic resonance imaging analysis in a canine model of aging. Prog Neuro-Psychopharmacology Biol. 2005;29:389–97.
42. Kimotsuki T, Nagaoka T, Yasuda M, Tamahara S, Matsuki N. Changes of magnetic resonance imaging on the brain in beagle dogs with aging. J Vet Med Sci. 2005;67:961–7.
43. Borras D, Ferrer I, Pumarola M. Age-related changes in the brain of the dog. Vet Pathol. 1999;36:202–11.
44. Szabo K, Poepel A, Pohlmann-Eden B, Hirsch J, Back T, Sedlaczek O, Hennerici M, Gass A. Diffusion-weighted and perfusion MRI demonstrates parenchymal changes in complex partial status epilepticus. Brain. 2005;128:1369–76.
45. Konermann S, Marks S, Ludwig T, Weber J, de Greiff A, Dörfler A, Leonhardt G, Wiedemayer H, Diener H-C, Hufnagel A. Presurgical evaluation of epilepsy by brain diffusion: MR-detected effects of flumazenil on the epileptogenic focus. Epilepsia. 2003;44:399–407.
46. Fatzer R, Gandini G, Jaggy A, Doherr M, Vandevelde M, Data E. Necrosis of hippocampus and Piriform lobe in 38 domestic cats with seizures: a retrospective study on clinical and pathologic findings. J Vet Intern Med. 2000;14:100–4.
47. Wall CJ, Kendall EJ, Obenaus A. Rapid alterations in diffusion-weighted images with anatomic correlates in a rodent model of status Epilepticus. Am J Neuroradiol. 2000;21:1841–52.
48. Zhong J, Petroff AC, Prichard JW, Gore JC. Changes in water diffusion and relaxation properties of rat cerebrum during status Epilepticus. Magn Reson Med. 1993;30:241–6.
49. Nakasu Y, Nakasu S, Kizuki H, Uemura S, Morikawa S, Inubushi T, Handa J. Changes in water diffusion of rat limbic system during status epilepticus elicited by kainate. Psychiatry Clin Neurosci. 1995;49:S228–30.
50. Nairism J, Kettunen MI, Nissinen J, Kauppinen RA, Pitk A. Progression of brain damage after status Epilepticus and its association with Epileptogenesis : a quantitative MRI study in a rat model of temporal lobe epilepsy. Epilepsia. 2004;45:1024–34.
51. Kim J, Chung J II, Yoon PH, Kim DI, Chung T, Kim E, Jeong E. Transient MR signal changes in patients with generalized Tonicoclonic seizure or status Epilepticus: Periictal diffusion-weighted imaging. Am J Neuroradiol. 2001; 22:1149–60.
52. Rosenow F, Lüders H. Presurgical evaluation of epilepsy. Brain. 2001;124(Pt 9): 1683–700.

Risk factors of brucellosis seropositivity in Bactrian camels of Mongolia

Chimedtseren Bayasgalan[1,3,4*], Tungalag Chultemdorj[1], Felix Roth[2], Jakob Zinsstag[3,4], Jan Hattendorf[3,4], Battsetseg Badmaa[1], Bayanzul Argamjav[1] and Esther Schelling[3,4]

Abstract

Background: More information on brucellosis epidemiology in Bactrian camels is needed due to their growing economic and livelihood importance for herders and renewed efforts in Mongolia to eliminate brucellosis through mass vaccination of ruminants excluding camels. Brucellosis prevalence in camels increased over the past two decades. Random multi-stage cluster surveys were done in the Eastern provinces of Dornod and Sukhbaatar in 2013 and 2014 and in the Southern & Western provinces of Dornogobi, Umnogobi and Khovd in 2014 and 2015. A total of 1822 camels, 1155 cattle, and 3023 small ruminant sera were collected and tested with the Rose Bengal Test. In addition, 195 vaginal swabs and 250 milk samples for bacteriological culture were taken from livestock with history of abortion.

Results: The overall apparent seroprevalence in camels was 2.3% (95% confidence interval 1.6–3.3). The main risk factor for camel seropositivity was being in an Eastern province when compared to Southern & Western provinces (odds ratio 13.2, 95% CI 5.3–32.4). Camel seroprevalences were stable over the two consecutive survey years, despite introduction of ruminant vaccination: 5.7% (95% CI 3.1–10.2%) and 5.8% (3.3–10.1%) in Eastern provinces and 0.4% (0.2–1.2%) and 0.5% (0.1–2.0%) in Southern & Western provinces. We isolated *Brucella abortus* from camels and cattle. Camel seropositivity was associated to keeping cattle together with camels. Monitoring of vaccination campaigns showed that coverage in cattle was insufficient because animals could not be adequately restrained.

Conclusions: The present study reveals that brucellosis is present with important seroprevalence in Mongolian camels and was endemic in Eastern provinces. Camel herd seropositivity was most closely associated to infection in cattle.

Longer term monitoring is needed to assess whether camel seroprevalance decreases with ongoing vaccination in Mongolia. This should be coupled with further confirmation on *Brucella* spp. isolates. To date, only *Brucella abortus* was isolated, but camels are also susceptible to *Brucella melitensis*. Clear verbal and written information on disease prevention in livestock and household members is important, particularly for remote camel herders who had only moderate knowledge on brucellosis epidemiology and preventive measures.

Keywords: Bactrian camel, Brucellosis, Epidemiology, Mongolia, Seroprevalence, *Brucella* spp., Risk factors

Background

The Bactrian camel (two humped) and the dromedary (one humped Arabian camel) represent the old-world domesticated camel species and are closely related [1, 2]. The Bactrian camel inhabits cold deserts in the southern areas of Russia, Mongolia, East-Central Asia and China [3].

Camel husbandry in Mongolia is practiced primarily by pastoralists in the Gobi Desert. Camels produce milk, wool and meat and are also used for racing and, less commonly now, for transportation of people and goods. In 2014, it was estimated that there were 367,900 camels in Mongolia [4]. The camel population resides in close contact with cattle, sheep, goats and occasionally horses, particularly at watering places (wells, branch-water, ditch-water, rivers, and lakes) and during calving and

* Correspondence: chimee_vet@muls.edu.mn
[1]School of Veterinary Medicine, Mongolian University of Life Sciences, PO Box 17024, Zaisan, Ulaanbaatar, Mongolia
[3]Swiss Tropical and Public Health Institute, PO Box, CH-4002 Basel, Switzerland
Full list of author information is available at the end of the article

wool shearing periods. Camels, unlike other domestic large animals, often travel up to 16 km daily in search of food [5]. They are less susceptible to some highly contagious livestock diseases, such as foot-and-mouth disease [6].

Brucellosis is a zoonosis caused by the intracellular, Gram negative bacteria of the genus *Brucella*. Sheep and goats are the main hosts for *Brucella melitensis*, while cattle are the main host for *Brucella abortus* and pigs are the main host for *Brucella suis*. These three species cause the majority of the disease burden in animals and are also the most important *Brucella* pathogens in people. However, other species (e.g. *Brucella canis*) are also potentially infectious to humans [7, 8].

Brucellosis is thought to be the most economically important zoonosis worldwide because it is endemic in many countries and impacts both human and livestock health [9–11]. Brucellosis is transmitted from animals to people often through consumption of unpasteurized milk and dairy products [12–15], but direct contact, particularly with livestock abortion material, is more important among livestock-keeping communities. The disease is rarely fatal in people but causes high morbidity in both animals and humans [16, 17].

Camels are susceptible to both *B. abortus* and *B. melitensis* [18–20]; however, camels are considered to be secondary hosts of *Brucella* spp. [3, 14]. Brucellosis was reported in camels as early as in 1931 by Solonitsiun in Russia [18, 21]. Since then, serological evidence of brucellosis has been reported from the most important camel-keeping countries [3, 18, 21–23]. Camels infected with brucellosis show fewer clinical signs than other livestock species, in particular less than domesticated cattle, sheep and goats [24]. This may be a reason why little information is available on epidemiology of brucellosis in camels and its impact on human health, notably in Mongolia [3, 25].

Brucellosis serological tests have rarely been validated for camels. Empirically, the Rose Bengal test is commonly used for diagnosis in camels and seems to give accurate results [24, 26].

Camels were included in mass screening surveys in Mongolia, but risk factors for exposure were not further evaluated. A screening survey in 2011 [27], which sampled between 6 and 3590 camel sera from each of the 22 Mongolian provinces, found a moderate correlation (Spearman's rho = 0.26) between camel and cattle brucellosis seropositivity at district level; however, sheep were very weakly correlated while goats were not at all correlated (unpublished data). There is almost no information on which *Brucella* spp. cause seropositivity in Mongolian camels due to a lack of strain isolation and characterization. Past and current mass livestock vaccination campaigns in Mongolia did not include camels or horses. Older reports from veterinary laboratories indicated that the serological prevalence of brucellosis in camels in different Mongolian localities was increasing [28]. Notably, in 2010 a 3% seroprevalence in camels was found in a population-based survey in Sukhbaatar province [29].

Camels may be a reservoir for *Brucella* spp., and other livestock are at risk for reinfection when vaccination campaigns are discontinued because they are kept together. However, effective control of brucellosis could be achieved by establishing diagnostic and surveillance systems, by estimating the cost-benefits of control measures to guide policy makers, by rigorously implementing control programs, and by policies to connect human health and veterinary services at demographic, socioeconomic and political levels. Ruminant (Bovidae) mass vaccination was estimated to be highly cost effective for Mongolia [30]. In a mobile context, test and slaughter is hardly feasible. Instead, vaccination of cattle and small ruminants over several years is the viable control measure for mobile livestock husbandry systems, where there is also no feasible individual animal tracking system. The required vaccination coverage to interrupt transmission, in cattle (minimum 60% truly immunized animals) and in small ruminants (minimum 40%), must be monitored [31]. Post-vaccination campaign monitoring in cattle and small ruminants is now undertaken. However, the role of Bactrian camels in brucellosis epidemiology must be more clearly understood for successful elimination efforts in Mongolia, in particular, the ability of camels to maintain an own infection cycle and reintroduce brucellosis to domesticated Bovidae.

The objectives of this study were to contribute to understanding the epidemiology of camel brucellosis in Mongolia and to identify the *Brucella* species involved before and after implementation of vaccination campaigns in cattle and small ruminants. We tested the hypotheses that the seroprevalence of camel brucellosis is below 5% in Mongolia and the most important risk factor of camel seropositivity was herding together with cattle.

Results

A total of 6000 serum samples (1822 camels, 1155 cattle, 1531 sheep, 1492 goats) were collected from 365 herds in five provinces over 3 years. In addition, 195 vaginal swabs (72 from camels, 51 from cattle, 29 from sheep, 43 from goats) and 250 milk samples (104 from camels, 68 from cattle, 46 from sheep, 32 from goats) were collected for bacteriological culture. In total, 310 out of the 365 herds sampled completed a questionnaire during the study, with 240 being completed at the first visit of a herd.

No camels were sampled in 9 herds, so the total camel herds was 356 (Table 1). The selected districts within

Table 1 Distribution of the 356 camel herds sampled in 5 provinces over 3 years of sampling. In a second year the number of re-sampled herds and (+) the number of newly sampled herds is shown

	Year 1 (2013)	Year 2 (2014)	Year 3 (2015)
Dornod	32	24 + 8	
Sukhbaatar	37	34 + 4	
Dornogobi		36	22 + 14
Umnogobi		37	24 + 12
Khovd		36	19 + 17

the 5 provinces and the sites of sampling for the first and second years are depicted in Figs. 1 and 2.

A total of 1822 camel sera were tested, of which 17, 10 and 10 sera showed +, ++ and +++ postive agglutination, respectively. The 37 seropositive camels were in 29 of the 356 camel herds, and in herds with more than one positive camel different strengths of agglutination were seen. The overall apparent brucellosis seroprevalence in camels was 2.3% (95% CI 1.6–3.3). The estimated true seroprevalence was 1.8%. About one fifth of the camel sera collected originated from male animals. The majority of camels sampled were adults (13.9% young vs. 86.1% of adult camels), and seroprevalences were comparable across age groups (Table 2).

Camel brucellosis seropositivity was highest in Sukhbaatar (6.1%, 95% CI 3.5–10.1%) followed by Dornod (5.3%, 2.9.-9.6%), Dornogobi (0.8%, 0.3–2.3%), Umnogobi (0.4%, 0.1–1.4%), and Khovd (0.3%, 0.04–1.9%). The camel seroprevalences remained steady between the first and second years of sampling with 5.7% (95% CI 3.1–10.2%), and 5.8% (95% CI 3.3–10.1%) in Eastern provinces, and, at much lower levels, in the Southern & Western provinces with 0.4% (0.2–1.2%) in 2014 and 0.5% (0.1–2.0%) in 2015 (Table 2).

Regarding risk factors, camel age and sex were not significantly associated with seropositivity. The Eastern provinces had significantly higher seropositive proportions than the Southern & Western provinces (Table 3). Keeping camels together with cattle was significantly associated to brucellosis seropositivity in camels, whereas the presence of small ruminants was not. Out of all camels sampled, 86.9%, 93.1%, and 94.4% were kept together with cattle, sheep and goats, respectively (Table 3).

We found no association between camel seropositivity and history of abortion or preventive biosafety measures such as destroying abortion material (Table 3). None of the biosafety measure (e.g., buying of live animals, safely disposing of abortion material) question outcomes were associated with seropositivity in camels, nor was the variable with distances of camel herds to the closest district centre (mean distance was 55 km).

Owners of seropositive camels had significantly more sources of information on brucellosis, indicating that

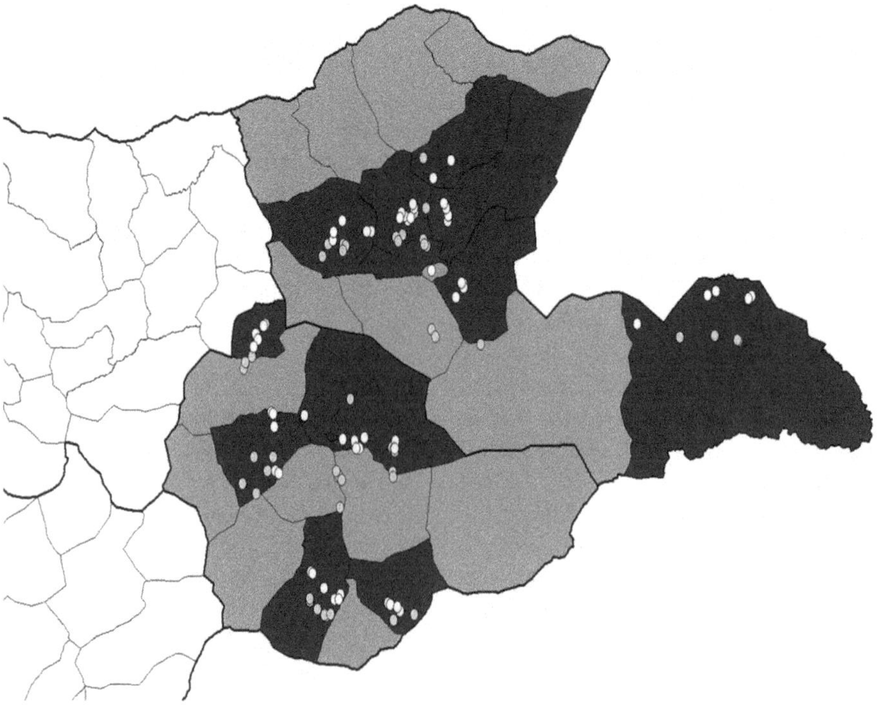

Fig. 1 Map of Eastern provinces Dornod and Sukhbaatar (shaded in grey) and showing the selected districts (in black). The location of camel herds at time of sampling in 2013 (white dots) and 2014 (grey dots) are shown

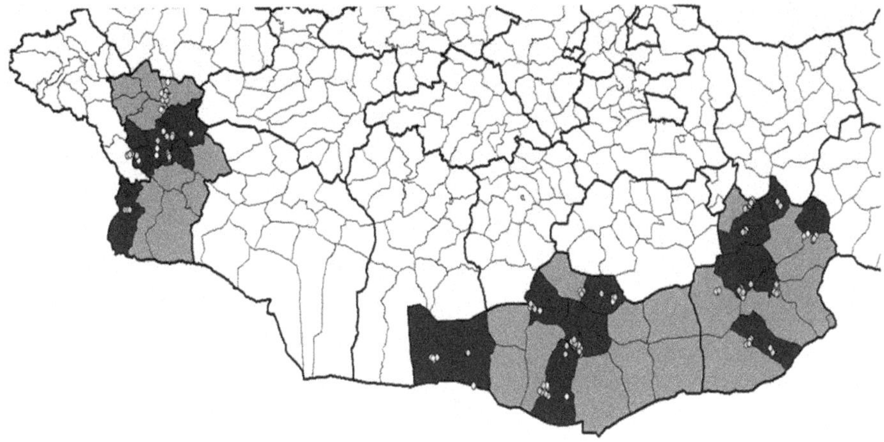

Fig. 2 Map of Southern & Western provinces Dornogobi, Umnogobi and Khovd (shaded in grey) and showing the selected districts (in black). The location of camel herds at time of sampling in 2014 (white dots) and 2015 (grey dots) are shown. Due to movement of *hot ails* not all herds were subsequently found in the district where they were first registered

they were informed about brucellosis in their herd. However, knowledge of herders on brucellosis can only be judged as moderate. From a total of 38 possible scores of the three knowledge themes with 19 questions, the median score achieved by participants was 23.

At the herd level, no significant correlations were found between camel and ruminant seroprevalences with the regression model using bootstrapping, regardless of considering all herds or considering only herds in provinces with no ruminant vaccination to ensure that seropositivity in ruminants was not a result of vaccination (even though there is little possibility of seropositivity persisting from previous vaccination) (Table 4). Goats in provinces and years with on vaccination were negatively correlated.

Variances of camel serpositivity were higher at herd level than province and district levels (Table 5). The ICC was estimated at herd level. For the cluster sample size calculation we assumed an ICC of 0.1 at herd level. In the Eastern provinces, this was nearly the case; however, the ICC was much lower in the Southern & Western provinces, where there were rarely seropositive camels. Clustering in herds is higher than in provinces or districts, therefore, correlation within herds (as the ecological unit) was accounted for in the statistical analysis.

Brucella spp. were isolated from the milk of one camel and from three vaginal swabs of cattle. The four isolated *Brucella* strains were identified as *B. abortus* (Fig. 3).

Table 2 Results of camel seroprevalences by the Rose Bengal Test (RBT) stratified by sex, age class, province and sampling year

Variable	Category	n	n pos	Seroprevalence[b]	95% CI[b]
Province	Dornod	241	13	5.3	2.9–9.6
	Sukhbaatar	298	18	6.1	3.5–10.6
	Dornogobi	388	3	0.8	0.3–2.3
	Umnogobi	526	2	0.4	0.1–1.4
	Khovd	369	1	0.3	0.04–1.9
Sex	Female	1429	26	2.2	1.4–3.4
	Males	332	10	3.0	1.6–5.5
Age class	≤ 4 years	253	5	2.0	0.8–4.7
	> 4 years	1569	32	2.3	1.6–3.4
Year	Eastern provinces 2013	237	13	5.7	3.1–10.2
	Eastern provinces 2014	302	18	5.8	3.3–10.1
	Southern & Western provinces 2014	897	4	0.4	0.2–1.2
	Southern & Western provinces 2015	386	2	0.5	0.1–2.0

[a]Positive with RBT, [b]95% confidence interval (CI) calculated with the panel variable on the level of herd to consider potential clustering within herds; Eastern provinces: Sukhbaatar and Dornod Southern & Western provinces: Dornogobi, Umnogobi and Khovd

Table 3 Analysis of risk factors for camel seropositivity, multivariable analysis showing odds ratios using a generalized estimating equation (GEE) model considering the panel variable at herd level

		n neg	% neg	n pos	% pos	OR	95% CI	*p*-value
Province	Dornogobi	385	99.2	3	0.8	ref		
	Dornod	228	94.6	13	5.4	7.9	2.1–30.1	0.003
	Khovd	368	99.7	1	0.3	0.4	0.05–3.2	0.4
	Sukhbaatar	280	94.0	18	6.0	10.2	2.7–38.6	0.001
	Umnogobi	524	99.6	2	0.4	0.5	0.1–2.4	0.4
Age class	≤ 4 years	248	98.2	5	1.8	ref		
	> 4 years	1537	98.0	32	2.0	1.2	0.4–3.2	0.7
Sex	Female	1403	99.2	26	1.8	ref		
	Male	322	97.0	10	3.0	0.8	0.3–1.8	0.5
Year	2013	224	94.5	13	5.5	ref		
	2014	1177	98.2	22	1.8	1.0	0.4–2.4	1.0
	2015	384	99.5	2	0.5	1.0	0.2–5.6	1.0
Cattle present	no	238	100	0	0.0	ref		
	yes	1547	97.7	37	2.3	8.1	1.5-inf	0.01[ǂ]
Sheep present	no	126	100	0	0.0	ref		
	yes	1659	97.8	37	2.2	4.0	0.7- inf	0.1 [ǂ]
Goats present	no	102	100	0	0.0	ref		
	yes	1683	97.8	37	2.2	3.2	0.6- inf	0.2 [ǂ]

[ǂ] -exact logistic regression, * $p \leq 0.05$

Discussion

A mass screening survey in all 22 provinces of Mongolia in 2011 reported seroprevalences of brucellosis in camels between 0.2 and 5.9% [28]. A previous (2010) population-based randomized survey in Sukhbaatar of Eastern Mongolia found a seroprevalence of 3% in camels [29]. In this study, we assessed seroprevalence and risk factors of camel seropositivity, in consideration of previous exposure to *Brucella* spp. There are shortcomings of using a serological test to define an outcome, as there will be false seronegative and false seropositive results, particularly when specificity of the test is low. Results subsequently need to be interpreted cautiously. In consideration of false positives, many authors set the cut-off for a seropositive herd as having at least two positive animals. In a complementary study on serological test characteristics comparing five different tests for use in camels, we concluded that the RBT is valid to assess brucellosis exposure status of Mongolian camels given its high specificity. However, due to lower sensitivity in camels when compared to other livestock species, we do not recommend it as a screening test for brucellosis monitoring in camels [26].

Between 2013 and 2015, seroprevalences in provinces showed high variation ranging from 0.3 to 6.1%, but the prevalences in regions were stable between the two sampling years. The ICC depends on the degree of clustering

Table 4 Regression coefficients using bootstrap re-sampling technique for camel herd seropositivity and within herd seropositivity of cattle, sheep and goats (all herds) and only for herds in a province without vaccination (no vaccination), [a] significant negative correlation

		N herds	Intercept (95% confidence interval [CI])	Slope (95% CI)
Ruminants	All herds	348	0.02 (−0.01–0.03)	0.06 (−0.07–0.21)
	No vaccination	137	0.03 (0.01–0.05)	0.08 (−0.14–0.5)
Cattle	All herds	292	0.03 (0.01–0.04)	0.06 (−0.02–0.2)
	No vaccination	103	0.04 (0.01–0.06)	0.06 (−0.06–0.3)
Sheep	All herds	333	0.03 (0.02–0.04)	0.03 (– 0.04–0.1)
	No vaccination	127	0.03 (0.01–0.05)	0.1 (– 0.2–0.7)
Goats	All herds	341	0.03 (0.02–0.04)	−0.003 (– 0.07–0.1)
	No vaccination	133	0.03 (0.01–0.05)	−0.1 (– 0.27 - -0.04)[a]

Table 5 The variances and intraclass correlation coefficients (ICC) of camel seropositivity at different levels. The greater the variances between herds compared to the overall total variance, the higher the ICC

Eastern provinces	2013	2014	Both years
Variance at herd level	2.1	2.0	1.2
Variance at district level	0.16	0.48	0.4
Variance at province level	< 0.01	< 0.01	< 0.01
Calculated ICC for camel herds	0.2	0.12	0.06
Southern & Western provinces	2014	2015	Both years
Variance at herd level	5.6	2.85	2.2
Variance at district level	2.0	1.3	1.1
Variance at province level	< 0.01	< 0.01	< 0.01
Calculated ICC for camel herds	< 0.001	0.04	< 0.001

and also on the prevalence. The ICC used for the sample size calculation (0.1) was appropriate for the Eastern provinces; however, since a much lower ICC at herd level was calculated for the Southern & Western provinces, we may have slightly oversampled there [32, 33].

Brucellosis seroprevalences above 5% in livestock species are important, indicating endemic status [34]. Eastern provinces had significantly higher seroprevalences than Southern & Western provinces. Being in an Eastern province was the most important risk factor of camel brucellosis seropositivity, with an OR of 13.2 when compared to the Southern & Western provinces. The same result was seen when the cut-off value of camel seropositivity was set at higher agglutination (++ positivity). The majority of serological studies on brucellosis report higher seroprevalences in older animals [20, 35], which we did not see among camels. Nonetheless, another study reported that brucellosis infection began early in life, probably through suckling, and persisted into adulthood [14].

Public health education campaigns should continue among herders to inform them about brucellosis prevention practices and herd and human health management. Past surveys in the framework of monitoring vaccination outcomes coupled with human brucellosis prevalence found that all information sources (veterinarians, radio/TV, newsletters to herders, information brochures and newspapers) significantly improved herder knowledge on brucellosis epidemiology, prevention and clinical signs in both people and livestock. Since Mongolian herders are literate, both oral and written information material is appropriate.

Musa et al. [36] reported that cattle were a possible source of infection for camels because all small ruminants tested in their study were negative. Hadush et al. [20] reported that camel herds with close contact in pastures with cattle and small ruminants were 3.6 and 2.3 times, respectively, more at risk to be brucellosis seropositive than those with no contact. We found an association between camel seropositivity and cattle, but not small ruminants, keeping. The fact that our camel isolate was *B. abortus* further supports a linkage of brucellosis in cattle and in camels. This finding is consistent with the screening in all Mongolian provinces with a correlation of camel and cattle seropositivity at district level, as well as previous reports of identification on *Brucella* spp. from camels in Asia, where another isolate from a Mongolian camel also was *B. abortus* [37]. Monitoring surveys of achieved vaccination coverage from 2012 to

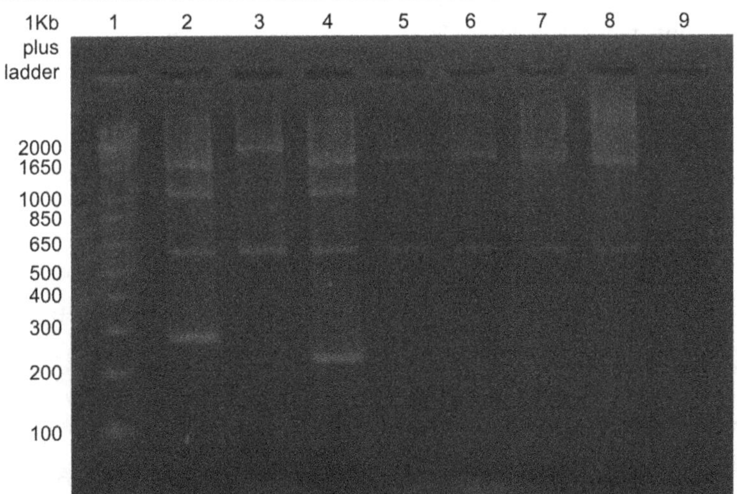

Fig. 3 Agarose gel electrophoresis PCR products. Lane 1: DNA ladder; Lane 2: positive control *Brucella suis;* Lane 3: positive control *Brucella abortus* (vaccine strain RB51) with two bands at 2524 and 587 bp; Lane 4: positive control *Brucella melitensis* (vaccine strain Rev1); Lane 5: the isolate from a camel; Lanes 6–8: isolates from cattle; Lane 9: negative control

2015 indicate that sufficient coverage was achieved in small ruminants, but coverage was critically low in cattle. Veterinarians reported that cattle were difficult to restrain adequately to administer conjunctival vaccination. Achieving insufficient vaccination coverage in cattle in the first year of newly introduced ruminant vaccination campaigns could explain why camel seropositivity remained stable between the years, both without and with cattle vaccination.

Conclusions

The results of this survey confirm the presence of *Brucella* spp. in camel herds in Mongolia. Camel seropositivity was significantly higher in Eastern than in Southern & Western provinces and was associated with keeping cattle together with camels. Decrease of camel brucellosis seropositivity was not observed despite ongoing ruminant vaccination. Repeated studies are needed to see if seroprevalences in camels drop over time with ongoing vaccination in other livestock species. Close attention should be given to achieve and monitor sufficient vaccination coverage in cattle in Mongolia. More isolates are needed to confirm that seropositivity in camels is limited to infection with *B. abortus*.

Materials and methods

Study design and selection of herds

We purposely selected the two Eastern provinces Sukhbaatar and Dornod for the first year of the study in 2013. The seroprevalence of brucellosis was high (> 3%) in camels in the multi-disease screening survey in Dornod in 2011 [27] and in Sukhbaatar during an epidemiological survey in 2010 [29]. Both provinces had a substantial number of camels and had not yet been included in the livestock (cattle, sheep and goats) brucellosis vaccination campaigns initiated in September 2013. Therefore, it was possible to sample before and after introduction of vaccination in 2014 in both Eastern provinces. The selection of three additional provinces in 2014 (second year of the study) was proportional to the size of their respective camel population as available from the annual livestock census [38]. Selection of provinces and districts proportional to size better ensured equal probability of camels to be enrolled in the study. The selected provinces had on average 32,500 camels per province. The Southern and Eastern provinces (Umnogobi, Dornogobi and Khovd) were surveyed in year 2 (2014) and year 3 (2015) (Fig. 4 and Table 1). During the study period, Umnogobi was the only province (out of 22) with no livestock brucellosis vaccination due to the large proportion of camels and vast size of the province. In areas using conjunctival vaccination of cattle and small ruminants, sampling was more than 5 months after vaccination campaigns, so the animals would no longer be seropositive due to vaccination [39, 40]. In each province, six districts were selected proportional to size of the camel population.

Repeated surveys using multi-stage cluster sampling were done in all provinces. Households with camels were randomly selected from lists of families registered with the district governor's office. The epidemiological sampling unit in rural zones was the *hot ail*, typically 2–3 families which pasture their livestock together and share watering places during certain times of the year. The entire *hot ail* herd of a selected family was included. District veterinarians indicated the zone where a selected *hot ail* was at the time of sampling, then the study team would travel to the zone and ask encountered herders about precise locations for the selected *hot ail*. Six and 30 % of initially selected *hot ails* could not be sampled in Eastern and Southern & Western provinces, respectively. Reasons for non-participation were family moved

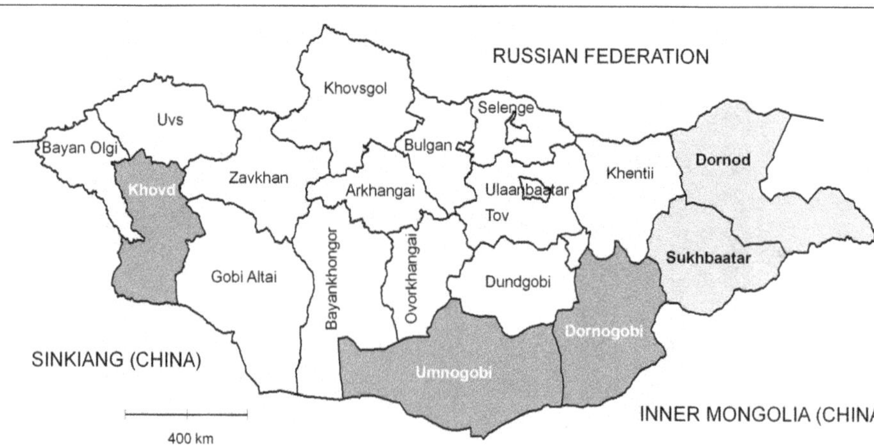

Fig. 4 Map of Mongolia showing the surveyed provinces. The light grey provinces of Dornod and Sukhbaatar (Eastern provinces) were sampled in 2013, and a second survey was done in 2014. Surveys in the darker grey provinces of Khovd, Umnogobi and Dornogobi (Southern & Western provinces) started in 2014 and were repeated in 2015

too far away, family was preparing to move and did not have time or family's camel herd was located too far from the *hot ail*. In such cases of non-participation, a replacement *hot ail* was enrolled which was either additionally selected from the district family list (the initial selection assumed that not all families would be found in a district) or from the nearest *hot ail* located in a northern direction from where the team determined that a selected *hot ail* could not be enrolled. For second year sampling in the same province, herders selected the previous year were contacted by mobile phone to establish their location and schedule the sampling. Reasons for non-participation were the same as for the first enrollment, and revisits were not possible in 10% and 40% in Eastern and Southern & Western provinces, respectively, so replacements were enrolled (Table 1).

Sample size

The sample size calculation assumed an intraclass correlation coefficient (ICC) of 0.1 for all livestock species. The ICC is the ratio of the variance between clusters over the total variance [41]. An ICC of 0.1 was reported for a range of endemic zoonoses [42] and was assumed, based on previous livestock brucellosis serological surveys in Mongolia [43]. This led to a design effect D of 1.2 and 1.4, when 3 and 5 animals, respectively, were sampled per cluster (herd).

The sample size calculation aimed to estimate the prevalence in each province with a precision, defined as one half-length of the 95% confidence interval, of 5%-points. We assumed seroprevalences of the different livestock species as were reported by Sukhbaatar in 2010 (3% for camels, 5% for goats, 7% for sheep, 8% for cattle). The calculated sample size for a province was to sample 30 herds each with at least 3 camels, 3 cattle, 5 sheep and 5 goats.

Selection of animals and sampling

In a selected herd, sheep and goats were selected when exiting an enclosure using the sampling interval i: total number of animals divided by 5. The first animal was selected with a random number and then every i^{th} sheep and goat was sampled. Camels and cattle were selected in the direction of the bottle head after the bottle was spun and a random number to tell which animals were to be included in that direction. Species, sex, age, breed, and main use for each animal were recorded on a data sheet, where any noted clinical symptoms (e.g. abortions) in the herd within the past months were also registered.

Blood samples were collected from the jugular vein using a Vacutainer® tube with disposable needle. Tubes were centrifuged for 5–10 min at 1000–1500 rpm, then serum was aliquoted into two 2 mL Eppendorf tubes®, which were stored on ice in a cool box and transported regularly to the Veterinary Laboratory at the Province Center, where they were kept at − 20 °C until transported to the School of Veterinary Medicine (SVM), Ulaanbaatar, and again stored at − 20 °C until further processing.

Vaginal swabs and/or milk samples for bacteriology were collected from individual animals with history of abortion. Swabs were placed in transport medium tube (BD BBL™Culture swab plus, Amies without Characoal, Becton Dickinson, France) and transported to the State Central Veterinary Laboratory (SCVL) in cool boxes. Milk samples consisted of 10–20 mL of milk taken from each teat. The first streams were discarded and then the milk sample was collected into a sterile vessel [44].

Serological testing

All serum samples were tested by the Rose Bengal Test (RBT) using RBT antigen (Biocombinate, Mongolia). Camel and cattle sera were tested with a serum:RBT reactive ratio of 1:1 (25 μL 25 μL) and small ruminant sera were tested with a serum:RBT reactive ratio of 3:1 (75 μL, 25 μL), all for 4 min, as recommended by the World Organization for Animal Health [45] and according to Mongolian national standards [46]. Results were recorded as agglutination negative (−), doubtful (+/−), or positive (+, ++ or +++) according to the strength and time to reaction. All tests and readings were performed by the same person. The serological test results were transformed to a binary outcome with the cut-off of seropositivity set at positive + agglutination. The RBT test with camel sera performed with 99% specificity, which is comparable to other livestock, however, with a rather low sensitivity of 75% [47].

Bacteriological examination

Milk samples were centrifuged to concentrate bacteria, at 6000–7000 g for 15 min in sealed tubes to avoid potential for aerosolization [7, 44]. A mixture of cream and deposit was streaked both on petri dishes with Farrell's medium (*Brucella* medium base, CM0169; antibiotic supplement, SR0083, Oxoid™) and with CITA medium (blood agar base number 2, CM0271, Oxoid™; and antibiotic supplements vancomycin, colistin, nystatin, nitrofurantoin, amphotericin B, Sigma™, as well as containing 5–10%, inactivated horse serum, SR0035, Oxoid™). The inoculated plates were incubated at 37 °C in absence and presence of 10% CO_2 for up to 2 weeks [44, 48]. A bacteriologist selected colonies based on *Brucella* colony morphology. These were stained by Gram stain (K001, Himedia) and modified Ziehl-Neelsen stain (21,820 Sigma™). In addition, reactivity to oxidase strips (MB0266A, Oxoid) was tested and both urea agar and urea broth were used for urease tests (urea agar 211,795,

BD BBL™; Bacto agar 214,010 BD and Urease Test Broth 221,719, BBL™). Colonies positive for these tests were passaged to obtain pure cultures, from which DNA was extracted using G-Dex™llc Genomic DNA Extraction kit (iNtRON Biotechnology, Inc).

To identify *Brucella* species, the Bruce-Ladder multiplex PCR, using INgene Bruce-ladder (V R.10.BRU.k5) kits, was used. The PCR products were analyzed by 1.5% agarose gel electrophoresis (GelRed reagent used in place of Etidiumbromid, GelRed™ Nucleic Acid Gel Stain Biotium), and fragment sizes were estimated using the 1 kb plus DNA ladder as molecular size marker (Invitrogen). Gel images were captured with G-Box (G:Box F3 Syngene, USA).

Questionnaires

The questionnaires were written in English and translated to Mongolian before pre-testing with 3 herder families in the vicinity of Ulaan Bator. The member of each selected camel-keeping family with the best knowledge on management of the camel herd was interviewed to obtain information about the herd, household and individual risk factors for brucellosis (Additional file 1). The interview included questions on i) knowledge of epidemiology of brucellosis ii) history of brucellosis in the household, iii) herd risk factors (including buying/selling of animals, sharing of pasture and watering places), iv) herd and human health management (including disposal of aborted fetuses/placentas), v) vaccination of cattle and small ruminants (Additional file 2). Questionnaires were not filled in on second visits to the same household. The coordinates of the household (*hot ail)* at time of the visit was recorded with a GPS. The mobile phone number of each participant was recorded for dissemination of results and to establish contact for second visits.

Data management and analysis

Questionnaire and sample data were double entered in Microsoft Access® and compared and corrected using Epi-Info 3.5.3 (Centers for Disease Control and Prevention, USA). An identification system was used to uniquely identify all samples and individuals and facilitated merging data sets at province, district, household/herd and individual levels. Data analyses were done using Stata 14 (StataCorp IC, USA).

We calculated seroprevalences for brucellosis in camels using generalized estimating equations (GEE, Stata command xtgee) to account for clustering at herd level, which expands the confidence interval compared to simple binary confidence intervals (CI). The apparent seroprevelance was converted to an estimated true seroprevalence using the formula developed by Rogan and Gladen [49] to account for the fact that the apparent seroprevalence might be over- or underestimated. A multivariable GEE model accounting for clustering was used to assess the association of biologically plausible risk factors to the serological outcome. Since vaccination of other livestock was highly linked to province and year it was not included in the multivariable analysis. Exact logistic regression was used for explanatory variables, with zero cell counts in two-by-two tables. Other variables, such as knowledge of herders or preventive measures, were not tested as risk factors in the multivariable model in order to keep the model simple. Other variables were tested with univariable GEE models. Age categorization of camels was based on breeding maturity: young camels were ≤ 4 years and adult camels were > 4 years. The variance components at different sampling levels were determined with the generalised linear latent and mixed models (gllamm) command in Stata for hierarchical models. The ICC at the *hot ail* level was estimated with ANOVA. The ICC was estimated at the herd level because the variance components indicated that correlation within clusters was highest at this level, so it was used for the sample size calculation. Correlations between camel and other livestock herd seropositivity was done with linear regression models in R version 3.3.2. The 95% confidence intervals of the intercepts and slopes of the regressions were constructed using bootstrap re-sampling technique and the information on total number of livestock per herd and species.

We assigned scores to the questions on knowledge within three themes: transmission of brucellosis between herds, transmission from livestock to people, and clinical signs of livestock brucellosis. Correct answers were scored as 2, 'Do not know' as 0, and wrong answers as −1. All scores within a knowledge theme were summed and the median taken to classify those with lower and higher scores.

Additional files

Additional file 1: Hot ail questionnaire. The interview included Hot ail questions on herd risk factors (including buying/selling of animals, sharing of pastures and watering places), herd and human health management (including disposal of aborted fetuses/placentas), vaccination of cattle and small ruminants. (DOCX 29 kb)

Additional file 2: Herder questionnaire. The interview included questions on knowledge on epidemiology of brucellosis and history of brucellosis in the household. (DOCX 28 kb)

Abbreviations

CI: Confidence Interval; GEE: Generalized estimating equation; ICC: Intraclass correlation coefficient; OR: Odds ratio; RBT: Rose Bengal Test; SCVL: State Central Veterinary Laboratory; SVM: School of Veterinary Medicine

Acknowledgements

The authors would like to thank provincial and private veterinarians, staff at local governor's offices, and colleagues at the laboratory facilities for their field and technical support. Many thanks also to all herders who have participated in this research by allowing interviews and strongly assisting in the sampling of their livestock.

Funding
This research was funded by the Animal Health Project Mongolia, the Swiss Agency for Development and Cooperation, the stipend commission of the City of Basel-Stadt and funding from the Swiss TPH.

Authors' contributions
CB performed most of the research work. BB and BA assisted in serological and bacteriological analysis and data management. CB, ES and TC drafted the manuscript. FR, JZ, JH, ES and TC contributed to study conception and design, data analysis and interpretation of data. ES contributed to manuscript editing. All authors read and approved the final version of the manuscript.

Consent for publication
Not applicable.

Competing interests
The authors declare that they have no competing interests.

Author details
[1]School of Veterinary Medicine, Mongolian University of Life Sciences, PO Box 17024, Zaisan, Ulaanbaatar, Mongolia. [2]Basel, Switzerland. [3]Swiss Tropical and Public Health Institute, PO Box, CH-4002 Basel, Switzerland. [4]University of Basel, Basel, Switzerland.

References
1. Santis Rd, Ciammaruconi A, Pomponi A, Fillo S, Lista F. Brucella: molecular diagnostic techniques in response to bioterrorism threat. J Bioterrorism and Biodefense. 2011;5(Special Issue), S2:004. https://doi.org/10.4172/2157-2526.
2. Buyankhishig D. Mongolian nomadic livestock husbandry, vol. VI. Ulaanbaatar: Sodpress; 2011.
3. Gwida M, El-Gohary A, Melzer F, Khan I, Rosler U, Neubauer H. Brucellosis in camels. Res Vet Sci. 2012;92(3):351–5.
4. NSO: Annual official data of National Statistical Office of Mongolia. 2015.
5. Chuluunbat B, Charruau P, Silbermayr K, Khorloojav T, Burger PA. Genetic diversity and population structure of Mongolian domestic Bactrian camels (Camelus bactrianus). Anim Genet. 2014;45(4):550–8.
6. Wernery U, Kinne J. Foot and mouth disease and similar virus infections in camelids: a review. Rev Sci Tech. 2012;31(3):907–18.
7. Poester FP, Nielsen K, Samartino LE, Yu WL. Diagnosis of brucellosis. Open Vet Sci J. 2010;4:46–60.
8. de Oliveira MZ, Vale V, Keid L, Freire SM, Meyer R, Portela RW, Barrouin-Melo SM. Validation of an ELISA method for the serological diagnosis of canine brucellosis due to *Brucella canis*. Res Vet Sci. 2011;90(3):425–31.
9. McDermott J, Grace D, Zinsstag J. Economics of brucellosis impact and control in low-income countries. Rev Sci Tech Off Int Epiz. 2013;32(1):249–61.
10. Gul ST, Khan A. Epidemiology and epizootology of brucellosis: a review. Pak Vet J. 2007;27(3):145–51.
11. Schelling E, Diguimbaye C, Daoud S, Nicolet J, Boerlin P, Tanner M, Zinsstag J. Brucellosis and Q-fever seroprevalences of nomadic pastoralists and their livestock in Chad. Prev Vet Med. 2003;61(4):279–93.
12. Cooper CW. Risk factors in transmission of brucellosis from animals to humans in Saudi Arabia. Trans R Soc Trop Med Hyg. 1992;86(2):206–9.
13. Wanjohi M, Gitao CG, Bebora L. The prevalence of *Brucella* spp. in camel milk marketed from north Eastern Province, Kenya. Res Opin Animal & Vet Sci. 2012;2(7):425–34.
14. Dawood HA. Brucellosis in camels (Camelus dromedorius) in the south province of Jordan. Am J Agri Biol Sci. 2008;3(3):623–6.
15. Shimol SB, Dukhan L, Belmaker I, Bardenstein S, Sibirsky D, Barrett C, Greenberg D. Human brucellosis outbreak acquired through camel milk ingestion in southern Israel. Israel Med Assoc J : IMAJ. 2012;14(8):475–8.
16. Pappas G, Papadimitriou P, Akritidis N, Christou L, Tsianos EV. The new global map of human brucellosis. Lancet Infect Dis. 2006;6(2):91–9.
17. Schelling E, Grace D, Willingham AL, Randolph T. Research approaches for improved pro-poor control of zoonoses. Food Nutr Bull. 2007;28(2):S345–56.
18. Abbas B, Agab H. A review of camel brucellosis. Prev Vet Med. 2002;55(1): 47–56.
19. Kaltungo BY, Saidu SNA, Musa IW, Baba AY. Brucellosis: a neglected zoonosis. Brit Microbiol Res J. 2014;4(12):1551–74.
20. Hadush A, Pal M, Kassa T, Zeru F. Sero-epidemiology of camel brucellosis in the Afar region of Northeast Ethiopia. ©2013 Acad J. 2013;5(9):269–75.
21. Mustafa IE. Bacterial diseases of dromedaries and bactrian camels. Rev sci tech Off int Epiz. 1987;6(2):391–405.
22. Fatima S, Khan I, Nasir A, Younus M, Saqib M, Melzer F, Neubauer H, El-Adawy H. Serological, molecular detection and potential risk factors associated with camel brucellosis in Pakistan. Trop Anim Health Prod. 2016; 48(8):1711–8.
23. Wernery U. Camelid brucellosis: a review. Rev sci tech Off int Epiz. 2014; 33(3):839–57.
24. Gwida MM, El-Gohary AH, Melzer F, Tomaso H, Rösler U, Wernery U, Wernery R, Elschner MC, Khan I, Eickhoff M, et al. Comparison of diagnostic tests for the detection of *Brucella* spp. in camel sera. BMC Res Notes. 2011;4:525.
25. Azwai S, Carter S, Woldehiwet Z, MacMillan A. Camel brucellosis: Evalution of field sera by conventional serological tests and ELISA. J Camel Prac Research. 2001;8(2):185–93.
26. Bayasgalan C, Chultemdorj T, Felix R, Argamjav B, Badmaa B, Vanabaatar B, Zinsstag J, Hattendorf J, Schelling E. Serological test comparison for brucellosis in Mongolian camels, forthcoming
27. SCVL (State Central Veterinary Laboratory): Report of the mass livestock screening for eight diseases. Report of unpublished results: State Central Veterinary Laboratory 2011.
28. Myagmar N. Brucellosis situation in Mongolia and Result of Bovine Brucellosis Proficiency Test. In: 4th FAO-APHCA/OIE/DLD Regional Workshop on Brucellosis Diagnosis and Control in Asia-Pacific Region - Proficiency Test and Ways Forward: 2014. Chiang Mai; 2014. http://www.fao.org/fileadmin/templates/rap/files/meetings/2014/140318-cr.mongolia.pdf.
29. Baljinnyam Z, Dorj G, Dashzevge E, Roth F, Zinsstag J, Schelling E. Representative sero-prevalence of livestock Brucellosis in two Mongolian provinces. In: Brucellosis 2011 International Research Conference: 21–23 September 13 2011. UCA Auditorium, Puerto Madero Buenos Aires - Argentina: Organizer by the Argentine Association for Microbiology; 2011. p. 40.
30. Roth F, Zinsstag J, Orkhon D, Chimed-Ochir G, Hutton G, Cosivi O, Carrin G. Human health benefits from livestock vaccination for brucellosis: case study. Bull World Health Organ. 2003;81(12):867–76.
31. Zinsstag J, Roth F, Orkhon D, Chimed-Ochir G, Nansalmaa M, Kolar J, Vounatsou P. A model of animal-human brucellosis transmission in Mongolia. Prev Vet Med. 2005;69(1–2):77–95.
32. Twisk JWR. Basic principles of multilevel analysis. In: Applied Multilevel Analysis: A Practical Guide edn. Cambrigde: University Press; 2013. p. 6–29.
33. Wu S, Crespi CM, Wong WK. Comparison of methods for estimating the Intraclass correlation coefficient for binary responses in Cancer prevention cluster randomized trials. Contemp Clin Trials. 2012;33(5):869–80.
34. McDermott JJ, Arimi SM. Brucellosis in sub-Saharan Africa: epidemiology, control and impact. Vet Microbiol. 2002;90(1–4):111–34.
35. Mohammed MA, Shigidy MT, Al-juboori AY. Sero-prevalence and epidemiology of brucellosis in camels, sheep and goats in Abu Dhabi emirate. Int J Anim Veter Adv. 2013;5(2):82–6.
36. Musa MT, Eisa MZ, El Sanousi EM, Abdel Wahab MB, Perrett L. Brucellosis in camels (Camelus dromedarius) in Darfur, Western Sudan. J Comp Pathol. 2008;138(2–3):151–5.
37. Kim J-Y, Kang S-I, Janchivdorj E, Batbaatar V, Ulziisaikhan G, Khursbaatar O, Lee K, Ju Lee J, Sung S-R, Chan Jung S, et al. Distinctive phenotypic and molecular characteristics of Brucella abortusstrains isolated from Mongolia. Turk Vet J Anim Sci. 2016;40(5):562–68.
38. NSO: Annual official data of National Statistical Office of Mongolia. 2012.
39. Chand P, Chhabra R, Nagra J. Vaccination of adult animals with a reduced dose of *Brucella abortus* S19 vaccine to control brucellosis on dairy farms in endemic areas of India. Trop Anim Health Prod. 2015;47(1):29–35.
40. Fensterbank R. Brucellosis in cattle, sheep and goats: diagnosis, control and vaccination. Rev Sci Tech Off Int Epiz. 1986;5(3):605–18.
41. Bennett S, Woods T, Liyanage WM, Smith DL. A simplified general method

for cluster-sample surveys of health in developing countries. World Health Stat Q. 1991;44(3):98–106.
42. Otte MJ, Gumm ID. Intra-cluster correlation coefficients of 20 infections calculated from the results of cluster-sample surveys. Prev Vet Med. 1997;31:147–50.
43. Baljinnyam Z, Tsend S, Tsegeen N, Dorj G, Dashzevge E, Zinsstag J, Schelling E. Representative Seroprevalences of human and livestock brucellosis in two Mongolian provinces. EcoHealth. 2014;11:356–71.
44. OIE. Bovine Brucellosis. In: Manual of Diagnostic Tests and Vaccine For Terrestrial Animals, vol. II. Paris: World Organization for Animal Health; 2008. p. 629–53.
45. OIE. Bovine brucellosis. In: Manual of Diagnostic Tests and Vaccines for Terrestrial Animals, vol. II. Paris: World Organization For Animal Health; 2009. p. 130.
46. MASM. Animal brucellosis, serological diagnostic method (MNS5198:2002). In: Mongolian Agency for Standardization and Metrology; 2002.
47. Nielsen K, Gall D, Smith P, Balsevicius S, Garrido F, Ferrer MD, Biancifiori F, Dajer A, Luna E, Samartino L, et al. Comparison of serological tests for the detection of ovine and caprine antibody to *Brucella melitensis*. Rev Sci Tech Oie. 2004;23(3):979–87.
48. Junior GN, Megid J, Vicente AF, Listoni FJP, Morato MF, Lara GHB, Motta RG, Chacur MGM, Ribeiro MG. Comparison of *Brucella* agar, CITA and Farrell media for selective isolation of *Brucella abortus* from semen of bovine bulls. Afr J Microbiol Res. 2015;9(9):617–20.
49. Rogan WJ, Gladen B. Estimating prevalence from the results of a screening test. Am J Epidemiol. 1978;107(1):71–6.

24

Peripheral mononuclear blood cell apheresis in a preclinical ovine model

Helen Lydon[1], Roger Brooks[1], Andrew McCaskie[1] and Frances Henson[1,2*]

Abstract

Background: Recent research has demonstrated that circulating peripheral blood mononuclear fractions (PBMC) containing haematopoietic stem (HSC)/progenitor cells have the potential to play a crucial role in regenerative medicine strategies. Work in our laboratory has shown that a peripheral blood mononuclear cell fraction (PBMC) enhances cartilage repair in an osteochondral defect model in sheep and has a significant effect on cells in the joint niche. In order to obtain PBMC rich blood containing HSCs for further studies, we have performed, for the first time, apheresis on adult sheep.

Results: Subcutaneous granulocyte-colony stimulating factor (G-CSF) was used to mobilise white blood cells and continual flow apheresis was performed on 8 sheep under general anaesthetic. There were no observable side effects, although a marked tendency for blood clotting during the procedure was noted. The administration of G-CSF for 3 days increased the white blood cell (WBC) count in the peripheral blood from to $6.7 \pm 2.1 \times 10^6$/ml to $16.1 \pm 5.0 \times 10^6$/ml. Following apheresis, the WBC numbers in the apheretic product increased to $38.5 \pm 27.6 \times 10^6$/ml, comprised of a significant increase in neutrophils and PBMC (from $5.25 \pm 1.8 \times 10^6$/ml following G-CSF stimulation to $27.5\ 5 \pm 27.6 \times 10^6$/ml). There was a mean of 2.1% CD34 + ve cells and 95.5% CD45 + ve cells in the apheretic product.

Conclusions: This study describes the administration of G-CSF and subsequent apheresis in adult sheep. The technique is safe when performed as described with no observable side effects. The technique permits collection of an increased WBC fraction containing neutrophils and PBMC in adult sheep. This apheretic product contains CD34 + ve cells, representing an HSC/progenitor population for use in *in vivo* and *in vitro* experiments.

Keywords: G-CSF, Apheresis, Haematopoetic stem cells, CD34, Ovine, Sheep

Background

The repair of articular cartilage defects remains challenging and all currently available methods have their disadvantages. In addition to autologous chondrocytes, a number of cell types have been proposed as stimulators or contributors to repair either alone or in combination. We have described the successful use of a peripheral blood mononuclear cell fraction (PBMC) to enhance cartilage repair in an ovine osteochondral defect model [1]. This study showed that isolated PBMC had effects on migration and differentiation of both chondrocytes and mesenchymal stromal cells (MSC) [2, 3]. PBMC populations contain a number of cell types, including peripheral haematopoietic stem cells (HSC) [4], derived from the bone marrow. CD34 + ve HSC are widely used in regenerative medicine to treat malignant and non malignant haematopoetic disorders [5] and, increasingly, are being used in regenerative medicine strategies to treat disorders of other body systems [6]. Traditionally HSC were harvested directly from the bone marrow for bone marrow transplantation; however, automated retrieval of a peripheral blood progenitor cell (PBPC) fraction for this purpose using an apheresis procedure is now standard clinical practice [7]. The technique is based on the mobilisation of bone marrow cells into the peripheral blood by the administration of exogenous granulocyte colony stimulating factor (G-CSF) [8]. Many studies have described the use of apheresis to collect G-CSF stimulated PBMC in man and apheresis has been described in a number of animal species including dogs [9, 10], monkeys [11] and swine [12].

* Correspondence: fmdh1@cam.ac.uk
[1]Department of Surgery, University of Cambridge, Hill's Road, Cambridge, UK
[2]Department of Veterinary Medicine, University of Cambridge, Madingley Road, Cambridge, UK

In order to continue investigating the effect of PBMC and PBPC on the healing of joint surface defects in experimental ovine models, we have performed apheresis in adult sheep to provide concentrated populations of peripheral blood cells for in vitro and in vivo research. In this paper we describe the use of G-CSF to stimulate the bone marrow niche, the method of apheresis in sheep and the cell types harvested.

Methods

Animals

Eight 3 year-old (adult) healthy Welsh Mountain female sheep weighing 40-42 kg underwent apheresis. The animals were purchased from a Licenced Supplier specifically for this study. All animal procedures were carried out in accordance with the regulations as set out in the Animal [Scientific Procedures] Act 1986. This study received approval from both the Animal Welfare and Ethical Review Board, Cambridge University and the UK Home Office (Project Licence number 70/8165).

Donor preparation

Animals were treated with rhG-CSF (Neupogen, Amgen) 5 mg/kg subcutaneously once a day for 3 days prior to apheresis with the final dose being administered 2 h before apheresis commenced [13]. Blood samples collected into EDTA were obtained prior to commencing rhG-CSF administration and immediately prior to apheresis and complete blood counts (CBC) were performed to establish haematological values using an automated haematology analyser.

Apheresis

A 20 g intravenous catheter was placed into the cephalic vein and anaesthesia induced with a single intravenous bolus of 3 mg/kg alfaxalone (Alfaxan, Jurox). This catheter was secured and subsequently used as the fluid return portal during apheresis. Sheep were intubated and maintained on isofluorane. Animals were placed in dorsal recumbency and jugular venous access obtained via the integral cannula of the closed system apheresis tubing kit. At the completion of apheresis, the jugular cannula and cephalic catheter were removed and the animals were allowed to recover normally, prior to being replaced into their pens.

Apheresis was performed using a Cobe Spectra (Terumo-BCT) with a disposable double needle closed system apheresis tubing kit. The tubing kit and collection chambers were primed with 50 ml acid-citrate-dextrose A (ACD-A, Biomet, USA) anticoagulant and 0.9% saline. PBPC collections were performed on the basis of individual data (body weight and haematocrit). This data, fed into the CobeSpectra at the start of the procedure, automatically established each animal's total blood volume, the optimal and maximal pump rates and anticoagulant flow rate. Manually varying the plasma pump speed allowed adjustments of the collection product colour and flow rate. A colourgram was used to verify collection of PBMC products.

Throughout apheresis, the body temperature of the animals was monitored to ensure that the temperature remained within normal limits (38.3–39.8). Animals were positioned on a heat retaining mat to reduce heat loss onto the underlying surface and maintain temperature in the physiological range; also, animals were covered with blankets to retain body heat. To avoid ACDA-A solution induced hypocalcaemia, 40 ml of a 10% calcium gluconate solution was administered either subcutaneously during apheresis ($n = 4$) or mixed with blood and returned intravenously throughout the procedure via the cephalic vein ($n = 3$). Apheresis was stopped when 35 ml apheretic product and 30 ml plasma had been collected. Once the flow-back was completed the animal was allowed to recover.

Apheretic product analysis

A CBC was made of the apheretic product and flow cytometry was used to quantify CD34 and CD45 positive cells in the apheretic samples. Cells were stained with mouse anti-sheep CD45 FITC (0.001 mg mL^{-1}; MCA2220F, AbD Serotec, UK) and mouse anti-sheep CD34 (0.005 mg mL^{-1}; (AM32448PU-N, Acris/Origene Europe, Germany) [14] conjugated to FITC using FITC Fast Conjugation Kit (Abcam, UK) in staining buffer. Cells were also stained with an equivalent concentration of IgG controls: mouse IgG1-FITC (MCA928F, AbD Serotec, UK) and mouse IgG2a FITC (ab81197, Abcam, UK). Dead cells were excluded based on fluorescence using a viability stain (AquaZombie, Biolegend). Cellular staining was measured using a BD LSR-Fortessa with BD FACSDiva software. Data was analysed using Beckman Coulter Kaluza software (v1.2).

Statistical analysis

Results are expressed as mean ± standard deviation. Comparisons between cell numbers at different experimental points in the animals was determined by one way ANOVA using Graph Pad prism. A p value of < 0.05 was considered statistically significant.

Results

Effects of rhG-CSF treatment

No obvious signs of any adverse effects that have been reported in humans [15] were observed in the sheep i.e. there was no allergic reaction, lameness reflecting bone pain or reduction in food or water intake.

CBC were performed in peripheral blood before G-CSF administration and immediately prior to apheresis. Prior to G-CSF administration, the mean WBC concentration was $6.74 \pm 2.06 \times 10^6$/ml. Following the administration of G-CSF the mean WBC concentration was $16.1 \pm 5.0 \times 10^6$/ml, a statistically significant 238% increase (Fig. 1). Mean red blood cell (RBC) concentrations prior to G-CSF administration were $7.7 \pm 1.7 \times 10^6$/ml, with RBC concentrations post-G-CSF administration significantly decreasing to $6.4 \pm 1.6 \times 10^6$/ml (Fig. 2).

Individual WBC types were quantified to identify which cell types were being stimulated by G-CSF. Neutrophils and PBMC (lymphocytes + monocytes) were significantly increased following G-CSF treatment, no significant alteration was seen in the granulocyte population (eosinophils + basophils). Neutrophils increased from $3.1 \pm 2 \times 10^6$/ml pre-treatment to $10.5 \pm 4.2 \times 10^6$/ml post-treatment, whilst PBMC increased from 3.4 ± 0.6 pre-treatment to 5.2 ± 1.8 post-treatment. (Fig. 3).

One animal did not apparently respond to the administration of G-CSF. In this animal, the pre-G-CSF WBC count was 7.10×10^6/ml but, following the administration of G-CSF, the WBC count had fallen to 3.9×10^6/ml.

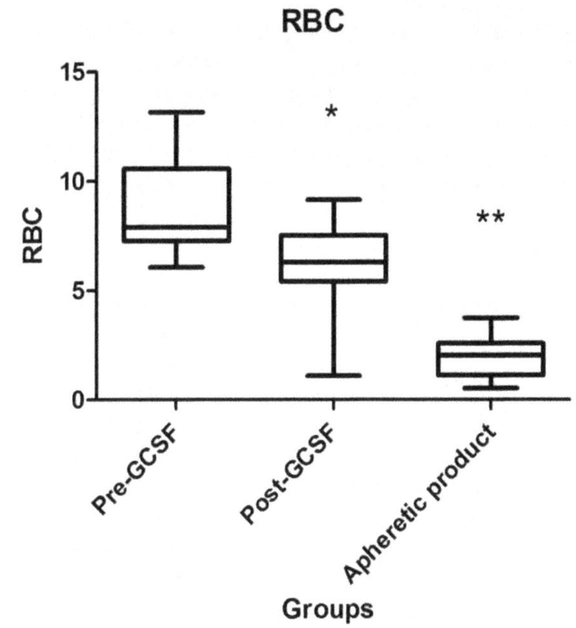

Fig. 2 Total red blood cell (RBC) numbers in whole blood before (Pre-GCSF) ($n = 8$) and after administration of G-CSF (Post-GCSF) ($n = 8$) and in the apheretic product ($n = 7$). *Significantly different from Pre-GCSF value, **Significantly different from Pre- and Post- GCSF values. $P < 0.05$. Values $\times 10^6$/ml blood

Apheresis procedure

Seven of the eight animals completed the apheresis. In one sheep, rapid and repeated clotting of venous blood within the cannula and tubing at the start of apheresis necessitated abandoning the procedure. In addition, 2 further animals produced blood clots in the cannula and/or tubing immediately upon starting blood withdrawal by the Cobe Spectra. In these animals, replacement catheters and heparin saline flushes were required to continue the apheresis procedure in the initial stages. The mean time required for collection in the 7 sheep was 93 min ± 12 min to obtain 35 ml apheresis product and 30 ml plasma.

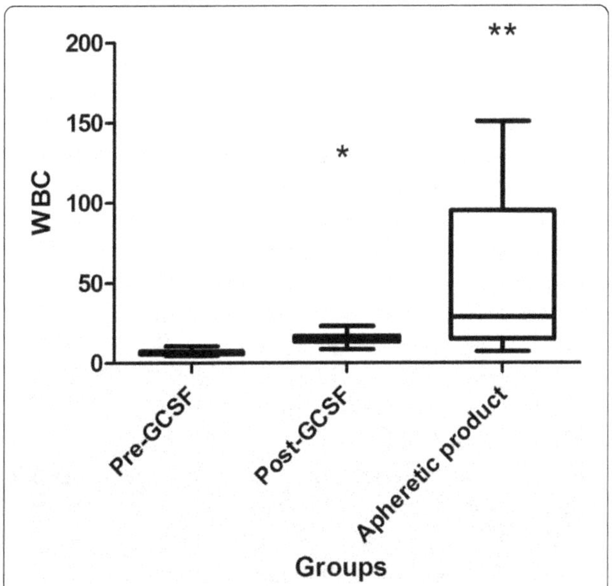

Fig. 1 Total white blood cell (WBC) numbers in whole blood before (Pre-GCSF) ($n = 8$) and after administration of G-CSF (Post-GCSF) ($n = 8$) and in the apheretic product ($n = 7$). *Significantly different from Pre-GCSF value, **Significantly different from Pre- and Post- GCSF values. $P < 0.05$. Values $\times 10^6$/ml blood

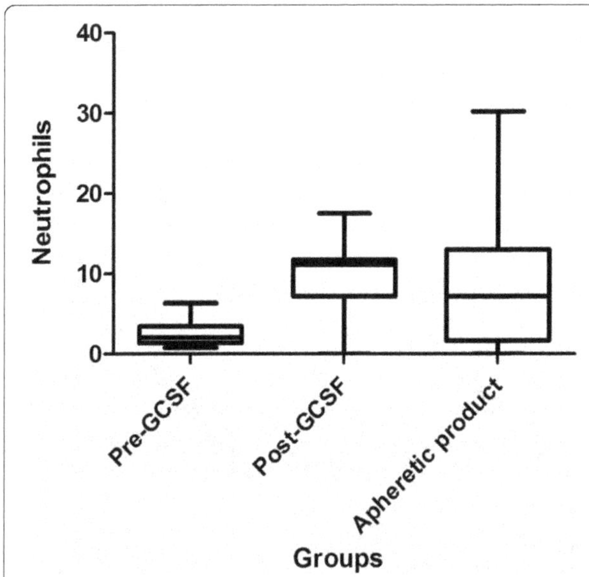

Fig. 3 Numbers of neutrophils in in whole blood before (Pre-GCSF) ($n = 8$) and after administration of G-CSF (Post-GCSF) ($n = 8$) and in the apheretic product ($n = 7$)

Effects of apheresis

Hypothermia was present in 1/7 sheep upon cessation of the procedure. This animal was immediately covered with blankets and placed into a warmed recovery area until stable. No signs of hypocalcaemia (licking, agitation or tremors in the absence of low body temperature) were detected in any sheep during the procedure or post-procedure.

Apheresis cell yields

The final collection volume was approximately 35 ml in all animals. Following apheresis WBC concentrations had risen significantly from a pre-apheresis value of $16.1 \pm 5.03 \times 10^6$/ml to $38.5 \pm 27.6 \times 10^6$/ml and RBC concentration had significantly decreased from $6.4 \pm 1.6 \times 10^6$/ml to $1.9 \pm 1.0 \times 10^6$/ml. When individual cell types were quantified, the concentration of neutrophil in the apheretic product was reduced pre-apheresis ($10.5 \pm 4.2 \times 10^6$/ml compared to post-apheresis of 6.4 ± 4) (Fig. 3). However, a significant increase in PBMC was seen. When all 7 animals were included in the analysis, including the non-responder, PBMC concentrations rose from $5.2 \pm 1.8 \times 10^6$/ml pre-apheresis to $27.5 \pm 23.9 \times 10^6$/ml post-apheresis. (Fig. 4).

Using flow cytometry, the number of CD34+ and CD45+ cells in the apheresis product was measured. In the apheretic product $2.71 \pm 2.3\%$ of nucleated cells were CD34 + ve (Fig. 5.)

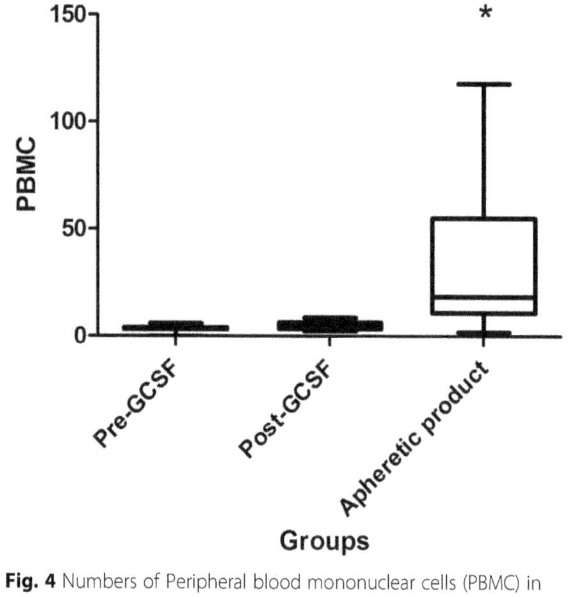

Fig. 4 Numbers of Peripheral blood mononuclear cells (PBMC) in whole blood before (Pre-GCSF) ($n = 8$) and after administration of G-CSF (Post-GCSF) ($n = 8$) and in the apheretic product ($n = 7$). *Significantly different from Pre- and Post- GCSF values. $P < 0.05$. Values $\times 10^6$/ml blood

Discussion

This report documents for the first time the successful concentration and collection of PBMC in sheep using automated apheresis and demonstrates that the procedure is a clinically safe method of obtaining a cell product enriched for PBMC containing CD34+ cells that did not pose significant technical difficulties.

Venous access was obtained via the jugular vein with the cephalic vein acting as the return portal. The apheresis machine was primed with saline rather than pre-collected blood as recommended in paediatric patients and small animal apheresis [9, 16]. In these smaller patients, priming with blood is required for successful apheresis as the extracorporeal circulating blood is a significant percentage of blood volume. In this study the sheep were sufficiently large (40-42 kg) that the haemodilution caused by the addition of saline to the circulation at the commencement of the cellular collection was not significant.

In 1/8 animals rapid repeated clotting of blood led to abandonment of the procedure in that individual. In 2 other animals clotting at the start of the procedure necessitated rapid placing of alternate catheters and/or flushing of tubing with heparin to remove blood clots before the pump could draw in the blood with sufficient pressure for effective centrifugation. The reason for such vigorous coagulation in 3/8 animals is not known. A study on interspecies difference in coagulation profiles reported that sheep had a similar clotting time and endogenous thrombin potential to humans [17] and so the response to the initial connection to the Cobe Spectra could not have been predicted. The appearance of clots coincided with the initial pressure from the machine within the vein to draw blood from the animal. Clotting is more likely at the beginning of the procedure as this is when the least amount of anticoagulant is distributed systemically. We recommend that particular attention is paid to the placing of the withdrawal portal in sheep undergoing apheresis and that all catheters/cannulas/tubing are primed with heparin prior to drawing blood.

In order to increase the numbers of circulating WBC containing the desired PBMC fraction, G-CSF was administered to the sheep prior to apheresis. G-CSF is a haematopoetic cytokine produced primarily by bone marrow stromal cells that acts, at higher doses, by stimulating the differentiation of several haematopoetic progenitors including CD34+ cells. In this study we administered 5 mg/kg rhG-CSF subcutaneously, daily for 3 days prior to apheresis. In a previous report this was the optimum dose for mobilisation of ovine WBC [13] and gave a peak response on day 3 of mobilisation, after which time, the total WBC dropped markedly. In this study, the sheep had a starting WBC count of 4.45×10^6/ml, which rose to a post-GCSF value of approximately 13.5×10^6/ml)

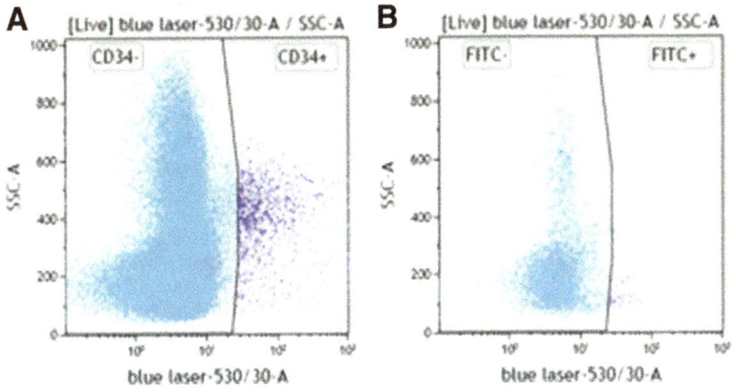

Fig. 5 **a** Representative light-scatter (SSC-A) vs fluorescence (CD34-FITC) plot of CD34 expression on cells from ovine apheresis samples using two-colour flow cytometry. **b** IgG control

[13]. These blood results mirror very closely the values we report in this paper and, coupled with the observation that rhG-CSF did not cause any adverse clinical effects in any of our sheep, support the use of commercially available rhG-CSF for the mobilisation of sheep WBC cells in the circulation. Of the 8 sheep treated with rhG-CSF one animal did not show an increase in WBC. In the other publication that reports the use of rhG-CSF in sheep, 1/3 animals did not respond. It has been reported that G-CSF based mobilisation regimes have a 5–30% failure rate among healthy individuals [18], with various factors being associated with a poor response to G-CSF in human patients, including age of patient, type of G-CSF used and prior exposure to other drugs. The reasons for poor mobilisation in animals are unknown, although they are likely to be similar.

Stimulation of the bone marrow using G-CSF and subsequent apheresis lead to a significant increase in WBC numbers and a significant decrease in RBC numbers in the apheretic product compared to unstimulated peripheral blood and peripheral blood obtained immediately prior to the apheresis technique. However, we did not find that the post-G-CSF WBC concentration was a predictor of apheretic product WBC concentration as has been reported in the dog [9]. Analysis of the cell types contributing to the increase in WBC numbers in the sheep reported here showed that neutrophils and PBMC were the cell types that were significantly increased in the apheretic product.

The PBMC fraction of blood is of particular interest in regenerative medicine as it contains HSC and progenitor cell populations. Whilst these progenitor cells have traditionally been used to treat malignant and non malignant haematopoetic disorders [5], they have also been used in regenerative medicine strategies to treat disorders of other body systems, including orthopaedic disease [6, 19] However, the identification of stem and progenitor cell populations in peripheral blood and apheretic products in veterinary species is not straightforward, due both to potential differences in stem cell CD designation and function between species and the availability of suitable reagents to characterise CD markers. In man, there is a recognised population of CD34 + ve cells that have stem/progenitor potential and are used for clinical transplantation [14]. In the sheep CD34 + ve cells have also been shown to have haematopoetic potential [20] and so CD34 appears to be an appropriate marker in this species, as well as man, for HSC. In this study, using flow cytometry and a sheep specific anti-CD34 antibody [14], we have shown that, 2.7% of the apheretic product was CD34 + ve. This figure is similar to the 1.5% reported in other studies [21] and supports our methodology.

Conclusions

In conclusion this study has demonstrated that apheresis can be used in the sheep safely and without risk to the animal. The administration of G-CSF and subsequent apheresis provides a neutrophil and PBMC rich collection product containing > 2% of CD34 + ve cells that can be used for further in vivo or in vitro experimental investigations.

Abbreviations

ACD-A: Acid-citrate-dextrose A; CBC: Complete blood counts; CD: Cluster designation; EDTA: Ethylenediaminetetraacetic acid; FITC: Fluorescein isothiocyanate; GCSF: Granulocyte colony stimulating factor; HSC: Haematopoetic stem cells; IgG: Immunoglobulin G; MSC: Mesenchymal stromal cells; PBMC: Peripheral blood mononuclear cell fraction; PBPC: Peripheral blood progenitor cell; RBC: Red blood cell; WBC: White blood cell

Acknowledgements

We would like to acknowledge Mrs. Gill Pout for her technical expertise, and the Cambridge NIHR Cell Phenotyping Hub for advice and assistance with flow cytometry.

Funding
This study was funded by the Arthritis Research UK. The funders did not play any role in the design, conclusions or interpretation of the study.

Authors' contributions
HL collected the apheretic products, performed the flow cytometry, and was involved in data analysis. RB was involved in the study design and apheresis procedure. AWM was involved in the study design and securing funds for performing this work. FH was involved in the study design, apheresis procedure, data analysis and manuscript writing. All authors read and approved the final manuscript.

Consent for publication
Not applicable.

Competing interests
None of the authors have any competing interests.

References

1. Hopper N, Wardale J, Brooks R, Power J, Rushton N, Henson F. Peripheral blood mononuclear cells enhance cartilage repair in in vivo Osteochondral defect model. PLoS One. 2015;10:e0133937.
2. Hopper N, Henson F, Brooks R, Ali E, Rushton N, Wardale J. Peripheral blood derived mononuclear cells enhance osteoarthritic human chondrocyte migration. Arthritis Res Ther. 2015;17:199.
3. Hopper N, Wardale J, Howard D, Brooks R, Rushton N, Henson F. Peripheral blood derived mononuclear cells enhance the migration and chondrogenic differentiation of multipotent mesenchymal stromal cells. Stem Cells Int. 2015;2015:323454.
4. Kato K, Radbruch A. Isolation and characterization of CD34+ hematopoietic stem cells from human peripheral blood by high-gradient magnetic cell sorting. Cytometry. 1993;14:384–92.
5. Tripura C, Pande G. Applications of human haematopoetic stem cells isolated and expanded from different tissues in regenerative medicine. Regen Med. 2013;8:783–95.
6. Muller AM, Huppertz S, Henschler R. Haematopoietic stem cells in regenerative medicine: astray or on the path? Transfus Med Hemother. 2016;43:247–54.
7. Weaver CH, Buckner CD, Longin K, Appelbaum FR, Rowley S, Lilleby K, Miser J, Storb R, Hansen JA, Bensinger W. Syngeneic transplantation with peripheral blood mononuclear cells collected after the administration of recombinant human granulocyte colony-stimulating factor. Blood. 1993;82:1981–4.
8. Bendall LJ, Bradstock KF. G-CSF: from granulopoietic stimulant to bone marrow stem cell mobilizing agent. Cytokine Growth Factor Rev. 2014;25:355–67.
9. Lupu M, Gooley T, Zellmer E, Graves SS, Storb R. Principles of peripheral blood mononuclear cell apheresis in a preclinical canine model of hematopoietic cell transplantation. J Vet Intern Med. 2008;22:74–82.
10. Lee R, Shorb R, Little M-T, Joslyn A, Spectr M, Kuhr CS. Percutaneous central dual-lumen catheter for apheresis in the canine. J Investig Surg. 2002;15:337–41.
11. Ageyama N, Hanazono Y, Shibata H, Ono F, Ogawa H, Nagashima T, Ueda Y, Yoshikawa Y, Hasegawa M, Ozawa K, et al. Safe and efficient collection of cytokine-mobilized peripheral blood cells from cynomolgus monkeys (Macaca Fascicularis) with human newborn-equivalent body weights. Exp Anim. 2005;54:421–8.
12. Horner BM, Cina RA, Wikiel KJ, Lima B, Ghazi A, Lo DP, Yamada K, Sachs DH, Huang CA. Predictors of organ allograft tolerance following hematopoietic cell transplantation. Am J Transplant Off J Am Soc Transplant Am Soc Transplant Surg. 2006;6:2894–902.
13. Almeida-Porada G, Porada C, Gupta N, Torabi A, Thain D, Zanjani ED. The human-sheep chimeras as a model for human stem cell mobilization and evaluation of hematopoietic grafts' potential. Exp Hematol. 2007;35:1594–600.
14. Porada CD, Harrison-Findik DD, Sanada C, Valiente V, Thain D, Simmons PJ, Almeida-Porada G, Zanjani ED. Development and characterization of a novel CD34 monoclonal antibody that identifies sheep hematopoietic stem/progenitor cells. Exp Hematol. 2008;36:1739–49.
15. McCullough J, Clay M, Herr G, Smith J, Stroncek D. Effects of granulocyte-colony-stimulating factor on potential normal granulocyte donors. Transfusion. 1999;39:1136–40.
16. Michon B, Moghrabi A, Winikoff R, Barrette S, Bernstein ML, Champagne J, David M, Duval M, Hume HA, Robitaille N, et al. Complications of apheresis in children. Transfusion. 2007;47:1837–42.
17. Siller-Matula JM, Plasenzotti R, Spiel A, Quehenberger P, Jilma B. Interspecies differences in coagulation profile. Thromb Haemost. 2008;100:397–404.
18. Gertz MA, Wolf RC, Micallef IN, Gastineau DA. Clinical impact and resource utilization after stem cell mobilization failure in patients with multiple myeloma and lymphoma. Bone Marrow Transplant. 2010;45:1396–403.
19. Filardo G, Perdisa F, Roffi A, Marcacci M, Kon E. Stem cells in articular cartilage regeneration. J Orthop Surg Res. 2016;11:42.
20. Shaw SW, Blundell MP, Pipino C, Shangaris P, Maghsoudiou P, Ramachandra DL, Georgiades F, Boyd M, Thrasher AJ, Porada CD, et al. Sheep CD34+ amniotic fluid cells have haematopoeitic potential and engraft after autologous in utero transplantation. Stem Cells. 2015;33:122–32.
21. Olivero S, Alario T, Ladaique P, Haccoun M, Viens P, Blaise D, Chabannon C. CD34+ cell enumeration in peripheral blood and apheresis samples, using two laboratory diagnostic kits or an institutional protocol. Bone Marrow Transplant. 1999;23:387–94.

25

Brucellosis seroprevalence in ovine and caprine flocks in China during 2000–2018

Xuhua Ran, Xiaohong Chen†, Miaomiao Wang†, Jiajia Cheng, Hongbo Ni, Xiao-Xuan Zhang* and Xiaobo Wen*

Abstract

Background: Brucellosis remains one of the most common zoonotic diseases globally, with more than half million human cases reported annually. Brucellosis is an emerging and re-emerging disease in China since the 1990s. An infectious reservoir constituted by domestic animals with brucellosis, especially ovine and caprine herds, poses a significant threat to public health. The seroprevalence of brucellosis in sheep and goat flocks in a national context is unavailable so far. Therefore, we conducted this systematic review and meta-analysis to assess the overall status of brucellosis in sheep and goats in China in almost two decades.

Results: The pooled prevalence of brucellosis in ovine and caprine flocks in China increased in 2000–2009 (1.00%; 95% CI, 0.70–1.30) to 2010–2018 (3.20%; 95% CI, 2.70–3.60). The seroprevalence of brucellosis in sheep and goat flocks was higher in Eastern China, with 7.00% of positive rate, than that in any other region, especially Shandong province (18.70%). Brucellosis is highly endemic in some local regions. The high prevalence of brucellosis in agricultural regions is suggestive of a shift of geographic distribution. The pooled prevalence of brucellosis is higher in goat flocks than in sheep flocks in China.

Conclusions: The overall data in this meta-analysis demands comprehensive intervention measures and further surveillance to facilitate the control of brucellosis in livestock. Further studies aimed at evaluating the risk factors associated with spreads of brucellosis in domestic animals unaddressed so far, and sufficient epidemiological data is important to the exploration and understanding of the prevalent status of brucellosis throughout the country and to disease control.

Keywords: Brucellosis, Prevalence, Systematic review, Meta-analysis, China, Ovine and caprine

Background

Brucellosis is a highly contagious zoonotic disease caused by various species of the genus *Brucella* and poses a threat to public health; over half a million cases of the disease are reported annually [1, 2]. Meanwhile, brucellosis causes significant economic losses to the animal industry worldwide because it usually results in abortion, infertility and decrease in milk and meat production [3]. Brucellosis is effectively controlled in developed countries, [4, 5], but it remains endemic in some developing countries and regions, especially in Middle East [6, 7], Africa [8–10], Central America [11] or Latin America [12] and Asia including China [13–15], where the seroprevalence and incidence of human brucellosis are also increasing or even highly prevalent despite great efforts for the prevention and control of disease [16].

To date, brucellosis has been reported in 30 of the 32 provinces or autonomous regions of China [17, 18], where northeast China and northwest China appear to be severely afflicted by brucellosis that affects humans [19, 20] and domestic animals [21, 22]. In the last decade, the increasing demand of dairy products, including goat milk and corresponding material for industrial production, and the blind expansion of farming scale, have promoted investments in domestic animal ranching in mainland China and have dramatically increased the frequency of transport of breeding animals, which may

* Correspondence: zhangxiaoxuan1988@126.com; wenxiaobo1977@163.com
†Xiaohong Chen and Miaomiao Wang contributed equally to this work.
College of Animal Science & Veterinary Medicine, Heilongjiang Bayi Agricultural University, No.5, XinFeng Rd., Saertu District, Daqing City 163319, Heilongjiang Province, China

have accelerated the spread of *Brucella* and increased the prevalence of brucellosis. Thus, humans, especially herdsmen and veterinarians, are at increased risk of being exposed to *Brucella* [23–25]. Additionally, a study has confirmed that 79.4% of the patients with brucellosis had histories of having close contact with domestic animals [26]. During the past decade, new cases of human brucellosis have been reported, and the disease had a dramatic geographic expansion from Northern China [27]. Furthermore, non-occupational exposure may have been common because of the easy movement of animals and acquirement of animal food from brucellosis-endemic regions. Presently, brucellosis in domestic animals is the major cause of human infection. Thus, a substantial decline in the incidence rate of human brucellosis is expected when the prevalence of brucellosis is controlled by eliminating positive-animal reservoirs [1].

Human brucellosis is mainly caused by exposure to *Brucella*-infected livestock, aborted materials or their products or by consuming unpasteurized food contaminated by *Brucella* spp., especially milk or milk products of sheep and goats [28]. Moreover, the high incidence of human brucellosis is associated with the high density of sheep and goats and not with the high density of swine and cattle [29]. Among the nine known *Brucella* species, *B. melitensis* is the most virulent and invasive [30]. The epidemiological studies revealed that 84.5% of the 634 strains isolated from the patients with brucellosis are *B. melitensis* [31]. Therefore, the prevention and control of brucellosis in small ruminants will contribute to decline of human brucellosis incidence, especially in the endemic regions of China. However, epidemiological data is the first prerequisite for the implementation of a comprehensive campaign aimed at controlling brucellosis throughout the country. To the best of our knowledge, no study has estimated the seroprevalence of brucellosis in ovine and caprine flocks in China. Therefore, we conducted this systematic review and meta-analysis to evaluate the incidence of brucellosis in ovine and caprine herds in China. Our study may facilitate the prevention and control of the diseases associated with various species of *Brucella*.

Results

Studies included

A total of 1627 relevant articles related to *Brucella* infection were retrieved, from which 66 articles were selected for quantitative analysis (Fig. 1 and Additional file 1). Then, 51 papers were excluded because the species in the studies were not described. The quality of the articles was evaluated according to the following criteria: content of articles, prevalence of brucellosis, purpose of research, and comprehensiveness of data presented in the selected studies, 25 papers were scored to be high quality (3 or 4 points), 20 scored medium quality (2 points), and the 21 papers were classified into the low quality (0 or 1 point) (Additional file 1).

Publication Bias

The extent of publication bias in the selected studies was measured and demonstrated by the funnel plot (Additional file 1, Figs. 2 and 3, respectively). The medium asymmetry was confirmed. Each of the selected paper had a slight publication bias, which may have likely affected the analysis (Table 1).

Pooled seroprevalence of brucellosis in ovine and caprine in China

Our systematic review and meta-analysis based on 66 studies with 1,634,742 clinical samples demonstrated

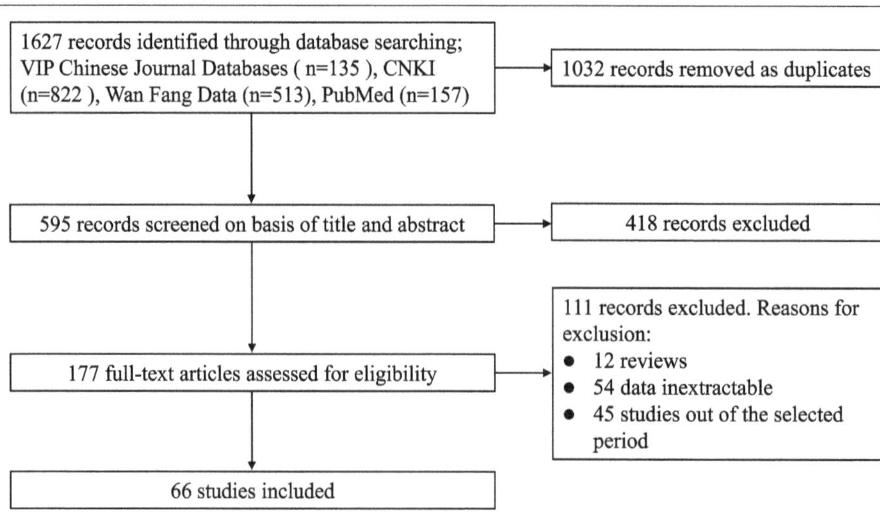

Fig. 1 Flow diagram of literature search and selection

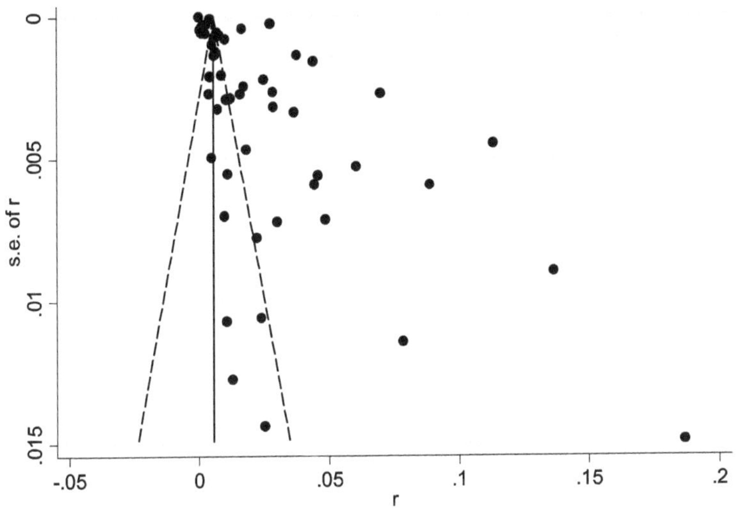

Fig. 2 Funnel plot with pseudo 95% confidence limits for examination of publication bias

that seroprevalence of brucellosis in ovine and caprine flocks at the country level was 2.30% (95% CI 2.00–2.60) from 2000 to 2018 when the samples were harvested in various studies (Table 1). The prevalence rate of brucellosis between 2000 and 2009 was 1.00% (95% CI 0.70–1.30). Meanwhile, between 2010 and 2018, the seroprevalence reached 3.20% (95% CI 2.70–3.60), demonstrating significantly increasing infection by *Brucella* spp. in ovine and caprine flocks in China ($P < 0.001$).

Pooled brucellosis seroprevalence in administrative districts or provinces of China

We aimed to evaluate the seroprevalence of *Brucella* spp. and distribution of brucellosis in China. However, most studies or sample origins were focused on northwest (42/66) and southwest China (10/66), where the populations of sheep and goats accounts for an overwhelming majority compared with the populations in other regions in China. The distribution of the samples covered 16 provinces or the regions of 32 provinces of China. Epidemiological data regarding the seroprevalence of brucellosis in other provinces are currently unavailable because the distribution of ovine and caprine herds in China is unbalanced during decades.

Our analysis demonstrated that the pooled brucellosis positive rate in ovine and caprine flocks in Eastern China was 7.00% (95% CI 0–17.40%), higher than that in other regions of China (Table 1). Comparatively, the regions where the positive rate of brucellosis was higher than 5.00% included Northeast China and Southwest China (5.60 and 5.30%, respectively). At the province level, the seroprevalence in Shandong province was the highest (18.70, 95% CI 15.80–21.60%), followed by Jilin, Guizhou and Yunnan (8.90, 5.80 and 5.30%, respectively; Table 2 and Additional file 1 Fig. 4).

Brucellosis seroprevalence based on various of diagnostic tests

The majority of studies included in this systematic review and meta-analysis evaluated positive rate by using SAT (48/66) with pooled 2.20% seroprevalence during 2000–2018, and 18 of the 66 studies conducted assessment by using RBPT and pooled 2.80% positive rate during the period.

Seroprevalence of brucellosis in ovine or caprine flocks

The seroprevalence of brucellosis was significantly higher in goats than in sheep (3.50% vs. 1.80%, $P < 0.001$). Sheep is the predominant breeding species in some regions, especially in Inner Mongolia, which has the largest sheep population in China (18.2% of flocks) [32]. In this meta-analysis, the number of samples from sheep was approximately 8 times of that of goats (Table 1 and Additional file 1), and the number of samples from sheep of Inner Mongolia accounted for more than half of the total samples tested (Table 1 and Additional file 1).

Discussion

Brucellosis is one of the most widespread zoonoses globally, especially in undeveloped countries and regions, and causes significant social and economic burden to humans or livestock industry annually [33]. Brucellosis in domestic animals is the major source of human infection, and high incidence of human brucellosis is associated with high density of sheep and goats rather than of swine and cattle [29]. Therefore, detailed knowledge of the epidemiological status of brucellosis in sheep and goats has become crucial to the assessment of effective prevention measures against brucellosis in human or domestic animals. To the best of our knowledge, the study

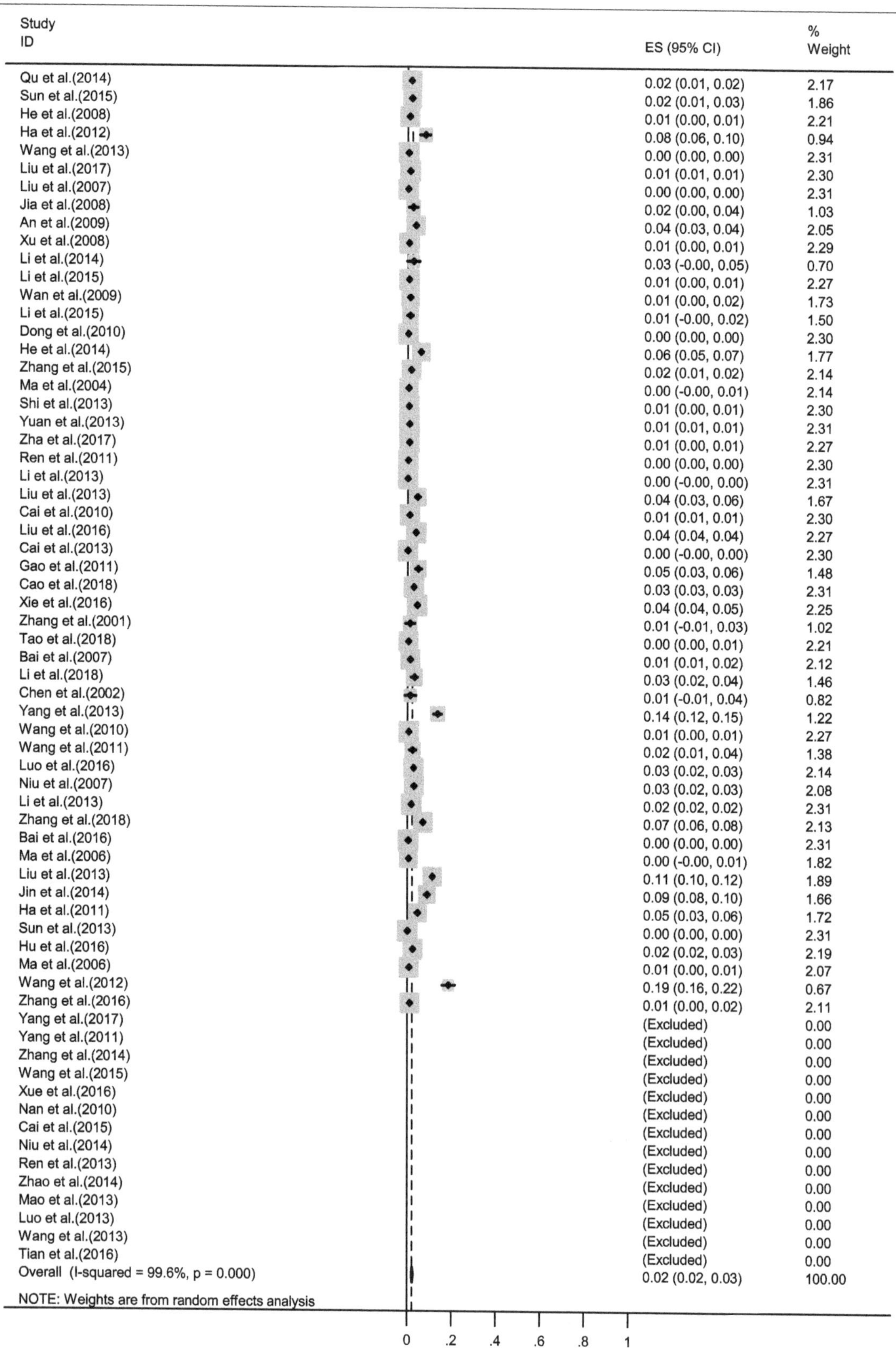

Fig. 3 Forest plot of prevalence of brucellosis in ovine and caprine flocks amongst studies conducted in China

Table 1 Association of different variables in the seroprevalence of brucellosis in ovine and caprine in China

	Variables	No. studies	No. samples	No. Positive	Rate (%) (95% CI)	Heterogeneity		
						χ^2	*P*-value	I^2 (%)
Region	Northeast China*	2	2651	211	5.60 (0-12.10)	46.10	0.000	97.8%
	Northern China	3	846759	3663	3.20 (0-6.60)	84.81	0.000	97.6%
	Northwest China	42	644113	13592	1.40 (1.00-1.80)	8545.14	0.000	99.6%
	Eastern China	4	1066	130	7.00 (0-17.40)	106.33	0.000	98.1%
	Southern China	3	6296	129	2.00 (0.50-3.60)	17.10	0.000	94.2%
	Central China	2	1796	30	1.90 (0-3.80)	6.39	0.012	84.3%
	Southwest China	10	132061	3814	5.30 (3.60-7.10)	1286.40	0.000	99.5%
Sampling year	2010-2018	47	1474801	19540	3.20 (2.70-3.60)	11402.65	0.000	99.7%
	2000-2009	24	159941	2029	1.00 (0.70-1.30)	1367.24	0.000	98.4%
Method	SAT	48	1607691	21115	2.20 (1.90-2.50)	12495.11	0.000	99.7%
	RBPT	18	27051	454	2.80 (1.90-3.80)	219.96	0.000	95.5%
Species	Goat	28	188687	4246	3.50 (2.80-4.10)	2835.30	0.000	99.3%
	Sheep	45	1446055	17323	1.80 (1.50-2.20)	9705.32	0.000	99.6%
	Total	66	1634742	21569	2.30 (2.00-2.60)	12732.79	0.000	99.6%

CI Confidence interval, *SAT* Serum agglutination test; *RBPT* Rose Bengal plate test
*Northeast China: Heilongjiang, Jilin, Liaoning; Northern China: Inner Mongolia, Shanxi, Hebei, Beijing, Tianjin; Northwest China: Xinjiang, Qinghai, Gansu, Ningxia, Shaanxi; Eastern China: Shandong, Anhui, Jiangxi, Jiangsu, Zhejiang, Shanghai, Fujian; Southern China: Guangxi, Guangdong, Shenzhen, Hainan, Macao, Hong Kong; Central China: Henan, Hunan, Hubei; Southwest China: Tibet, Yunnan, Guizhou, Sichuan, Chongqing

is the first to report the seroprevalence of brucellosis in ovine and caprine flocks in China.

In this systematic review and meta-analysis, we demonstrated that Eastern China has the highest seroprevalence of brucellosis in sheep and goat flocks. This region is considered a Type II general epidemic region implicated by brucellosis. Thus, a shift in the geographic distribution of brucellosis occurred from the traditional pastoral regions of Northern China to agricultural or semi-agricultural regions. In Eastern China, sheep and goat flocks in Shandong province represented the highest seroprevalence of the diseases (18.70%) [34]. Only one study regarding the prevalence of brucellosis that included in this analysis was conducted in Shandong

Table 2 Estimated pooled seroprevalence of brucellosis in ovine and caprine by provincial regions in China

Province	Region	No. tested	No. positive	Rate (%)	95% CI
Liaoning	Northeast China	360	8	2.20	0.70–3.70
Jilin	Northeast China	2291	203	8.90	7.70–10.00
Inner Mongolia	Northern China	846,759	3663	3.20	0–6.60
Gansu	Northwest China	432,433	11,697	2.40	0.80–4.10
Shaanxi	Northwest China	43,443	131	0.30	0.20–0.40
Ningxia	Northwest China	4000	0	0	–
Xinjiang	Northwest China	75,658	1292	2.40	1.60–3.20
Qinghai	Northwest China	88,579	472	0.60	0.40–0.80
Henan	Central China	1796	30	1.90	0–3.80
Shandong	Eastern China	685	128	18.70	15.80–21.60
Anhui	Eastern China	93	1	1.10	0–3.20
Fujian	Eastern China	288	1	1.30	0–3.80
Yunnan	Southwest China	98,895	2160	5.30	0.70–9.80
Guizhou	Southwest China	16,639	928	5.80	2.20–9.30
Guangxi	Southern China	6296	129	2.00	0.50–3.60
Chongqing	Southern China	16,527	726	4.40	4.10–4.70

CI Confidence interval

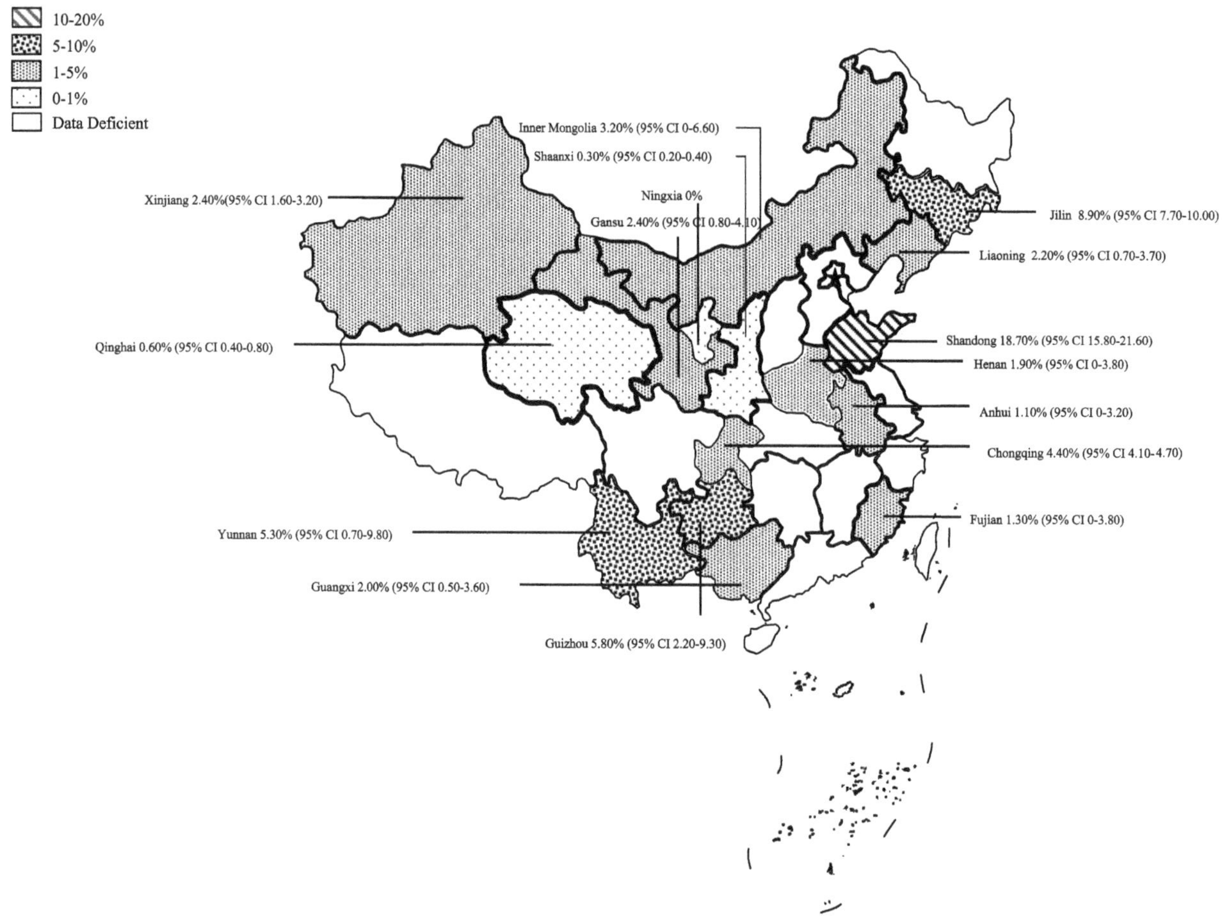

Fig. 4 Map of prevalence of brucellosis in ovine and caprine flocks in China

province during the selected period. In that study, the number of sheep and goats was 685 (sheep 315 and goats 370, respectively) (Additional file 1). Moreover, the seropositive rate in the local area reached 32.3%, and the overall seropositive rates were 27.6 and 11.1% in sheep and goat flocks, respectively. Our systematic review indicates that brucellosis is highly endemic in some local regions, and thus a comprehensive surveillance of wide geographic regions is required for understanding the overall seroprevalence of brucellosis in domestic animals in this region. Livestock vaccination in endemic regions might be effective in controlling brucellosis according to the National Mid-Term and Long-Term Animal Disease Control Plan of China (2012–2020) [35]. Meanwhile, throughout China, the pooled seroprevalence of brucellosis was lower in sheep herds than in goat flocks (1.80% vs. 3.50%; Table 1), though the seroprevalence of brucellosis in sheep flocks was higher in some local areas. Some epidemiological surveys demonstrated that the prevalence of the disease was higher in goat flocks than in sheep herds in some countries [36–38]. Furthermore, the data represented that the prevalence in flocks with sheep and goats was two times higher than flocks with sheep or goats alone [36]. Given that caprine brucellosis is a neglected disease in some countries, including China, especially in agricultural regions, breeding ovine is exclusively predominant in some regions or local areas in China. However, caprine brucellosis might pose a significant threat to public health and animal industry.

In China, some indigenous sheep or goat species are the exclusive species of livestock breeding for local ranches or farms, especially in Xinjiang and Qinghai provinces of China. Species related to brucellosis prevalence monitored in numerous studies were not elucidated, and thus these papers were excluded. Therefore, the authentic incidence of brucellosis might be underestimated in some regions. Moreover, sheep populations are overwhelmingly predominant in major pasturing areas in China similar to Inner Mongolia, Xinjiang and Qinghai provinces, which are categorized as Type I brucellosis severe epidemic regions in China. In these regions, most human brucellosis cases were transmitted by sheep-type *Brucella*, and the dominant strain was *B. melitensis*. Epidemiological data revealed that 84.5% of

Brucella strains isolated from the patients with brucellosis in China are *B. melitensis* [31]. From 1996 to 2010, 90.25% or more of the total 78,246 human brucellosis cases were caused by sheep-originated *Brucella* [21]. Furthermore, epidemiological studies confirmed that 99% of patients in Italy were infected by *B. melitensis* [30], indicating that sheep with brucellosis pose much more threat to humans than other species. Therefore, the prevention and control of brucellosis in sheep flocks are expected to reduce the incidence of human brucellosis in endemic areas, including Inner Mongolia of China, which accounts for 47.2% of new cases of human brucellosis in China in 2010 [21].

Additionally, Heilongjiang province was considered a Type I brucellosis severe epidemic region in Northern China besides Inner Mongolia and Jilin province. The incidence of human brucellosis in Heilongjiang province was 5.92 per 100,000 population in 2004, although the annual incidence of human brucellosis dramatically reached 19.45 per 100,000 population in 2012, which is the second highest after Inner Mongolia in China [20]. Notwithstanding the high prevalence of human brucellosis in Heilongjiang province of China and the importance of sheep and goat reservoirs to the spread of brucellosis, epidemiological data on the seroprevalence of brucellosis in sheep and goats in Heilongjiang province is deficient, suggesting that comprehensive epidemiological surveillance combined with intervention measures in domestic animals, especially in sheep and goat flocks, is necessary for disease control. Additionally, the milk goat industry in Heilongjiang province has been developing, and thus the comprehensive surveillance of disease in domestic animals and humans, especially diseases associated with occupational exposure, has become increasingly important.

The systematic review revealed that the selected studies for brucellosis surveillance in ovine and caprine flocks were implemented with SAT or RBPT, both of which have lower specificity and sensitivity compared with the methods recommended by WHO (indirect ELISA and fluorescent polarization assay) [39, 40]. The pooled seroprevalence based on our meta-analysis may not be consistent with the authentic incidence of brucellosis in some regions or provinces because of the limitation in the serological test used in the selected studies and agglutination tests, including SAT and RBPT, are commonly used for diagnosing acute brucellosis, which are not suitable for chronic brucellosis and infection caused by *B. canis* [41]. Therefore, the seroprevalence of brucellosis in sheep and goats in the selected regions might have been underestimated. However, we believe that this meta-analysis presented the status and tendency of brucellosis in ovine and caprine flocks in China during the periods.

Our meta-analysis has several limitations. First, there are chances that not all the publications related to sheep and goat brucellosis were included during document retrieval from the selected databases, although numerous searching MeSHs were used, partially because of the keyword selection in publication itself. Second, the risk factors associated with the incidence of brucellosis widespread of *Brucella* spp. were unavailable in the majority of the selected papers. Thus, the associated risk factors involved in brucellosis in sheep or goat flocks in China can not be further analyzed in this study.

Conclusion

We conducted a systematic review and meta-analysis to assess the prevalence of brucellosis in ovine and caprine flocks in China. The prevalence of brucellosis in ovine and caprine flocks in China shows a tendency to rise and highly endemic in some regions in China. The higher prevalence of brucellosis in agricultural regions is suggestive of a shift of geographic distribution. The pooled prevalence of brucellosis is higher in goat flocks than in sheep in China. The overall data demands intervention measures, including vaccination and enhanced public awareness, and further surveillance for the control of brucellosis in livestock. Further studies that are aimed at evaluating the risk factors associated with the spread of brucellosis in domestic animals and sufficient epidemiological data are crucial to the exploration of the epidemiology of the disease throughout the country.

Methods

Search strategy

We performed a systematic search across four electronic databases: VIP Chinese Journal Databases, China National Knowledge Infrastructure (CNKI), Wan Fang Data and PubMed with the following Mesh terms and key word subject heading “brucellosis”, "*Brucella*" or their various short terms in Chinese, or synonymous terms “brucellosis” and synonymous terms of brucellosis, “Malta fever”, “Mediterranean fever”, “Mediterranean remittent fever”, “Undulant fever”, “Gibraltar fever”, “Rock fever” or “Neapolitan fever” and “seroprevalence”, “prevalence”, “surveillance” “epidemiological survey”, “sheep or ovine”, “goat or caprine” and “China” were included during searching in PubMed. We focused on studies about the brucellosis seroprevalence of natural infection in ovine and caprine flocks in China. The samples in these studies were collected from January 1, 2000 to June 1, 2018. The reviews, duplicate reports, studies for other species (e.g., human, cattle, swine, bison, dog, water buffalo, yak, deer and takins) and evaluation of vaccine efficacy in herds were excluded, as well as studies and reports that only reported seroprevalence without primary data, had sample size of < 30, included regions out of China and modelling studies. Additionally, the studies in which the diagnostic methods or species were not clearly described was also excluded from this analysis.

Literature screening and data extraction

Reviewers independently extracted and recorded data from each selected study. Any disagreement between the reviewers or uncertainty about the eligibility of a study was further evaluated by additional reviewers. Information was recorded as follows: the first author, the year of sample isolation, year of publication, location of flocks, diagnostic tests, the number of tested sheep or goats, and the number of seropositive animals. Moreover, we neither contacted the authors of the original studies for additional information nor identified unpublished data. The data collection form that was used for this analysis is presented in Additional file 1.

Quality assessment

The quality of the eligible publications was estimated according to the criteria derived from the Grading of Recommendations Assessment, Development and Evaluation method. The quality of the publications was graded by using a scoring approach. Briefly, the score for each of the following items was determined as 1 point when information was elaborated: object, detection method used, sampling time and classification of a subgroup in a study. Papers would be assigned 0–4 points on the basis of score criterion. Studies with 3–4 points were considered high quality, those with 2 points were deemed moderate and those with scores of 0–1 point was designated as low quality.

Statistical analysis

The pooled seroprevalence of brucellosis in ovine and caprine based on publications by numerous studies were calculated by meta-analysis. Heterogeneity in the qualified studies was expected, and thus a random-effects model was used for the calculation and preparation of the forest plots with the code of "generate ser=sqrt(r*(1-r)/n); metan r ser, random label (namevar=study)" with Stata 12 (Stata Corp. College station, Texas). The heterogeneity was anticipated in advance, and statistical methods with I^2 and Cochrane Q (represented as χ^2 and P values) statistics were used for the assessment of the variations. The potential sources of heterogeneity were further investigated by subgroup and meta-regression analyses. The factors associated with heterogeneity in this study were examined on the basis of an individual model or multiple-variable models. Basically, the factors include sampling year (comparison between sample harvesting time of before 2010 [2000–2009] with that of 2010 or later [2010–2018]), administrative districts or regions, diagnostic methods (serum agglutination test [SAT] VS. Rose Bengal plate test [RBPT]). The meta-analysis was performed according to the PRISMA guideline [42] and the confidence intervals of the seroprevalence of brucellosis were calculated using Woolf's method with Stata program.

Abbreviations

ELISA: Enzyme-linked immunosorbent assay; RBPT: Rose Bengal plate test; SAT: Serum agglutination test

Acknowledgments

Not Applicable.

Funding

This work was supported by National Key R&D Program of China (2018YFD0500900). The funder had no role in the design of the study and collection, analysis, and interpretation of data and in preparation of this manuscript.

Author's contributions

XR and XXZ contributed to conception and design of this analysis. XC and MW reviewed records, JC and HN analyzed the data. XXZ and XW re-analyzed the disagreements. XXZ conducted statistical analysis. XR and XW prepared the manuscript. All authors reviewed the manuscript and approved the submission.

Author's information

Not Applicable.

Consent for publication

Not Applicable.

Competing interests

The authors declare no competing interests.

References

1. Seleem MN, Boyle SM, Sriranganathan N. Brucellosis: a re-emerging zoonosis. Vet Microbiol. 2010;140(3–4):392–8.
2. Pappas G, Papadimitriou P, Akritidis N, Christou L, Tsianos EV. The new global map of human brucellosis. Lancet Infect Dis. 2006;6(2):91–9.
3. Rossetti CA, Arenas-Gamboa AM, Maurizio E. Caprine brucellosis: a historically neglected disease with significant impact on public health. PLoS Negl Trop Dis. 2017;11(8):e0005692.
4. Savini L, Candeloro L, Conte A, De Massis F, Giovannini A. Development of a forecasting model for brucellosis spreading in the Italian cattle trade network aimed to prioritise the field interventions. PLoS One. 2017;12(6): e0177313.
5. Aznar MN, Samartino LE, Humblet MF, Saegerman C. Bovine brucellosis in Argentina and bordering countries: update. Transbound Emerg Dis. 2014; 61(2):121–33.
6. Refai M. Incidence and control of brucellosis in the near east region. Vet Microbiol. 2002;90(1–4):81–110.
7. Musallam II, Abo-Shehada MN, Hegazy YM, Holt HR, Guitian FJ. Systematic review of brucellosis in the Middle East: disease frequency in ruminants and humans and risk factors for human infection. Epidemiol Infect. 2016;144(4): 671–85.
8. Maurice NA, Wungak SY, Gana BA, Nanven MB, Ngbede EO, Ibrahim A, et al. Seroprevalence of bovine brucellosis in northern plateau state, north Central Nigeria. Asian Pacific Journal of Tropical Disease. 2013;3(5):337–40.

9. Ducrotoy M, Bertu WJ, Matope G, Cadmus S, Conde-Alvarez R, Gusi AM, et al. Brucellosis in sub-Saharan Africa: current challenges for management, diagnosis and control. Acta Trop. 2017;165:179–93.
10. Vhoko K, Iannetti S, Burumu J, Ippoliti C, Bhebhe B, De Massis F. Estimating the prevalence of brucellosis in cattle in Zimbabwe from samples submitted to the central veterinary laboratory between 2010 and 2014. Vet Ital. 2018;54(1):21–7.
11. Moreno E. Brucellosis in Central America. Vet Microbiol. 2002;90(1–4):31–8.
12. Lucero NE, Ayala SM, Escobar GI, Jacob NR. Brucella isolated in humans and animals in Latin America from 1968 to 2006. Epidemiol Infect. 2008;136(4): 496–503.
13. Erdenebaatar J, Bayarsaikhan B, Yondondorj A, Watarai M, Shirahata T, Jargalsaikhan E, et al. Epidemiological and serological survey of brucellosis in Mongolia by ELISA using sarcosine extracts. Microbiol Immunol. 2004; 48(8):571–7.
14. Wee SH, Nam HM, Kim CH. Emergence of brucellosis in cattle in the Republic of Korea. Vet Rec. 2008;162(17):556–7.
15. Yoon H, Moon OK, Lee SH, Lee WC, Her M, Jeong W, et al. Epidemiology of brucellosis among cattle in Korea from 2001 to 2011. J Vet Sci. 2014;15(4): 537–43.
16. Zolzaya B, Selenge T, Narangarav T, Gantsetseg D, Erdenechimeg D, Zinsstag J, et al. Representative seroprevalences of human and livestock brucellosis in two Mongolian provinces. EcoHealth. 2014;11(3):356–71.
17. Zhong Z, Yu S, Wang X, Dong S, Xu J, Wang Y, et al. Human brucellosis in the People's Republic of China during 2005-2010. Int J Infect Dis. 2013;17(5): e289–92.
18. Liu F, Li JM, Zeng FL, Zong Y, Leng X, Shi K, et al. Prevalence and risk factors of brucellosis, Chlamydiosis, and bluetongue among sika deer in Jilin Province in China. Vector Borne Zoonotic Dis. 2018;18(4):226–30.
19. Zhang J, Yin F, Zhang T, Yang C, Zhang X, Feng Z, et al. Spatial analysis on human brucellosis incidence in mainland China: 2004-2010. BMJ Open. 2014;4(4):e004470.
20. Zhang X, Wang Z, Mu G, Wang T. Brucellosis control in Northeast China: a long way to go. Public Health. 2015;129(8):1132–4.
21. Hou Q, Sun X, Zhang J, Liu Y, Wang Y, Jin Z. Modeling the transmission dynamics of sheep brucellosis in Inner Mongolia Autonomous Region, China. Math Biosci. 2013;242(1):51–8.
22. Zhou L, Fan M, Hou Q, Jin Z, Sun X. Transmission dynamics and optimal control of brucellosis in Inner Mongolia of China. Math Biosci Eng. 2018; 15(2):543–67.
23. Mufinda FC, Boinas F, Nunes C. Prevalence and factors associated with human brucellosis in livestock professionals. Rev Saude Publica. 2017;51:57.
24. Zhan BD, Wang SQ, Lai SM, Lu Y, Shi XG, Cao GP, et al. Outbreak of occupational brucellosis at a pharmaceutical factory in Southeast China. Zoonoses Public Health. 2017;64(6):431–7.
25. Ning C, Shuyi G, Tao Y, Hao Z, Zhang X. Epidemiological survey of human brucellosis in Inner Mongolia, China, 2010-2014: a high risk groups-based survey. J Infect Public Health. 2018;11(1):24–9.
26. Zheng R, Xie S, Lu X, Sun L, Zhou Y, Zhang Y, et al. A systematic review and meta-analysis of epidemiology and clinical manifestations of human brucellosis in China. Biomed Res Int 2018; 2018:5712920.
27. Chen JD, Ke CW, Deng X, Jiang S, Liang W, Ke BX, et al. Brucellosis in Guangdong Province, People's Republic of China, 2005-2010. Emerg Infect Dis. 2013;19(5):817–8.
28. Casalinuovo F, Ciambrone L, Cacia A, Rippa P. Contamination of bovine, sheep and goat meat with Brucella Spp. Ital J Food Saf. 2016;5(3):5913.
29. Li YJ, Li XL, Liang S, Fang LQ, Cao WC. Epidemiological features and risk factors associated with the spatial and temporal distribution of human brucellosis in China. BMC Infect Dis. 2013;13:547.
30. De Massis F, Di Girolamo A, Petrini A, Pizzigallo E, Giovannini A. Correlation between animal and human brucellosis in Italy during the period 1997-2002. Clin Microbiol Infect. 2005;11(8):632–6.
31. Deqiu S, Donglou X, Jiming Y. Epidemiology and control of brucellosis in China. Vet Microbiol. 2002;90(1–4):165–82.
32. Pu D, Li L, Zhao H, Cui B. Epidemic situation analysis of human brucellosis in Inner Mongolia during 1952 to 2007. Chin J Control Endem Dis 2009(4): 420–423.
33. Dean AS, Crump L, Greter H, Schelling E, Zinsstag J. Global burden of human brucellosis: a systematic review of disease frequency. PLoS Negl Trop Dis. 2012;6(10):e1865.
34. Wang Q. Seroepidemiology Survey of Brucellosis, Foot-and-Mouth disease and Hepatitis E in Sheep and Goats in part areas of Shandong. Master. Shandong Agricultural University; 2012 (In Chinese).
35. General Office of State Council, People's Republic of China: National mid-term and long-term animal disease control plan of China, 2012–2020. People's Republic of China. :http://www.gov.cn/zwgk/2012-05/25/content_2145581.htm. Accessed 14 Aug 2018.
36. Alhamada AG, Habib I, Barnes A, Robertson I. Risk factors associated with Brucella Seropositivity in sheep and goats in Duhok Province, Iraq. Veterinary sciences. 2017;4(4). https://doi.org/10.3390/vetsci4040065.
37. Sintayehu G, Melesse B, Abayneh D, Sintayehu A, Melaku S, Alehegne W, et al. Epidemiological survey of brucellosis in sheep and goats in selected pastoral and agro-pastoral lowlands of Ethiopia. Rev Sci Tech. 2015;34(3): 881–93.
38. Tadesse G. Brucellosis Seropositivity in animals and humans in Ethiopia. A meta-analysis. PLoS Negl Trop Dis. 2016;10(10):e0005006.
39. Franco MP, Mulder M, Gilman RH, Smits HL. Human brucellosis. Lancet Infect Dis. 2007;7(12):775–86.
40. Corbel MJ, Alton GG, Banai M, Diaz R, Dranovskaia BA. Brucellosis in humans and animals. In. Edited by FAO, WHO. Geneva: WHO Press; 2006.
41. Acha NP, Szyfres B. Zoonoses and communicable diseases common to man and animals, vol. 1, 3rd. EDN Washington, DC.: Pan American Health Organization (PAHO); 2003.
42. Shamseer L, Moher D, Clarke M, Ghersi D, Liberati A, Petticrew M, et al. Preferred reporting items for systematic review and meta-analysis protocols (PRISMA-P) 2015: elaboration and explanation. BMJ. 2015;350:g7647.

26

Preliminary reference intervals and the impact of citrate storage time for thrombelastography in cats including delta and the velocity curve

Carolin Engelen[1*], Andreas Moritz[1], Franziska Barthel[2] and Natali Bauer[1]

Abstract

Background: Thrombelastography is a useful tool in assessment of hemostasis. Beside the traditional variables, the velocity curve and the variable delta have lately earned attention. The velocity curve provides knowledge about the speed of clot formation including information about thrombin generation. Delta, which only reflects enzymatic coagulation, allows the determination of the origin of hypercoagulability when compared to clot rigidity, a variable that reflects both platelet and enzymatic activity. The aim was to establish preliminary reference intervals for feline thrombelastography including the velocity curve variables and delta obtained after 60 min of storage including the assessment of coefficients of variation. Furthermore, the effect of citrate storage time (30 versus 60 min) on feline thrombelastography will be determined.

Results: Prolonged storage times significantly reduced reaction (R) ($P = 0.019$) and clotting (K) ($P = 0.008$) times, split point (SP) ($P = 0.019$) and time to maximum rate of thrombus generation (TMRTG) ($P = 0.023$) values whereas maximum rate of thrombus generation (MRTG) significantly increased ($P = 0.040$). Preliminary reference intervals: R (min): 2.7–18.1; K (min): 0.8–3.9; alpha (°): 27.6–75.2; maximum amplitude (mm): 18.5–62.5; clot rigidity (dyn/cm^2): 1.2–8.2; coagulation index: −4.6 – 2.6; SP (min): 2.4–15.4; delta (min): 0.3–3.1; thrombus generation (mm/min): 255.3–751.2; MRTG (mm/min): 4.0–19.3; TMRTG (min): 3.5–22.0; maximum rate of lysis (mm/min): 0.0–4.7 and time to maximum rate of lysis (min): 0.4–55.8.

Conclusion: Storage for 60 versus 30 min induces hypercoagulable tracings including the velocity curve, some of which variables (MRTG, TMRTG) might function as sensitive markers for changes in the coagulation activity. Because of the impact of citrate storage time on thrombelastography, reference intervals have to be established using a specific and constant storage time in each laboratory.

Keywords: Feline, Hypercoagulable, TEG, Velocity curve

Background

Thrombelastography (TEG) is a global coagulation test that enables assessment of hemostatic function in whole blood combining plasma and cellular components of hemostasis [1–3]. Recently, the global integrity of the complex process of blood coagulation is preferably assessed by measurement of thrombin generation [4], which can be evaluated using the TEG velocity curve (VC) [4] thus gaining new attention in human and veterinary medicine. The VC is generated from the mathematical first derivative of TEG values and dynamically reflects the velocity of clot formation (positive curve above the horizontal axis) and clot dissolution (negative curve below the horizontal axis) [5, 6] as illustrated in Fig. 1. Variables generated from the curve of clot formation include the maximum rate of thrombus generation (MRTG) represented by the peak of this curve [5]. In human medicine, MRTG has been shown to increase exponentially compared with the non-exponential and thus less pronounced increase of TEG alpha as a traditional marker of clot

* Correspondence: Carolin.Engelen@vetmed.uni-giessen.de
[1]Department of Veterinary Clinical Sciences, Clinical Pathophysiology and Clinical Pathology, Justus-Liebig University Giessen, Frankfurterstraße 126, 35392 Giessen, Germany
Full list of author information is available at the end of the article

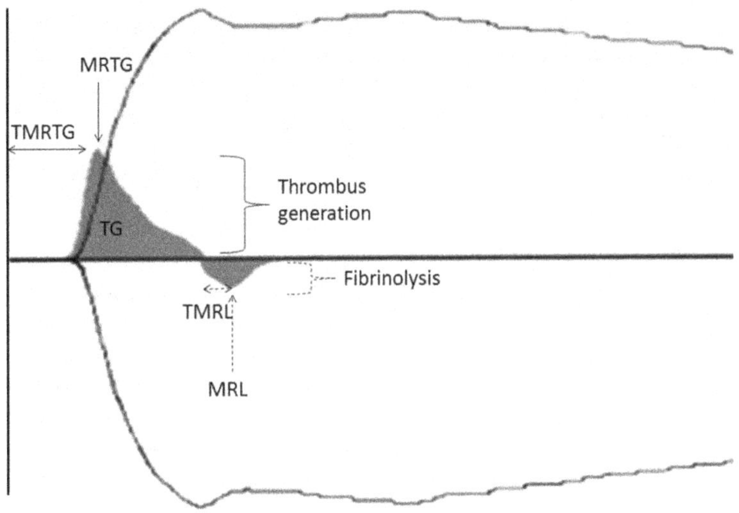

Fig. 1 Feline thrombelastography (TEG) showing the conventional tracing (black line) with superimposed velocity curve (gray solid curve). The gray curve above the horizontal axis reflects thrombus generation while the gray curve below represents fibrinolysis. Measurements that can be estimated include TMRTG (time to maximum rate of thrombus generation; min), MRTG (maximum rate of thrombus generation; mm/min), TG (thrombus generation; mm/min) from the area under the curve (AUC), TMRL (time to maximum rate of lysis; mm/min) and MRL (maximum rate of lysis; min)

formation, thus allowing a more precise evaluation of clot kinetics [7]. Other variables reflecting clot formation derived from the velocity curve include the time to maximum rate of thrombus generation (TMRTG), defined as the distance on the x-axis from zero to the peak of the curve, and the thrombus generation (TG), which is calculated from the area under the curve and represents an indirect measurement of clot strength [5]. TMRTG is also believed to be a good marker of thrombin generation in humans and shows a linear correlation with the TEG parameter delta [6]. Delta is easily obtained from the TEG tracing by calculating the difference between two parameters R and SP of the traditional TEG curve [6] as shown in Fig. 2. Delta represents the greatest clot growth depending on peak thrombin generation, thus allowing the assessment of thrombin generation [6]. In people, the variable TG has been shown to correlate with thrombin-antithrombin complex values which serve as a marker of thrombin generation [4]. Values that can be obtained from the curve below the horizontal axis reflect fibrinolysis and include the maximum rate of lysis (MRL) represented by the negative peak of this curve and the time to maximum rate of lysis (TMRL), which is the represented on the x-axis from the start of the fibrinolysis curve to its negative peak [5].

The TEG software provides two modes of calculating the VC variables: first, VC variables can be calculated on the basis of the maximum amplitude (MA), a traditional TEG variable. Second, VC variables can be derived from the clot rigidity (G), which itself is calculated from MA and represents the global coagulation activity. Like MA, G is dependent on factor XIII activity, concentration of fibrinogen and thrombin, the platelet count and function, and hematocrit [8].

Both versions (MA and G version) of calculation result in slightly different curves and subsequently different results. Furthermore, the variable names differ: G version variables have a "G" appended to the end of the name, i.e. MRTGG instead of MRTG [9].

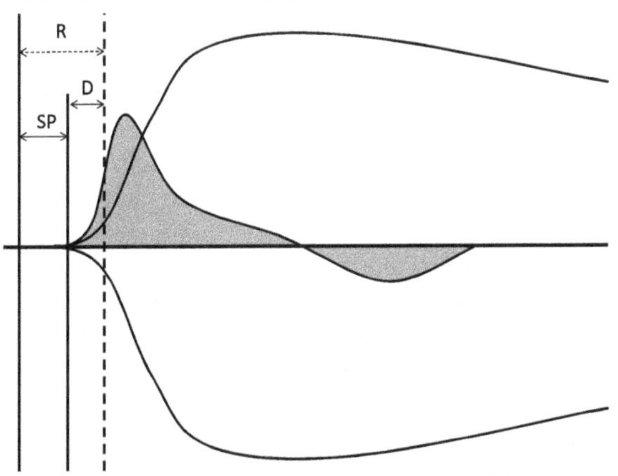

Fig. 2 Schematic representation of the variable delta (D; min; black arrow), which can be calculated from the difference between the reaction time (R; min; dotted arrow), i.e., the time from initiation of coagulation until the amplitude of the conventional TEG tracing reaches 2 mm and the split point (SP; min; longer black arrow), i.e., the time from starting the coagulation process until divergence of the TEG tracings from the zero line. The delta value = R - SP

From the clinical point of view, the TEG gained special interest for the evaluation of hypercoagulability [10], whereby it has an exceptional ability to detect individuals affected by or at risk for a thromboembolic event [10, 11]. In human medicine, hypercoagulable states measured by rapid thrombelastography have already been shown to be a good predictor of thromboembolic events [12]. To help differentiating the contribution of enzymatic activity (reflecting secondary hemostasis) and platelet reactivity (reflecting primary hemostasis) in hypercoagulable states, the novel variable delta which represents the enzymatic activity has been introduced [6]. In correlation with the variable G (reflecting both primary and secondary hemostasis), hypercoagulable states can be classified as predominantly caused by platelet hypercoagulability if the patients show a hypercoagulable G value and a normal delta [6]. Neither delta nor the VC variables have yet been evaluated in cats.

For interpretation of TEG results, pre-analytical factors such as the sample material and the time between sampling and TEG analysis have to be taken into account. Originally designed to be run with fresh whole blood [3, 13], TEG analysis in veterinary medicine is mostly done using re-calcified citrated whole blood [10, 14]. Because citrate does not entirely prevent thrombin generation since the generation of factor XIIa (via contact activation) is not dependent on calcium, contact activation is not inhibited in citrated samples and continues during storage, resulting in a certain degree of thrombin generation [8, 13]. Consequently, the citrate storage time has an impact on TEG results [13], as demonstrated previously for people, dogs and horses [3, 15–18]. The impact of citrate storage time on feline TEG is largely unknown. Even if a storage time of 30 min has been recommended [13] and has mostly been used in previous investigations in cats [19–24], a storage time of 60 min might be preferable in some clinical settings especially if samples are used for a variety of different coagulation tests.

Thus, one aim of this study was to establish preliminary reference intervals (RIs) including assessment of coefficients of variation (CVs) for traditional and novel feline TEG parameters using 60 min incubation. The second aim was to determine the effect of citrate storage time (30 versus 60 min) on TEG results which, to our knowledge, has not yet been done before in cats.

Methods

Study design

This prospective study was performed September 2015 and ethical approval has been given by the State Agency for Nature, Environment and Consumer Protection of North Rhine-Westphalia (LANUV NRW, reference number: 84–02.05.20.13.090, internal number: 200a176/232). Blood samples were collected from 21 clinically healthy adult domestic shorthair cats from Bayer Animal Health GmbH (Leverkusen, Germany) including 12 female and 9 male cats with a mean age of 12.3 months (range 12–13 months). The cats have been obtained from one breeder (Liberty Research, Waverly, US) and were kept under defined housing conditions in groups according to their gender. A commercially available food was fed (Josera Léger, Adult light, Kleinheubach, Germany) and water was available ad libitum.

Initial health status of the cats was determined through a routine physical examination. The blood was collected from the cephalic vein using a 21G needle (0.8 × 16.0 mm, Neolus needle, Terumo, Eschborn, Germany) and dropped into two 1.4-ml 3.2% sodium citrate tubes (S-Monovette®, 1.4-ml, 9NC, Sarstedt, Wedel, Germany) which were properly filled ensuring an ratio of blood to anticoagulant of 9:1. In a randomized order, one tube of citrated whole blood was used for TEG analysis. From the other tube, citrated plasma for a routine coagulation profile including thrombin time (TT), prothrombin time (PT), activated partial thromboplastin time (aPTT), fibrinogen concentration and D-Dimers was obtained within 20 min after sampling by centrifugation (Eppendorf 58 10 R, Eppendorf AG, Hamburg, Germany) for 10 min. The plasma was then transferred into plain tubes (Eppendorf Safe-Lock Tubes, Eppendorf AG, Hamburg, Germany) and frozen at −80 °C. For coagulation analyses, frozen samples were shipped on dry ice to the department of Veterinary Clinical Sciences, Clinical Pathophysiology and Clinical Pathology (Justus-Liebig University, Giessen, Germany), and stored at −80 °C until measurements were performed as batch on the automated coagulation analyzer STA Compact ® (Stago Germany, Düsseldorf, Germany) within a year after sample collection as described previously for dogs [25].

One week prior to the study, a complete blood count (CBC) measured with the automated hematology analyzer ADVIA® 120 Hematology System (Siemens HealthCare GmbH, Erlangen, Germany; software version: no. 1) which has been evaluated previously for cats [26] and a biochemistry profile (IDEXX Catalyst Dx®, IDEXX GmbH, Ludwigsburg, Germany) were performed. Results were compared with RIs provided by the manufacturer of the clinical chemistry analyzer. Cats were included in our study when they were considered healthy based on the physical examination and the absence of clinically relevant abnormalities of the hematological and blood chemical examination.

The hematocrit and platelet count were reevaluated from citrated blood at the day of blood sampling for TEG analysis. Results were corrected by the factor 1.1 to take the dilution of the sample with citrate into consideration. The hematocrit value was evaluated with the microhematocrit method after centrifugation of 5 min at

31,689 G using a microhematocrit-centrifuge ("Haematokrit 24", Hettich, Tuttlingen, Germany). The platelet count was estimated semiquantitatively by counting platelets in the monolayer of a May-Grünwald-Giemsa stained blood smear, whereby the mean of 10 high power fields (100× objective) was calculated and multiplied by a factor of 20 as previously recommended [27] to obtain the approximate platelet count ($\times 10^3/\mu l$). Thrombocytopenia was defined as values below 200 ($\times 10^3/\mu l$) [26]. When moderate to marked platelet clumping was seen, the assessed count was judged falsely low. Moderate to marked platelet clumping was defined as a high number of platelets within clumps that did not allow accurate counting of individual platelets [27]. As an addition to the size of clumps, the number of clumps was used to further classify the platelet clumping as low, moderate or high grade clumping. According to this classification, 13 cats were categorized as having low grade, 2 cats as moderate and 5 cats as having high grade platelet clumping.

TEG analysis

The analyses were always performed by the same person (CE) using three computerized TEG 5000 analyzers (Thrombelastograph, Haemonetics Corporation, Braintree, MA, USA). TEG analyses were done with recalcified whole blood stored at room temperature and according to the manufacturer recommendations. Briefly, standard TEG cups (Haemoscope Corporation) were placed in the 37 °C prewarmed instrument holder and filled with 20 µl of 0.2 M calcium chloride. After specific storage times of either 30 and/or 60 min respectively, 340 µl citrated whole blood was added and analysis was started. Each TEG analysis was performed for approximately 60 min and an electric internal quality control (e-test) was performed at least three times a day.

Blood from the first 10/21 cats was stored for 60 min before TEG analysis, which was run in duplicates using blood from the same tube to assess the variance. TEG assays for the remaining 11/21 cats were performed with blood taken from the same tubes after 30 and 60 min of storage time respectively to assess sample stability. One of these 11 cats had to be excluded from the study since TEG analysis only showed flat lines.

Evaluated TEG variables include the traditional variables: reaction time (R), clotting time (K), alpha, maximum amplitude (MA), clot rigidity (G), coagulation index (CI) and clot lysis at 30 min after MA is reached (LY30) as well as the novel measurements: SP, delta and the values from the velocity curve (TG, MRTG and TMRTG reflecting thrombin generation and MRL and TMRL reflecting clot lysis). The VC parameters used for all statistical analyses and figures were obtained from the MA version of calculation. For the sake of better comparison with other studies and potential future use by other investigators, reference intervals of VC parameters will be provided for both the G and MA version of calculation.

Statistical analysis

Preliminary RIs were established for a citrate storage time of 60 min. If samples were measured in duplicates (as done for assessment of variance), the first result was used. Data distribution regarding normality was assessed by reviewing the histogram and the QQ plot as well as using the Anderson-Darling test or a symmetry test for Robust provided by the software (Reference Value Advisor 2.1 [28]). For all variables except for TG and TMRL, a robust method after Box-Cox transformation (Reference Value Advisor 2.1 [28]) was used. For TG, the RI was calculated with a parametric method after Box-Cox transformation and RI for TMRL was established by use of a parametric method of untransformed data respectively. Mean, median, minimum and maximum values as well as standard deviation was determined from untransformed data. Pooled variance was used to assess the percentage of total variation that occurred between the duplicates.

For all statistical comparisons, a Shapiro-Wilk test was done in advance to evaluate the assumption of normality. The impact of citrate storage times was assessed using a paired t-test for alpha, G, CI, TG, MRTG and TMRTG and a Wilcoxon test for R, K, MA, LY30, SP, delta, TMRL, MRL respectively. Because of the low number of cats in the group of high grade clumping the assessment of normality is limited so the influence of platelet clumps on the results was assessed by a nonparametric test (Mann-Whitney U test) for all variables. For all analyses, a *p*-value <0.05 was considered significant.

Results

Hematological analyses

The platelet count (PLT) estimated from the blood smear showed a thrombocytopenia ($36–124 \times 10^3/\mu l$) in five cats, four of which (PLT: $44–124 \times 10^3/\mu l$) had marked aggregation on the blood smear so the count was considered falsely low. The remaining cat showing a thrombocytopenia ($36 \times 10^3/\mu l$) only had a moderate degree of platelet clumping. This cat did not show a thrombocytopenia on the CBC 1 week earlier and was clinically healthy without a history of bleeding so it was still included in the study.

Re-evaluation of the corrected hematocrit on day of sampling demonstrated no major abnormalities.

Analyses of plasmatic hemostasis

Mean, median, range and standard deviation for TT, PT, aPTT, fibrinogen and D-dimers are shown in Table 1.

Table 1 Results of the traditional coagulation profile obtained from 21 cats

Variable	TT (sec)	PT (sec)	aPTT (sec)	Fibrinogen (g/l)	D-dimers (μg/ml)
Mean	15.37	10.8	11.92	1.46	0.18
Median	15.4	10.8	12	1.48	0.2
Range	14–16.9	10.1–12.8	10.8–13	1.04–1.7	0.09–0.26
SD	0.82	0.56	0.74	0.17	0.05
RI (laboratory-internal[a])	13.4–19.1	9.9–12.2	10.8–14.0	0.6–2.2	0.0–0.3

Abbreviations: *SD* standard deviation, *RI* reference interval, *TT* thrombin time, *PT* prothrombin time, *aPTT* activated partial thromboplastin time, *sec* seconds
[a]For interpretation of the values, laboratory-internal reference intervals (RIs) established from 40 clinically healthy domestic shorthair cats using a robust method of untransformed data are additionally listed

Compared to the laboratory internal RIs which are also listed in Table 1, all values were considered normal denoting a physiological secondary hemostasis in all cats.

Preliminary RIs

One cat (1/21) had to be excluded because no TEG tracing could be obtained. This cat showed a marked aggregation of platelets on the blood smear and an estimated PLT count of $44 \times 10^3/\mu l$. The routine coagulation parameters were unremarkable in this cat.

Preliminary RIs, CVs as well as the mean, median, the standard deviation, minimum and maximum for the investigated TEG variables of citrated whole blood samples stored for 60 min are shown in Table 2.

Histograms of the distribution of all evaluated variables after Box Cox transformation (LY30) or untransformed data (all but LY30) are shown in Figs. 3 and 4. In one cat (1/20), the CI and K value were not reported by the TEG software and in another cat (1/20) no results for MRL and TMRL were obtained. For LY30, data distribution did not allow the calculation of a reliable RI.

The CV was <20% for the variables R, K, alpha, MA, G, SP, TG and MRTG. For the other evaluated variables (CI, LY30, delta, TMRTG, MRL and TMRL) CVs were ranging between 23.6% (delta) and 83.6% (CI) respectively. Statistical analysis did not reveal a significant difference between the first and the second measurement performed after a citrate storage time of 60 min for all assessed variables.

Impact of citrate storage time

As seen in Figs. 5 and 6, citrate storage time had a significant impact on many traditional and novel TEG variables. When evaluating the traditional TEG variables (Fig. 5), prolonged citrate storage time (60 versus 30 min) induced a significant decrease in median values of R (7 min. vs. 12.8 min., $P = 0.019$) and K (2.5 min. vs. 3.4 min., $P = 0.008$) respectively. Interestingly, a marked increase in inter-individual variation of LY30 was noted with increasing citrate storage time. Regarding the novel variables (Fig. 6), the TMRTG was significantly shorter (8.92 min. vs. 15.17 min., $P = 0.023$), the MRTG was significantly larger (8.03 mm/min vs. 6.26 mm/min, $P = 0.04$) and the SP was significantly smaller (5.9 min. vs. 11.4 min., P = 0.019) after 60 min when compared to results after 30 min of storage. Overall, these results reflect

Table 2 Shows preliminary reference intervals (RI) for all investigated trombelastography (TEG) variables

Variable (unit)	R (min)	K (min)	alpha (degree)	MA (mm)	G (dyn/cm²)	CI (unitless)	LY30 (%)	SP (min)	delta (min)	TG[a] (mm/min)	MRTG[a] (mm/min)	TMRTG[a] (min)	MRL[a] (mm/min)	TMRL[a] (min)
Number of cats (n)	20	19	20	20	20	19	20	20	20	20	20	20	19	19
RI	2.7–18.1	[b] 0.8–3.9	27.6–75.2	18.5–62.5	1.2–8.2	[b] −4.6 – 2.6	[c]	2.4–15.4	0.3–3.1	255.3–751.2	4.0–19.3	3.5–22.0	0.0–4.7	0.4–55.8
Minimum	2.8	1	26.1	18.2	1.1	−4.6	2.4	2.4	0.3	244.87	3.48	3.67	0.13	9.58
Maximum	18.7	3.6	74.9	61.4	8	2.5	15.8	15.8	2.9	735.09	19.28	22.5	4.37	56.08
Mean	7.6	2.3	57.6	46.3	4.6	−0.2	11.1	6.6	1.0	563.1	9.4	9.8	1.8	28.1
Median	6.6	2.3	58.1	47.3	4.5	0.1	6.6	5.8	0.9	588.5	8.5	8.8	1.8	22.4
SD	3.8	0.7	10.7	10.0	1.7	1.6	11.6	3.2	0.6	112.9	3.5	4.5	1.1	12.8
CV(%)	15.2	4.7	13.2	8.4	19.5	83.6	57.2	15.3	23.6	8.9	11.5	27.1	33.9	35.7

Abbreviations: *RI* reference interval, *min* minutes, *SD* standard deviation, *CV* coefficient of variation, *R* reaction time, *K* clotting time, *MA* maximum amplitude, *G* clot rigidity, *CI* coagulation index, *LY30* clot lysis at 30 min, *SP* split point, *TG* total thrombin generation, *MRTG* maximum rate of thrombus generation, *TMRTG* time to maximum rate of thrombus generation, *MRL* maximum rate of lysis, *TMRL* time to maximum rate of lysis
[a]Velocity curve variables (TG, MRTG, TMRTG, MRL, TMRL) were obtained as MA version
[b]Reference intervals are not considered valid according to the ASVCP (American Society of Veterinary Clinical Pathology) guidelines as number of animals <20
[c]A valid reference interval could not be calculated with any statistical method

the development of a more hypercoagulable TEG tracing with increasing citrate storage time. For the variables of clot lysis, only MRL was significantly influenced by citrate storage time with values being higher at 60 min compared to 30 min (1.71 mm/min vs. 1.25 mm/min, $P = 0.049$). In contrast, there was no significant impact of citrate storage time on the other investigated TEG variables (alpha, MA, G, CI, delta, LY30, TG, TMRL).

Examples of two TEG tracings performed in a cat after a citrate storage time of 30 and 60 min respectively is depicted in Fig. 7 clearly demonstrating the decrease in R, K, SP and TMRTG as well as an increase in MRTG.

Impact of platelet clumping

No statistically significant differences could be found between the group of cats classified as having low grade clumping and those cats classified as showing high grade platelet clumping. Table 3 provides the range and median of the different groups as well as the *p*-value between these two groups.

Discussion

To the authors' knowledge, this is the first study evaluating novel TEG variables such as SP, delta and the VC variables for cats as well as the impact of storage time on feline TEG tracings.

There is no definite evidence why one cat (excluded from the study) only showed flat lines drawing the conclusion that no clot could be detected by the analyzer. Because the routine plasmatic coagulation parameters were unremarkable in this cat, a coagulation disorder seems unlikely. Relating to the TEG being a test of global hemostasis, a platelet origin might be the reason of undetectable clots in this cat. In fact, this cat showed marked aggregation of platelets on the blood smear, but since five different cats also showed moderate to marked platelet aggregation on the blood smear and TEG tracings could still be obtained, an aggregation of platelet might not be the only reason. Further studies should be obtained to verify this observation.

Our study demonstrated a significant impact of citrate storage time on several traditional and novel TEG variables. Consequently, RI's are also influenced by the citrate storage time and thus should be established for any citrate storage time intended to be used in the laboratory. However, when using the RI, the relatively high CVs of many TEG variables have to be taken into account.

One limitation of our study is the small number of cats included so that potential significant effects might have been missed. Moreover, the establishment of RIs is hampered by the small sample size and RIs determined here have to be considered as preliminary values. As recommended by the American Society of Veterinary Clinical Pathology (ASVCP) guidelines for reference samples $20 \leq x < 40$, a robust method was mostly used for the establishment [29]. Furthermore, these guidelines suggest that reference intervals should not be obtained when less than 20 samples are available [29] as was the case for K, CI, MRL and TMRL. For reference samples $10 \leq x < 20$, the ASVCP guidelines recommend to report histograms (Figs. 3 and 4) as well as

Table 3 Comparison of the TEG results of different groups of cats categorized by the grade of platelet clumping

Group of cats	Low grade of clumping			High grade of clumping			*p*-value
Variable (unit)	Number of cats	Range	Median	Number of cats	Range	Median	
R (sec)	13	3.3–18.7	6.5	5	5.8–9.6	8.1	0.29
K (sec)	12	1.4–3.4	2.4	5	1.7–3.4	2.3	0.67
Alpha (°)	13	26.1–70	57.8	5	49.3–66.4	58.3	0.94
MA (mm)	13	18.2–61.4	46.6	5	42.1–60.9	52.6	0.12
G (dyn/cm^2)	13	1.1–8	4.4	5	3.6–7.8	5.5	0.11
LY30 (%)	13	0–36.8	5.3	5	1.2–27.6	7.9	0.92
CI (unitless)	12	−2.3 – 2.5	−0.2	5	−1.5 – 2.1	0.3	0.34
SP (min)	13	3–15.8	5.7	5	5.2–8.6	7	0.25
Delta (min)	13	0.3–2.9	0.8	5	0.6–1.1	1	0.52
TMRTG (min)	13	4.7–22.5	8.8	5	7.1–11.9	10.3	0.62
MRTG (mm/min)	13	3.5–14.7	8.1	5	6.2–12.2	9.6	0.63
TG (mm/min)	13	244.9–735.1	565	5	517.5–734.3	636.3	0.12
TMRL (min)	12	15.7–56.1	21.2	5	22.3–46.3	34.1	0.08
MRL (mm/min)	12	0.1–4.4	1.8	5	0.3–2.5	1.4	0.59

Abbreviations: *SD* standard deviation, *R* reaction time, *K* clotting time, *MA* maximum amplitude, *G* clot rigidity, *CI* coagulation index, *LY30* clot lysis at 30 min, *SP* split point, *TG* total thrombin generation, *MRTG* maximum rate of thrombus generation, *TMRTG* time to maximum rate of thrombus generation, *MRL* maximum rate of lysis, *TMRL* time to maximum rate of lysis

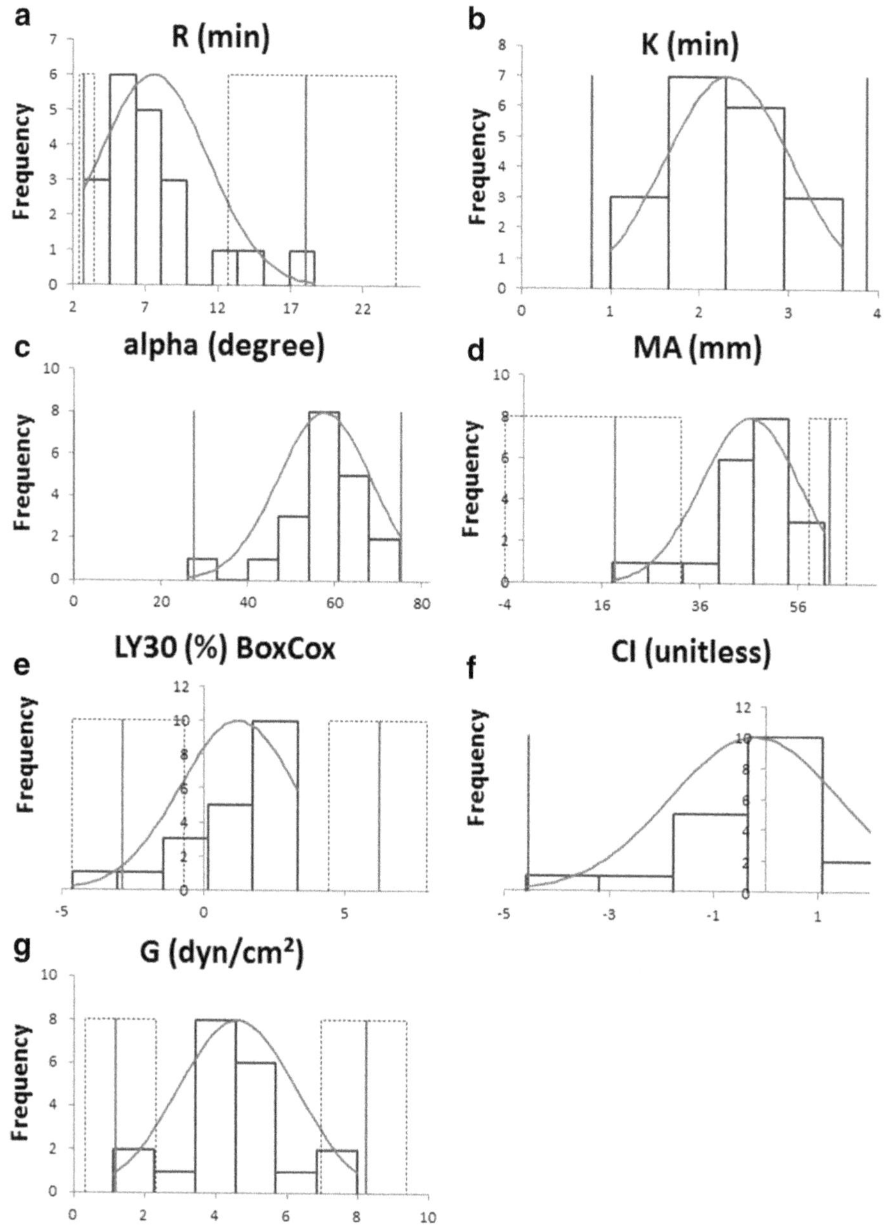

Fig. 3 Histograms showing distribution of untransformed (all but LY30) data obtained for calculation of the reference interval of the traditional TEG. Data for measurement included the first results of all samples after 60 min of storage time. The solid grey line represents the upper and the lower limit of the reference interval. The small black dotted line is consistent with the 90% confidence interval. The light grey line indicates the Gaussian curve. Abbreviations: R = reaction time (**a**), K = clotting time (**b**), Alpha = alpha angle (**c**), MA = maximum amplitude (**d**), LY30 = lysis at 30 min (**e**), CI = coagulation index (**f**), G = clot rigidity (**g**)

mean and median values (Table 2) to help facilitate interpretation of the values.

A direct comparison of RIs obtained in this study using a storage time of 60 min to the results of other studies cannot be made without serious limitations since other studies used a different citrate storage time (i.e., 30 min) [19, 21] or different modes of activation [19, 21] which also can affect TEG variables. With regard to the velocity variables, no other study evaluating the VC in feline thrombelastography was found. For better comparability, Table 4 provides the RIs of both the MA version and G version of the velocity curve variables, which are slightly different since the curves (MA version and G version) are minimally different.

Regarding the stability of citrated whole blood, our study shows that longer storage times induce a more hypercoagulable TEG tracing which is not only represented by a shorter R, K and SP but also can be

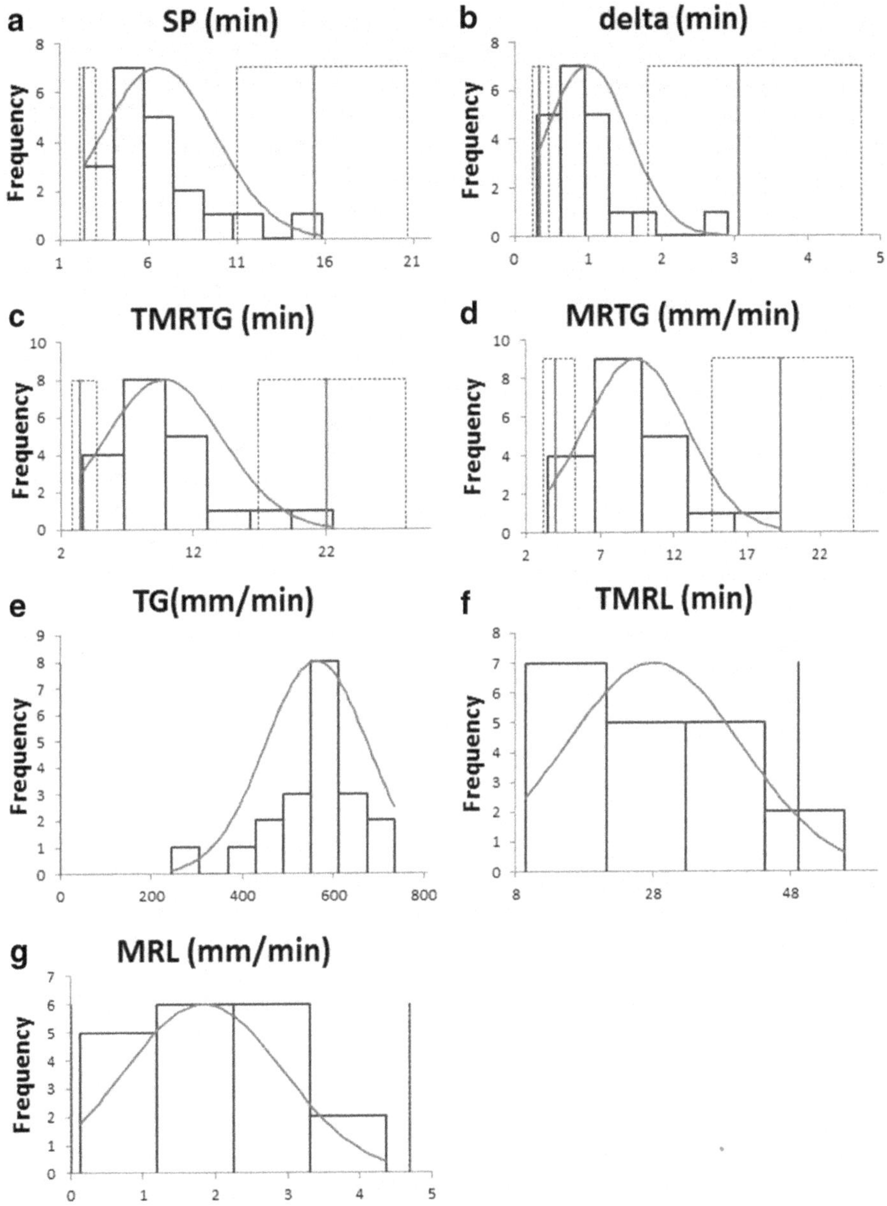

Fig. 4 Histograms showing the distribution of untransformed data for calculation of reference intervals of the novel TEG variables SP, delta, TMRTG, MRTG, TMRL and MRL respectively. Data for measurement included the first results of all samples after 60 min of storage time. The solid grey line represents the upper and the lower limit of the reference interval. The small black dotted line is consistent with the 90% confidence interval. The light grey line indicates the Gaussian curve. Abbreviations: SP = split point (**a**), D = delta (**b**), TMRTG = time to maximum rate of thrombus generation (**c**), MRTG = maximum rate of thrombus generation (**d**), TG = thrombus generation (**e**), TMRL = time to maximum rate of lysis (**f**), MRL = maximum rate of lysis (**g**)

seen on the velocity curve by reduced TMRTG and MRTG values.

The R value reflects the time from sample placement in the cuvette until an amplitude of 2 mm is reached on the TEG tracing. It is dependent on plasma clotting factors and circulating inhibitor activity and represents the initial fibrin formation rate [1]. The K value is a measurement from the point where 2 mm of amplitude is reached (R time) to the point of 20 mm amplitude. This time reflects the buildup and cross linking of fibrin, which is related to clotting factors such as factor II and VII, fibrinogen and platelets count and function [1].

Furthermore, alpha and delta show a non-significant trend towards hypercoagulability at 60 min. Alpha (°) is the angle formed by the TEG tracing between the R and the K value and reflects the speed of clot formation [1]. As alpha and MRTG reflect a similar item, a similarly significant change could have been expected between

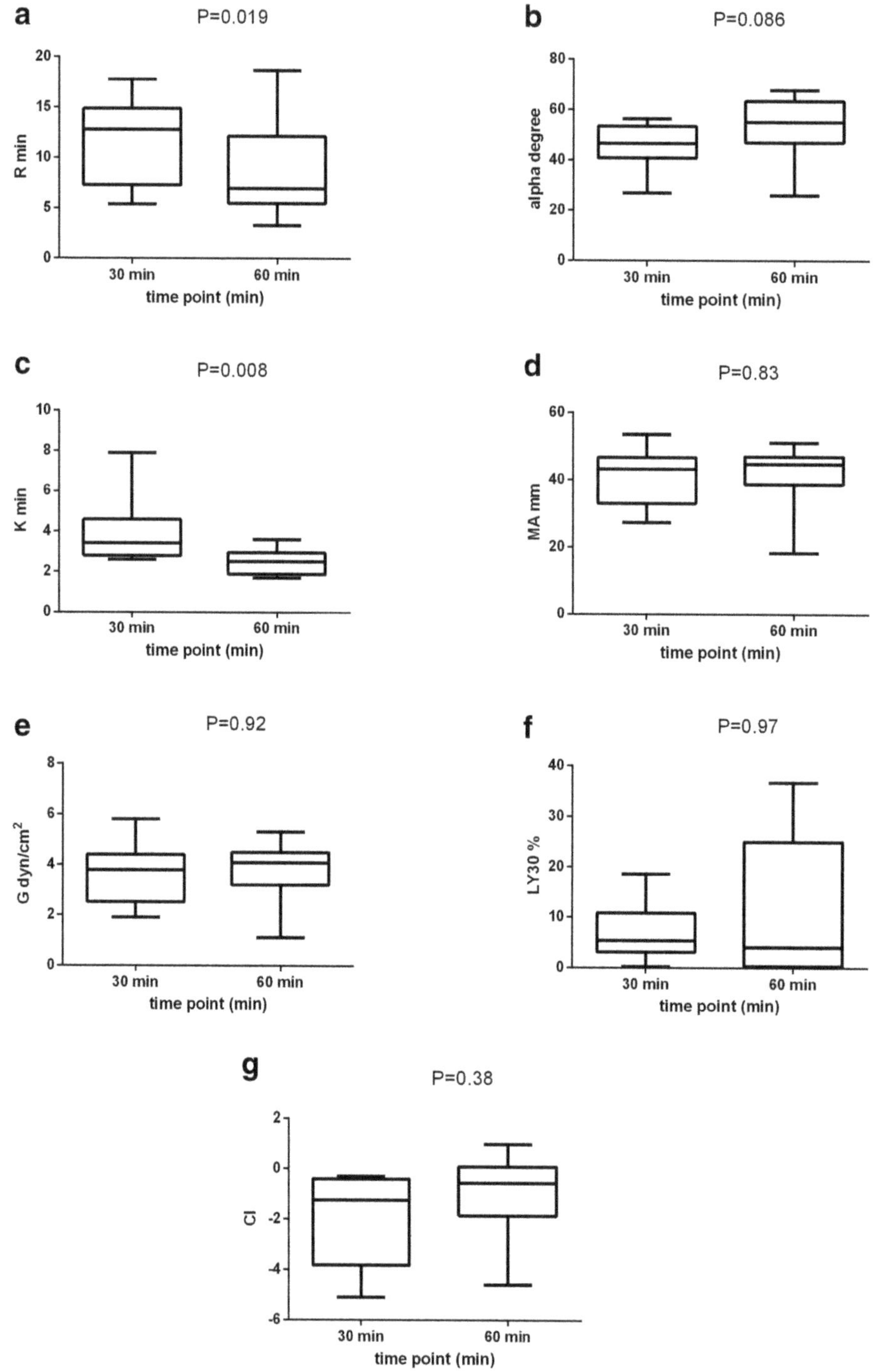

Fig. 5 Effect of citrate storage time (30 min versus 60 min) on the traditional thrombelastographic (TEG) variables expressed as box and whisker diagrams. The central box represents values from the lower (25th) to upper (75th) percentile, while the middle line is consistent with the median. The horizontal line depicts the minimum and maximum values. The level of significance was set at $P < 0.05$. Abbreviations: R = reaction time (**a**), alpha degree (**b**), K = coagulation time (**c**), MA = maximum amplitude (**d**), G = clot rigidity (**e**), LY30 = lysis at 30 min (**f**), CI = coagulation index (**g**)

the time points. However, alpha was not significantly altered while MRTG was significantly affected by different storage times. A possible explanation for this discrepancy could be their different mode of change during the coagulation process as described previously for humans [7]: compared to alpha which is variable of the traditional curve and shows a non-exponential behavior, MRTG as a parameter derived from the

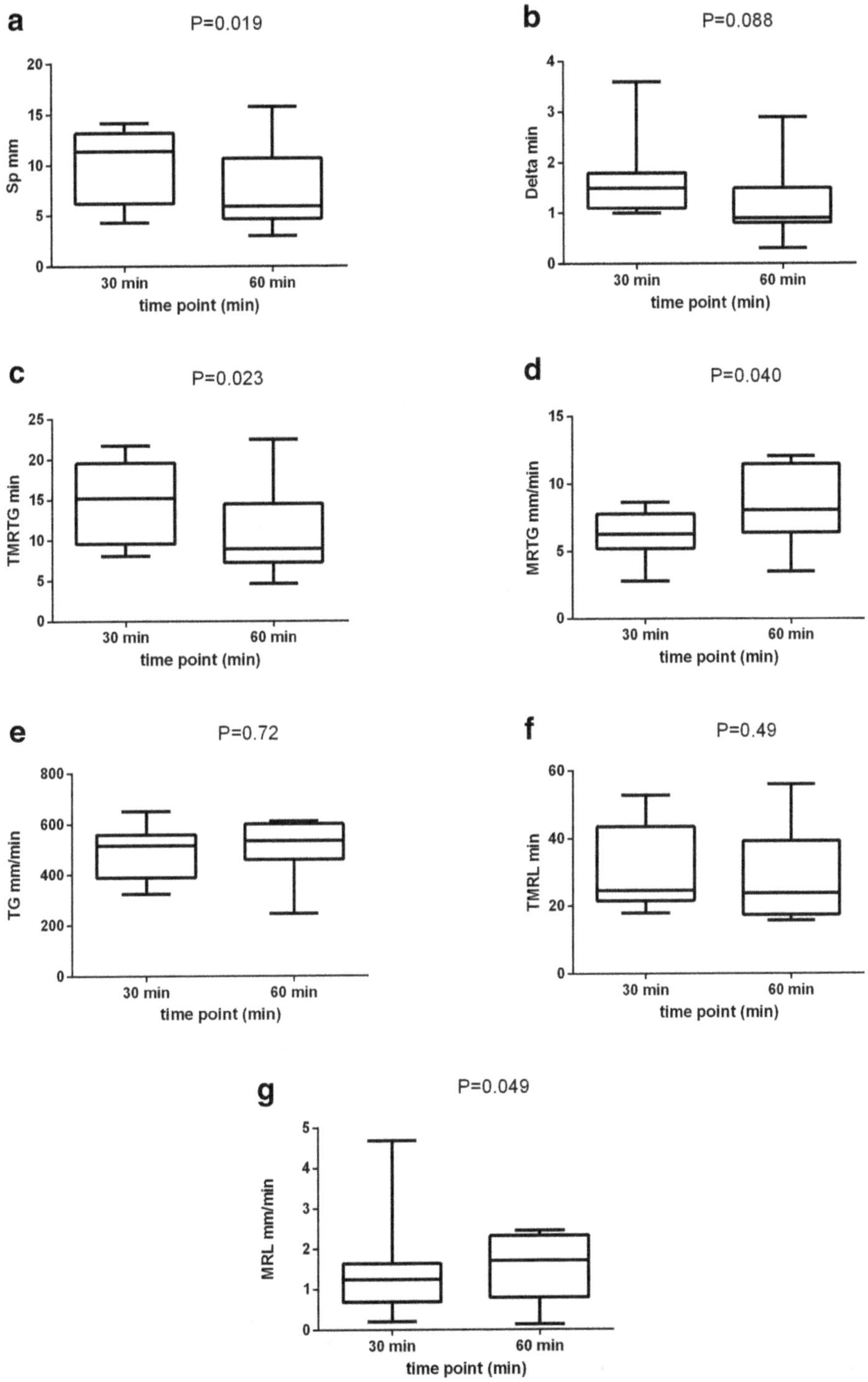

Fig. 6 Effect of citrate storage time (30 min versus 60 min) on the novel thrombelastographic (TEG) variables expressed as box and whisker diagrams. The central box represents values from the lower (25th) to upper (75th) percentile, while the middle line is consistent with the median. The horizontal line depicts the minimum and maximum values. The level of significance was set at $P < 0.05$. Abbreviations: SP = split point (**a**), D = delta (**b**), TMRTG = time to maximum rate of thrombus generation (**c**), MRTG = maximum rate of thrombus generation (**d**), TG = thrombus generation (**e**), TMRL = time to maximum rate of lysis (**f**), MRL = maximum rate of lysis (**g**)

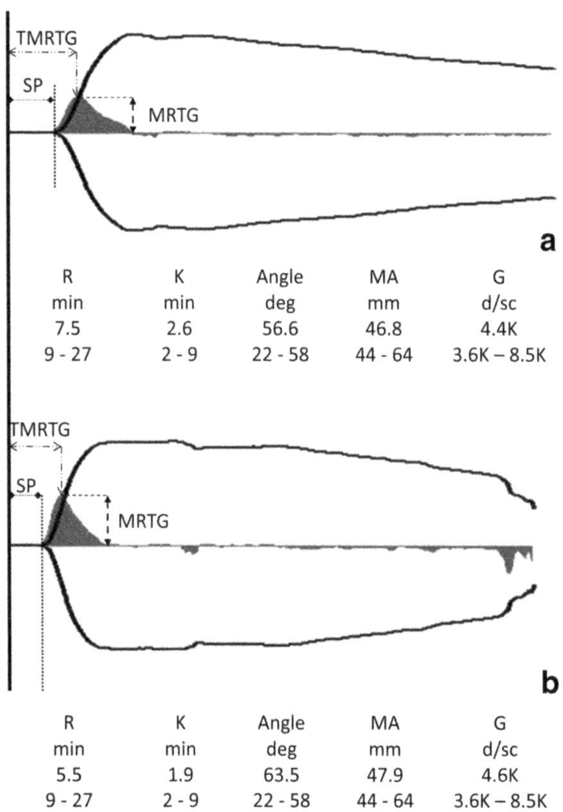

Fig. 7 Exemplarily illustration of the effect of citrate storage on the conventional thrombelastographic (TEG) tracing and the velocity curve (solid grey curve) in one cat included in the study. **a**: Analysis after 30 min, **b**: Analysis after 60 min. Note the shortening of the R-value and the K-value as well as the increase of MRTG and shortening of TMRTG consistent with a "hypercoagulable" TEG after increased incubation time. Abbreviations: TMRTG = time to maximum rate of thrombus generation, SP = split point, MRTG = maximum rate of thrombus generation.

velocity curve changes in an exponential and thus markedly pronounced way.

A similar effect was noticed here for TMRTG which in previous studies in human medicine has shown a linear correlation with delta [6] so that theoretically a similar impact of storage on both variables would have been expected. However, the citrate storage time only had a significant impact on the VC parameter TMRTG increasing exponentially but not on delta derived from the traditional TEG curve changing in a non-exponential mode. In conclusion, some VC variables (TMRTG, MRTG) might be a more sensitive marker of changes in coagulation activity like hypercoagulability than traditional TEG values. This hypothesis however, further has to be substantiated in future clinical studies.

A previous investigation in critically ill patients could further demonstrate a linear relationship between delta and TMRTG reflecting thrombin generation [6]. In our study evaluating the impact of citrate storage time in

Table 4 Comparison of the velocity curve reference intervals based on the maximum amplitude or clot rigidity

MA version		G version	
Variable (unit)	RI	Variable (unit)	RI
TMRTG (min)	3.5–22.0	TMRTGG (min)	4.1–23.0
MRTG (mm/min)	4.0–19.3	MRTGG (dsc)	2.1–11.9
TG (mm/min)	255.3–751.2	TGG (dsc)	138.8–828.5
TMRL (min)	0.4–55.8	TMRLG (min)	0.0–55.9
MRL (mm/min)	0.0–4.7	MRLG (dsc)	−1.6 – 7.7

For each variable, in both versions the same statistical method was used. G version variables show an appended "G"

Abbreviations: *MA* maximum amplitude, *G* clot rigidity, *RI* reference interval, *TMRTG(G)* time to maximum rate of thrombus generation, *MRTG(G)* maximum rate of thrombus generation, *TG(G)* (total) thrombus generation, *TMRL(G)* time to maximum rate of lysis, *MRL(G)* maximum rate of lysis, *min* minute, *mm* millimeter, *dsc* dyn/cm^2/s

TEG variables, the behavior of TMRTG resembled the findings observed for R more closely than those observed for delta. It thus could be hypothesized, that there is an even closer relationship between TMRTG and R than there is between TMRTG and delta. Reasons contributing to this difference in the current study compared to Gonzalez et al. [6] might be the different species, the different storage time, the different mode of activation and the prophylactic therapy with heparin potentially influencing the values as R partially depends on the activity of circulating inhibitors [1]. Further studies are needed to evaluate the relationship amongst this threesome (TMRTG, R and delta).

Regarding TG, previously investigated in humans as a marker of thrombin generation [4], the absolute amount of thrombus generated (TG) in our study in cats was interestingly not altered by prolonged citrate storage times. In conjunction with the changes in TMRTG and MRTG, citrate storage time apparently rather affects the speed of clot formation and thrombin generation (as TMRTG is believed to be a marker of thrombin generation [6]) than the total amount of thrombin generated.

In agreement with our findings in cats, significant differences with a tendency towards hypercoagulability with longer storage time have been observed in dogs [3] and horses [17]. In contrast to that, another study in horses reported sample (citrated whole blood) stability at room temperature for up to 20 h prior to TEG measurement, however, measurements were made after 2 and 19 to 48 h of citrate storage time so that changes prior 2 h of storage might have been missed [18].

Despite from an incomplete inhibition of thrombin formation during storage [3], repeated sampling from a single tube could function as a "contact activator" for the coagulation cascade via the pipette surface which in humans has been shown to alter TEG results [16]. The factor of repeated sampling has not been determined in our study but in other veterinary studies which used separate tubes for different time points to avoid repeated pipetting and still showed significant differences with a tendency towards hypercoagulability [3, 17]. Hypercoagulable TEG tracings with prolonged storage times might thus be resulting from different in vitro blood stability of different mammalian species [17].

Conclusion

Storage of citrated whole blood used for TEG analysis in cats has significant effects on both traditional and VC variables with a trend towards hypercoagulability with prolonged storage times. By that, some velocity curve variables (explicitly TMRTG, MRTG) might help in the early detection of changes in coagulation activity for example hypercoagulable states.

Because of the effect of citrate storage times on TEG analysis, RIs can only be used for a specific storage time which has to be established in each laboratory.

Abbreviations

aPTT: activated partial thromboplastin time; CI: coagulation index; cm: centimeter; CV: coefficients o variation; dsc: dyn/cm^2/s; G: clot rigidity; K: clotting time; LY30: lysis at 30 min after MA is reached; MA: maximum amplitude; min: minute; mm: millimeter; MRL: maximum rate of lysis; MRTG: maximum rate of thrombus generation; PT: prothrombin time; R: reaction time; RIs: reference intervals; sec: second; SP: split point; TEG: thrombelastography; TG: (total) thrombus generation; TMRL: time to maximum rate of lysis; TMRTG: time to maximum rate of thrombus generation; TT: thrombin time; VC: velocity curve

Acknowledgements

The authors would like to thank Bayer Animal Health GmbH, Leverkusen for kindly supporting this study.

Funding

The study was kindly supported by Bayer Animal Health GmbH by providing the equipment and material necessary for blood sampling and plasma preparation. No author received financial support for the authorship or publication of this article.

Authors' contributions

CE participated in the study design performed the plasma preparation and analyses, contributed to the statistical analysis, data interpretation and discussion of results and wrote the manuscript. FB collected the blood samples and helped in plasma preparation and analyzing the samples. AM conceived the study and participated in project planning and coordination. NB participated in project planning, performing the statistical analysis, data interpretation, discussing the results and writing the manuscript. All authors read and approved the final manuscript.

Consent for publication

Not applicable.

Competing interests

FB is employed by Bayer Animal Health GmbH, which has no financial interest with the subject matter, the materials used or the performance of the study. CE, AM and NB declare that they have no competing interests in the study.

Author details

[1]Department of Veterinary Clinical Sciences, Clinical Pathophysiology and Clinical Pathology, Justus-Liebig University Giessen, Frankfurterstraße 126, 35392 Giessen, Germany. [2]Bayer Animal Health GmbH, Alfred-Nobel-Straße 50, 40789 Monheim am Rhein, Germany.

References

1. Mallett SV, Cox DJ. Thrombelastography. Br J Anaesth. 1992;69:307–13.
2. Bauer N, Eralp O, Moritz A. Effect of hemolysis on canine kaolin-activated thromboelastography values and ADVIA 2120 platelet activation indices. Vet Clin Pathol. 2010;39:180–9.
3. Wiinberg B, Jensen AL, Rojkjaer R, Johansson P, Kjelgaard-Hansen M, Kristensen AT. Validation of human recombinant tissue factor-activated thromboelastography on citrated whole blood from clinically healthy dogs. Vet Clin Pathol. 2005;34:389–93.
4. Rivard GE, Brummel-Ziedins KE, Mann KG, Fan L, Hofer A, Cohen E. Evaluation of the profile of thrombin generation during the process of whole blood clotting as assessed by thrombelastography. J Thromb Haemost. 2005;3:2039–43. doi:10.1111/j.1538-7836.2005.01513.x.
5. Pommerening MJ, Goodman MD, Farley DL, Cardenas JC, Podbielski J, Matijevic N, et al. Early diagnosis of clinically significant hyperfibrinolysis using thrombelastography velocity curves. J Am Coll Surg. 2014;219:1157–66. doi:10.1016/j.jamcollsurg.2014.07.943.
6. Gonzalez E, Kashuk JL, Moore EE, Silliman CC. Differentiation of enzymatic from platelet hypercoagulability using the novel thrombelastography parameter delta (delta). J Surg Res. 2010;163:96–101. doi:10.1016/j.jss.2010.03.058.
7. Ellis TC, Nielsen VG, Marques MB, Kirklin JK. Thrombelastographic measures of clot propagation: a comparison of alpha with the maximum rate of thrombus generation [abstract]. Blood Coagul Fibrinolysis. 2007;18:45–8. doi: 10.1097/MBC.0b013e3280111a8e.
8. McMichael MA, Smith SA. Viscoelastic coagulation testing: technology, applications, and limitations. Vet Clin Pathol. 2011;40:140–53. doi:10.1111/j.1939-165X.2011.00302.x.
9. Haemonetics Corporation. TEG® 5000 System - User Manual - 2011.
10. Donahue SM, Otto CM. Thromboelastography: a tool for measuring hypercoagulability, hypocoagulability, and fibrinolysis. J Vet Emerg Crit Care (San Antonio). 2005;15:9–16. doi:10.1111/j.1476-4431.2005.04025.x.
11. Wiinberg B, Kristensen AT. Thromboelastography in veterinary medicine. Semin Thromb Hemost. 2010;36:747–56. doi:10.1055/s-0030-1265291.
12. Kashuk JL, Moore EE, Sabel A, Barnett C, Haenel J, Le T, et al. Rapid thrombelastography (r-TEG) identifies hypercoagulability and predicts thromboembolic events in surgical patients. Surgery. 2009;146:764–772; discussion 772-4. doi:10.1016/j.surg.2009.06.054.
13. Flatland B, Koenigshof AM, Rozanski E, Goggs R, Wiinberg B. Systematic evaluation of evidence on veterinary viscoelastic testing part 2: sample acquisition and handling. J Vet Emerg Crit Care (San Antonio). 2014;24:30–6. doi:10.1111/vec.12142.
14. Flint SK, Wood D, Abrams-Ogg AC, Kruth SA, Bersenas A. Comparison of citrated native and kaolin-activated samples for thrombelastographic analysis in healthy dogs. Vet Clin Pathol. 2012;41:249–55. doi:10.1111/j.1939-165X.2012.00431.x.
15. White H, Zollinger C, Jones M, Bird R. Can Thromboelastography performed on kaolin-activated citrated samples from critically ill patients provide stable and consistent parameters? Int J Lab Hematol. 2010;32:167–73. doi:10.1111/j.1751-553X.2009.01152.x.
16. Zambruni A, Thalheimer U, Leandro G, Perry D, Burroughs AK. Thromboelastography with citrated blood: comparability with native blood, stability of citrate storage and effect of repeated sampling. Blood Coagul Fibrinolysis. 2004;15:103–7.
17. Leclere M, Lavoie J, Dunn M, Bedard C. Evaluation of a modified thrombelastography assay initiated with recombinant human tissue factor in clinically healthy horses. Vet Clin Pathol. 2009;38:462–6. doi:10.1111/j.1939-165X.2009.00157.x.

18. Garreis K, Palmer S, Sommerey C, Klein R, Müller E. Investigation of sample stability of kaolin activated citrated whole blood and establishment of reference values for thromboelastography in healthy adult horses [abstract]. Tierarztl Prax Ausg K Kleintiere Heimtiere. 2015;2:A11.
19. Banerjee A, Blois SL, Wood D. Comparing citrated native, kaolin-activated, and tissue factor-activated samples and determining intraindividual variability for feline thromboelastography. J Vet Diagn Investig. 2011;23: 1109–13. doi:10.1177/1040638711425595.
20. Hall DJ, Rush JE, deLaforcade AM, Shaw SP. Kaolin-activated thromboelastography in echocardiographically normal cats. Am J Vet Res. 2012;73:775–8. doi:10.2460/ajvr.73.6.775.
21. Marschner CB, Bjørnvad CR, Kristensen AT, Wiinberg B. Thromboelastography results on citrated whole blood from clinically healthy cats depend on modes of activation. Acta Vet Scand. 2010;52:38. doi:10.1186/1751-0147-52-38.
22. Moldal ER, Kirpensteijn J, Kristensen AT, Haga HA, Nødtvedt A, Eriksen T. Evaluation of inflammatory and hemostatic surgical stress responses in male cats after castration under general anesthesia with or without local anesthesia. Am J Vet Res. 2012;73:1824–31. doi:10.2460/ajvr.73.11.1824.
23. Cöl R, Monthomery A, Iazbik MC, Defelice A, Saavedra PV, Couto CG. Whole-blood thrombelastography using calcium chloride activation in healthy cats. Turk J Vet Anim Sci. 2013;37:68–75.
24. Alwood AJ, Downend AB, Slensky KA, Fox JA, Simpson SA, Donahue SM, et al. Resident forum abstracts: evaluation of thrombelastography (TEG) in normal cats. J Vet Emerg Crit Care (San Antonio). 2004;14:S1–S17. doi:10. 1111/j.1476-4431.2004.04035.x.
25. Bauer N, Eralp Inan O, Moritz A. Reference intervals and method optimization for variables reflecting hypocoagulatory and hypercoagulatory states in dogs using the STA compact automated analyzer. J Vet Diagn Investig. 2009;21(6):803–14.
26. Moritz A, Fickenscher Y, Meyer K, Failing K, Weiss DJ. Canine and feline hematology reference values for the ADVIA 120 hematology system. Vet Clin Pathol. 2004;33:32–8. doi:10.1111/j.1939-165X.2004.tb00347.x.
27. Tasker S, Cripps PJ, Mackin AJ. Estimation of platelet counts on feline blood smears. Vet Clin Pathol. 1999;28:42–5.
28. Geffré A, Concordet D, Braun J-P, Trumel C. Reference value advisor: a new freeware set of macroinstructions to calculate reference intervals with Microsoft excel. Vet Clin Pathol. 2011;40(1):107–12. doi:10.1111/j.1939-165X. 2011.00287.x.
29. Friedrichs KR, Harr K, Freeman KP, Szladovits B, Walton RM, Barnhart KF, Blanco-Chavez J. ASVCP reference interval guidelines: determination of de novo reference intervals in veterinary species and other related topics. Vet Clin Pathol. 2012;41:441–53. doi:10.1111/vcp.12006.

Permissions

All chapters in this book were first published in VR, by BioMed Central; hereby published with permission under the Creative Commons Attribution License or equivalent. Every chapter published in this book has been scrutinized by our experts. Their significance has been extensively debated. The topics covered herein carry significant findings which will fuel the growth of the discipline. They may even be implemented as practical applications or may be referred to as a beginning point for another development.

The contributors of this book come from diverse backgrounds, making this book a truly international effort. This book will bring forth new frontiers with its revolutionizing research information and detailed analysis of the nascent developments around the world.

We would like to thank all the contributing authors for lending their expertise to make the book truly unique. They have played a crucial role in the development of this book. Without their invaluable contributions this book wouldn't have been possible. They have made vital efforts to compile up to date information on the varied aspects of this subject to make this book a valuable addition to the collection of many professionals and students.

This book was conceptualized with the vision of imparting up-to-date information and advanced data in this field. To ensure the same, a matchless editorial board was set up. Every individual on the board went through rigorous rounds of assessment to prove their worth. After which they invested a large part of their time researching and compiling the most relevant data for our readers.

The editorial board has been involved in producing this book since its inception. They have spent rigorous hours researching and exploring the diverse topics which have resulted in the successful publishing of this book. They have passed on their knowledge of decades through this book. To expedite this challenging task, the publisher supported the team at every step. A small team of assistant editors was also appointed to further simplify the editing procedure and attain best results for the readers.

Apart from the editorial board, the designing team has also invested a significant amount of their time in understanding the subject and creating the most relevant covers. They scrutinized every image to scout for the most suitable representation of the subject and create an appropriate cover for the book.

The publishing team has been an ardent support to the editorial, designing and production team. Their endless efforts to recruit the best for this project, has resulted in the accomplishment of this book. They are a veteran in the field of academics and their pool of knowledge is as vast as their experience in printing. Their expertise and guidance has proved useful at every step. Their uncompromising quality standards have made this book an exceptional effort. Their encouragement from time to time has been an inspiration for everyone.

The publisher and the editorial board hope that this book will prove to be a valuable piece of knowledge for researchers, students, practitioners and scholars across the globe.

List of Contributors

Alexander Grahofer and Heiko Nathues
Clinic for Swine, Department of Clinical Veterinary Medicine, Vetsuisse Faculty, University of Berne, Bremgartenstrasse 109a, CH-3012 Bern, Switzerland

Natalie Wiedemar and Cord Drögemüller
Institute of Genetics, Department of Clinical Research and Veterinary Public Health, Vetsuisse Faculty, University of Berne, Bremgartenstrasse 109a, CH-3012 Bern, Switzerland

Corinne Gurtner
Institute of Animal Pathology, Department of Infectious Diseases and Pathobiology, Vetsuisse Faculty, University of Berne, Länggassstrasse 122, CH-3012 Bern, Switzerland

María Dolores Contreras-Aguilar, Fernando Tecles, Silvia Martínez-Subiela, Luis Jesús Bernal and José Joaquín Cerón
Interdisciplinary Laboratory of Clinical Analysis (Interlab-UMU), Veterinary School, Campus of Excellence Mare Nostrum, University of Murcia, 30100, Espinardo, Murcia, Spain

Damián Escribano
Interdisciplinary Laboratory of Clinical Analysis (Interlab-UMU), Veterinary School, Campus of Excellence Mare Nostrum, University of Murcia, 30100, Espinardo, Murcia, Spain
Department of Food and Animal Science, School of Veterinary Medicine, Universitat Autònoma de Barcelona, 08193, Bellaterra, Barcelona, Spain

Trond M. Kortner and Åshild Krogdahl
Department of Basic Sciences and Aquatic Medicine, Faculty of Veterinary Medicine and Biosciences, Norwegian University of Life Sciences, Oslo, Norway

Michael H. Penn
Department of Basic Sciences and Aquatic Medicine, Faculty of Veterinary Medicine and Biosciences, Norwegian University of Life Sciences, Oslo, Norway
US Fish & Wildlife Service, Lamar, PA 16848, USA

Ingemar Björkhem
Department of Laboratory Medicine, Division for Clinical Chemistry, Karolinska University Hospital, Huddinge, Sweden

Kjell Måsøval
Biomar AS, Nordre gate 11, 7011 Trondheim, Norway

Alana Christina Gast, Julia Metzger and Ottmar Distl
Institute for Animal Breeding and Genetics, University of Veterinary Medicine Hannover, Bünteweg 17p, 30559 Hannover, Germany

Andrea Tipold
Department of Small Animal Medicine and Surgery, University of Veterinary Medicine Hannover, Bünteweg 9, 30559 Hannover, Germany

Franck Jolivet, Catherine Trumel and Simon Privat
Department of Clinical Sciences, ENVT, University of Toulouse, 31076 Toulouse, France

Armelle Diquélou and Olivier Dossin
Department of Clinical Sciences, ENVT, University of Toulouse, 31076 Toulouse, France
IRSD, INSERM 1220, INSERM, INRA, ENVT, UPS, University of Toulouse, 31024 Toulouse, France

Leslie A. Lyons
Department of Veterinary Medicine and Surgery, College of Veterinary Medicine, University of Missouri – Columbia, Columbia, MO 65211, USA

Robert A. Grahn
Veterinary Genetics Laboratory, School of Veterinary Medicine, University of California - Davis, Davis, CA, USA

Maria Longeri and Francesca Genova
Department of Veterinary Medicine, University of Milan, Milan, Italy

Michela Beccaglia
Ambulatorio Veterinario, Lissone, Monza e Brianza, Italy

John J. Hopwood
Lysosomal Diseases Research Unit, South Australian Health and Medical Research Institute, Adelaide, Australia

Marina S. R. Barreto and Cristina T. Andrade
Instituto de Macromoléculas Professora Eloisa Mano, Universidade Federal do Rio de Janeiro, Centro de Tecnologia, Bloco J, Rio de Janeiro, RJ 21941-598, Brazil

Luiz Cláudio R. P. da Silva and Lúcio M. Cabral
Universidade Federal do Rio de Janeiro, Faculdade de Farmácia, Av. Carlos Chagas Filho, 373, CCS, Bloco L, sala 24, Rio de Janeiro, RJ 21941-902, Brazil

Eduardo M. Del Aguila and Vânia M. Flosi Paschoalin
Instituto de Química, Universidade Federal do Rio de Janeiro, Av. Athos da Silveira, Ramos 149, Bloco A, sala 545, Rio de Janeiro 21941-909, Brazil

Jiafa Hou
College of Veterinary Medicine, Nanjing Agricultural University, Nanjing 210095, China

Xiaoping Ma
College of Veterinary Medicine, Nanjing Agricultural University, Nanjing 210095, China
College of Veterinary Medicine, Sichuan Agricultural University, Chengdu 611130, China

Changcheng Li
College of Veterinary Medicine, Sichuan Agricultural University, Chengdu 611130, China

Yu Gu
College of Life Sciences, Sichuan Agricultural University, Ya'an 625014, China

Irene A. Veladiano, Tommaso Banzato, Luca Bellini and Alessandro Zotti
Department of Animal Medicine, Production and Health, University of Padua, Viale dell'Università 16, Legnaro (PD) 35020, Italy

Alessandro Montani
Clinic for Exotic Animals, CVS, Rome 00137, Italy

Salvatore Catania
Avian Medicine Laboratory, Istituto Zooprofilattico Sperimentale delle Venezie, Legnaro 35020, Italy

Michelle L. Scott, Emily E. John, John C. H. Ching, Matthew E. Loewen and George W. Forsyth
Veterinary Biomedical Sciences, Western College of Veterinary Medicine, University of Saskatchewan, Saskatoon, SK S7N 5B4, Canada

Rebecca R. Bellone
Department of Biology, University of Tampa, Tampa, FL 33606, USA

Lynne S. Sandmeyer and Bruce H. Grahn
Small Animal Clinical Sciences, Western College of Veterinary Medicine, University of Saskatchewan, Saskatoon, Canada

Yaron Dekel
Shamir Research Institute, University of Haifa, 1290000 Kazerin, Israel
Zefat Academic College, Zefat, Israel
GGA - Galil Genetic Analysis Ltd, 12900 Kazerin, Israel

Oshrat Noked Partouche
Shamir Research Institute, University of Haifa, 1290000 Kazerin, Israel
Tel Hai College, 12210 Tel-Hai, Israel

Izhar Ben-Shlomo
Zefat Academic College, Zefat, Israel
Faculty of Medicine in the Galilee, Bar-Ilan University & Baruch Padeh Medical Center, Poria, Israel

Dani Bercovich
Tel Hai College, 12210 Tel-Hai, Israel
GGA - Galil Genetic Analysis Ltd, 12900 Kazerin, Israel

Aviad Stoler, Arava Aderet, Daniel Baumel, Efrat Kellerman and Yoram Plotsky
GGA - Galil Genetic Analysis Ltd, 12900 Kazerin, Israel

Yossy Machlu
Specialist in the Fields of Genetics, Epidemiology and Molecular Biology, Rehovot, Israel

Gal Elhalal
Vetmarket Ltd. Industrial Park Hevel Modiin, 6085001 Shoham, Israel

Takamasa Itoi, Yasuji Harada, Takuya Yogo, Yasushi Hara and Masahiro Tagawa
Division of Veterinary Surgery, Nippon Veterinary and Life Science University, 1-7-1 Kyonan-cho, Musashino, Tokyo 180-8602, Japan

Hiroyuki Irie and Michiko Sakamoto
HOYA Technosurgical orporation, 1-1-110 Tsutsujigaoka, Akishima, Tokyo 196-0012, Japan

Katsutoshi Tamura
Division of Animal and Clinical Regenerative Medicine, Kurashiki University of Science and Arts, 2640 Nishinoura, Tsurajima-machi, Kurashiki, Okayama 712-8505, Japan

Satoshi Soeta and Hajime Amasaki
Division of Veterinary Anatomy, Nippon Veterinary and Life Science University, 1-7-1 Kyonan-cho, Musashino, Tokyo 180-8602, Japan

Maria Vitale, Sergio Migliore, Maria La Giglia, Placido Alberti and Vincenzo Di Marco Lo Presti
Istituto Zooprofilattico Sperimentale of Sicily "A. Mirri", Palermo, Italy

Jan P. M. Langeveld
Department of Infection Biology, Central Veterinary Institute of Wageningen UR, Lelystad, The Netherlands

Yoann Mathevon, Gilles Foucras and Fabien Corbiere
IHAP, Ecole Nationale Vétérinaire de Toulouse, 23 chemin des Capelles, F-31076 Toulouse Cedex 3, France

Rémy Falguières
CAPEL Ovilot, 237 avenue Pierre Semard, 46000 Cahors, France

Anne Christine Claßen
Small Animal Veterinary Hospital Stommeln, D 50259 Pulheim, Germany

Sibylle Kneissl
Clinical Unit of Diagnostic Imaging, University of Veterinary Medicine, A 1210 Vienna, Austria

Johann Lang
Division of Clinical Radiology, Vetsuisse Faculty, University of Bern, CH 3012 Bern, Switzerland

Alexander Tichy
Department of Biomedical Sciences, University of Veterinary Medicine, A 1210 Vienna, Austria

Akos Pakozdy
Clinic for Internal Medicine, University of Veterinary Medicine, A 1210 Vienna, Austria

Ilaria Iacopetti, Anna Perazzi, Tamara Badon, Silvia Bedin, Barbara Contiero and Rebecca Ricci
Department of Animal Medicine, Production and Health, University of Padua, Legnaro (Padua), Italy

Getachew Mebrahtu Welay, Dawit Gebremichael Tedla, Gebreyohans Gebru Teklu and Shishay Kahsay Weldearegay
Department Animal Sciences, College of Agriculture, Aksum University, Shire Campus, Shire, Ethiopia

Mearg Belay Shibeshi
School of Geology, College of Agriculture, Aksum University, Shire Campus, Shire, Ethiopia

Haftom Hadush Kidane
Department of Biomedical Science, Aksum University, Aksum, Ethiopia

Berhe Beyene Gebrezgiabher
Department of Epidemiology & Biostatistics, School of Public Health, Aksum University, Aksum, Ethiopia

Teklehaymanot Huluf Abraha
Department of Reproductive Health, School of Public Health, Aksum University, Aksum, Ethiopia

Iuliu Scurtu, Flaviu Tabaran, Mircea Mircean, Gavril Giurgiu, Andras Nagy and Cornel Catoi
Universitatea de Stiinte Agricole si Medicina Veterinara din Cluj-Napoca, Calea Manastur 3-5, 400372 Cluj-Napoca, Romania

Dan G. Ohad
The Koret School of Veterinary Medicine, Robert H. Smith Faculty of Agriculture Food and Environment, Hebrew University of Jerusalem, 76100 Rehovot, Israel

Fanny Comblain
Bone and Cartilage Research Unit, Arthropôle Liège, University of Liège, Liège, Belgium

Yves Henrotin
Bone and Cartilage Research Unit, Arthropôle Liège, University of Liège, Liège, Belgium
Physical Therapy & Rehabilitation Department, Princess Paola Hospital, Vivalia, Marche-en-Famenne, Belgium

Nicolas Barthélémy, Michael Lefèbvre and Marc Balligand
Department of Clinical Sciences, Faculty of Veterinary Medicine, University of Liège, Liège, Belgium

Cédric Schwartz
Laboratory of Human Motion Analysis, University of Liège, Liège, Belgium

Samuel Serisier, Alexandre Feugier and Isabelle Lesponne
Royal Canin Research Center, Aimargues, France

Karina Retter, Dieter Steinhagen and Verena Jung-Schroers
Fish Disease Research Unit, Institute for Parasitology, University of Veterinary Medicine, Bünteweg 17, D-30559 Hannover, Germany

John Hellmann
Fish Disease Research Unit, Institute for Parasitology, University of Veterinary Medicine, Bünteweg 17, D-30559 Hannover, Germany
Landesamt für Natur, Umwelt und Verbraucherschutz Nordrhein-Westfalen (LANUV), Fisheries Ecology, Heinsberger Straße 53, D-57399 Kirchhundem, Albaum, Germany

Karl-Heinz Esser
Institute of Zoology, University of Veterinary Medicine, Bünteweg 17, D-30559 Hannover, Germany

Matthias Lüpke
Institute for General Radiology and Medical Physics, University of Veterinary Medicine, Bünteweg 17, D-30559 Hannover, Germany

Antje Hartmann
Department of Clinical Veterinary Medicine, Vetsuisse Faculty, University of Bern, Länggassstraße 128, 3012 Bern, Switzerland

Steffen Sager and Martin J. Schmidt
Department of Veterinary Clinical Sciences, Small Animal Clinic, Justus-Liebig-University Giessen, Frankfurter Straße 108, 35392 Giessen, Germany

Klaus Failing and Marion Sparenberg
Unit for Biomathematicsand Data Processing Faculty of Veterinary Medicine Justus Liebig University, Frankfurter Straße 95, 35392 Giessen, Germany

Tungalag Chultemdorj, Battsetseg Badmaa and Bayanzul Argamjav
School of Veterinary Medicine, Mongolian University of Life Sciences, Zaisan, Ulaanbaatar, Mongolia

Chimedtseren Bayasgalan
Swiss Tropical and Public Health Institute, CH-4002 Basel, Switzerland
University of Basel, Basel, Switzerland

Felix Roth
Basel, Switzerland

Jakob Zinsstag, Esther Schelling and Jan Hattendorf
Swiss Tropical and Public Health Institute, Basel, Switzerland
University of Basel, Basel, Switzerland

Helen Lydon, Roger Brooks and Andrew McCaskie
Department of Surgery, University of Cambridge, Hill's Road, Cambridge, UK

Frances Henson
Department of Surgery, University of Cambridge, Hill's Road, Cambridge, UK
Department of Veterinary Medicine, University of Cambridge, Madingley Road, Cambridge, UK

Xuhua Ran, Xiaohong Chen, Miaomiao Wang, Jiajia Cheng, Hongbo Ni, Xiao-Xuan Zhang and Xiaobo Wen
College of Animal Science & Veterinary Medicine, Heilongjiang Bayi Agricultural University, No.5, XinFeng Rd., Saertu District, Daqing City 163319, Heilongjiang Province, China

Carolin Engelen, Andreas Moritz and Natali Bauer
Department of Veterinary Clinical Sciences, Clinical Pathophysiology and Clinical Pathology, Justus-Liebig University Giessen, Frankfurterstraße 126, 35392 Giessen, Germany

Franziska Barthel
Bayer Animal Health GmbH, Alfred-Nobel-Straße 50, 40789 Monheim am Rhein, Germany

Index

www.ingramcontent.com/pod-product-compliance
Lightning Source LLC
LaVergne TN
LVHW080808220926
848485LV00011B/454
* 9 7 8 1 6 3 9 2 7 5 3 0 4 *